CLINICAL POSITRON EMISSION TOMOGRAPHY (PET)

Correlation with Morphological Cross-Sectional Imaging

CLINICAL POSITRON EMISSION TOMOGRAPHY (PET)

Correlation with Morphological Cross-Sectional Imaging

Editor

Gustav K. von Schulthess, M.D., Ph.D.
Professor and Director of Nuclear Medicine
University Hospital
Zurich, Switzerland

Coeditors

Alfred Buck, M.D., M.S.
Ivette Engel-Bicik, M.D.
Hans Ch. Steinert, M.D.
University Hospital, Zurich Switzerland

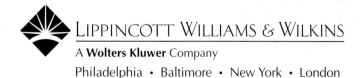

LIPPINCOTT WILLIAMS & WILKINS
A **Wolters Kluwer** Company
Philadelphia · Baltimore · New York · London
Buenos Aires · Hong Kong · Sydney · Tokyo

Acquisitions Editor: Joyce-Rachel John
Developmental Editor: Sara Lauber
Production Editor: Pauline Karakat
Manufacturing Manager: Tim Reynolds
Cover Designer: Catherine Lau Hunt
Compositor: Maryland Composition

Printed in and bound China

Library of Congress Cataloging-in-Publication Data
Clinical positron emission tomography (PET): correlation with
   morphological cross-sectional imaging / editor, Gustav K. von
   Schulthess.
      p.   cm.
   Includes bibliographical references and index.
   ISBN 0-7817-1756-6
   1. Tomography, Emission. I. Schulthess, Gustav Konrad von.
   [DNLM: 1. Tomography, Emission-Computed—methods. 2. Anatomy,
Cross-Sectional—methods. WN 206 C6413 1999]
   RC78.7.T62C565 1999
   616.07′575—dc21
   DNLM/DLC
   for Library of Congress   99-34436
                                           CIP

10 9 8 7 6 5 4 3 2

To Walter A. Fuchs,
who always said that imaging of morphology
asks for imaging of function and vice versa.

CONTENTS

CONTRIBUTING AUTHORS

Michele Arigoni, M.D., M.S.
Resident, Nuclear Medicine, University Hospital, Rämistr. 100, CH-8091 Zurich, Switzerland

Thomas Berthold, B.S.
Head Technician, Nuclear Medicine, University Hospital, Rämistr. 100, CH-8091 Zurich, Switzerland

Alfred Buck, M.D., M.S.
Senior Staff, Nuclear Medicine, University Hospital, Rämistr. 100, CH-8091 Zurich, Switzerland

Cyrill Burger, Ph.D.
Junior Staff, Nuclear Medicine, University Hospital, Rämistr. 100, CH-8091 Zurich, Switzerland

Ivette Engel - Bicik, M.D.
Junior Staff, Nuclear Medicine, University Hospital, Rämistr. 100, CH-8091 Zurich, Switzerland

Georg Kacl, M.D.
Junior Staff, Diagnostic Radiology and Nuclear Medicine, Spital Limmattal, CH-8902 Urdorf, Switzerland

Philipp A. Kaufmann, M.D.
Junior Staff, Nuclear Medicine and Cardiology, University Hospital, Rämistr. 100, CH-8091 Zurich, Switzerland

Stefan Kneifel, M.D.
Resident Nuclear Medicine, University Hospital, Rämistr. 100, CH-8091 Zurich, Switzerland

Rahel Kubik-Huch, M.D.
Junior Staff, Diagnostic Radiology, University Hospital, Rämistr. 100, CH-8091 Zurich, Switzerland

P. August Schubiger, Ph.D.
Professor and Director, Joint Center for Radiopharmaceutical Sciences of the Paul Scherrer Institute, CH-5232 Villigen PSI, Switzerland; and Swiss Federal Institute for Technology and University Hospital, Rämistr. 100, CH-8091 Zurich, Switzerland

Hans Ch. Steinert, M.D.
Senior Staff, Nuclear Medicine, University Hospital, Rämistr. 100, CH-8091 Zurich, Switzerland

Katrin D. M. Stumpe, M.D.
Resident, Nuclear Medicine, University Hospital, Rämistr. 100, CH-8091 Zurich, Switzerland

Gustav K. von Schulthess, M.D., Ph.D.
Professor and Director, Nuclear Medicine, University Hospital, Rämistr. 100, CH-8091 Zurich, Switzerland

Gerrit Westera, Ph.D.
Head, Radiopharmacy Group, Nuclear Medicine, University Hospital, Rämistr. 100, CH-8091 Zurich, Switzerland

Heinz-Gregor Wieser, M.D.
Professor of Neurology and Epileptology, University Hospital, Rämistr. 100, CH-8091 Zurich, Switzerland

Yasuhiro Yonehawa, M.D.
Professor and Director, Neurosurgery Department, University Hospital, Rämistr. 100, CH-8091 Zurich, Switzerland

FOREWORD

Positron emission tomography (PET) as the authors correctly point out, has been a remarkably successful research tool confined only to prestigious universities for close to 20 years, but has been conspicuously absent from nonuniversity clinical centers and diagnostic offices. The reasons for this have been mostly financial. To run PET and participate in meaningful research, it was essential to have the PET scanner, and a cyclotron, which is a well designed and secured pipe system for bringing short lived positron emitting isotopes to the patient preparation room, and a secure area for the storage of the decayed radioactive materials. In addition, there was a need for research technicians, radiopharmacists, physicists, engineers, physicians, and PET nuclear medicine specialists. Even institutions with generous research grants heavily subsidized the enterprise, and the latecomers, or those not successful in obtaining or renewing grant support, had to sacrifice other projects in order to support their PET effort. It is no wonder that PET became associated with financial disaster in the general clinical community and its potential for everyday clinical contributions was overlooked for many years. With the introduction of F-18 Fluorodeoxyglucose (FDG), better spatial resolution PET whole body scanners, smaller and less expensive cyclotrons producing FDG for several centers in a radius in which on time deliveries of the positron emitting isotopes can be feasible, significantly reduce the cost. Most importantly, precise clinical applications have resurrected PET and promise to bring it into the clinical arena. This book was written by experts and edited by a pioneer, not only in positron emission tomography, but also in magnetic resonance imaging, bringing forth the important point that for PET to become clinical, it cannot afford to ignore other cross-sectional imaging techniques with better spatial resolution with diminished functional specificity if it is to optimally localize lesions. Image fusion, made possible by the explosion of computer power in the last few years, provided an approach for better localization. Economic considerations allowing the PET containing department to remain financially solvent are an important part of the book, as the secret of other clinically successful cross-sectional techniques was a positive income balance. The authors discuss in clear detail the clinical indications for PET in the brain, heart, body oncology, and infectious diseases. It is clear that the oncologic applications in the brain and, particularly in the body, are going to be the clinical driving force for PET.

The book is written by members of a single department from the University Hospital in Zurich, who have state of the art equipment, unsurpassed experience with thousands of cases, and close cooperation with other cross-sectional imaging sections of the department, particularly with MR imaging in which Zurich is a world leader.

The clinical and practical approaches recommended by the authors does not confuse the practitioner with complicated algorithms; but fuses the PET findings with those of ultrasound, CT, or MRI (whichever give the best supplemental information); which make the running of the enterprise financially responsible. Above all, the proven clinical indications presented here will bring PET into every day clinical practice. The authors should be congratulated for their clear and constructive vision.

Alexander R. Margulis M.D., D.Sc.(hc)
Tiburon, CA

PREFACE

Positron emission tomography (PET) has existed for more than 20 years, yet the clinical relevance of this method has only started to be appreciated recently. The reasons for this are multiple. The most important includes efficient PET data acquisition technology, which has been around since the early nineties, and the method has long been dominated by research rather than clinically-oriented use. It is the aim of this book to familiarize the reader with PET applications of clinical relevance. Since medical imaging occurs within a context of multiple imaging methods, emphasis will be placed on the correlation of the PET examinations with other cross-sectional imaging examinations. Thus, the book is geared towards all members of Radiology departments who either perform PET studies themselves and want to understand how a PET finding may relate to morphological information, and towards radiologists and neuroradiologists confronted with PET scans as part of a patient's medical image portfolio. In addition, the book aims to educate clinicians—particularly those dealing with oncological problems (PET in tumor grading, staging and follow-up, and how to integrate PET findings with the findings of other cross-sectional imaging modalities). Sophisticated quantitative PET applications and the application of "esoteric" radiopharmaceutical compounds are not discussed in any detail, although some are briefly mentioned. This is intentional because few clinical PET users will be able to access such examinations in the near future. The data presented has been obtained chiefly with F-18 Fluorodeoxyglucose (FDG), O-15 water, and N-13 ammonia as radiopharmaceuticals. This makes sense from a clinical point of view, because FDG is the only clinically relevant compound at the moment which can be shipped widely, while water and ammonia studies can be replaced by SPECT nuclear medicine studies in satellite PET centers. In fact, cerebral perfusion can be imaged with Tc-99m-HMPAO or Tc-99m-ECD, and myocardial perfusion can be imaged with Tc-99m-MIBI, Tc-99m-Tetrofosmine, or Thallium. Alternatively, O-15 generators can be purchased and used for cerebral and cardiac perfusion studies.

It has been the guiding principle in our PET center over the last few years, that unless we can demonstrate that PET is relevant in a number of important clinical questions and can be run as a routine examination very much like CT and MR imaging, its future is doomed. In the current health care environment, PET is simply too costly, unless the expensive technology can be used around the clock on a large number of patients. Similar to MR imaging non-clinical research can be afforded only when the PET system is used clinically during much of the week and research is carried out during evenings and weekends. If PET studies should eventually have a reasonable price tag, a sizable number of patient studies must be carried out on a single scanner (i.e., in the order of eight studies per day, amounting to 1,500 to 2,000 paying examinations per year.) Furthermore, the cost of FDG and other routine compounds, such as water and ammonia, has to be affordable. The latter is only realistic if a cyclotron supplies several scanners and, therefore, the PET satellite concept is not only important for hospitals which cannot afford to run a cyclotron facility, but also to make the existing cyclotron facilities operate cost-effectively. For example, we are set up in Zurich so we can supply the whole German-speaking part of Switzerland with a population of around 4 million with FDG. Under these assumptions, a rough calculation shows that FDG costs of 400–500 dollars per hour and scanning costs of 500–600 dollars, PET can cover the cost even without an undue price tag in the range of 1,000–1,500 dollars, which is not prohibitive when compared to the other cross-sectional imaging modalities. To familiarize the reader with some of these calculations, a chapter deals with cost issues. The satellite PET concept is quickly becoming a reality because several manufacturers are now producing dual head SPECT cameras which have an added coincidence circuit, permitting PET data acquisition. With all of this, there is a growing need for clinicians worldwide to learn about clinical PET imaging.

Finally, a word about the books' contributors. We have decided to produce an "in-house" book with contributions from one institution. This may be a disadvantage. The advantage, however, is that the text can be written in a more consistent fashion. The imaging data is of consistent quality and acquired in a uniform way, so the text can be produced expediently. This assures timeliness in a quickly changing field. We hope this book will contribute to the understanding of clinical PET for imaging physicians and clinicians requiring medical imaging for patient management (particularly for the management of tumor patients, where PET is an excellent and, in many settings, probably the best imaging method). As the application of PET becomes more widespread, the costs of using it will surely decrease, and there is already considerable evidence that PET is a cost-effective method in many instances.

Gustav K. von Schulthess, M.D., Ph.D.

ACKNOWLEDGMENTS

The authors wish to acknowledge help from several individuals. Ms. S. Hess, U. Schaad, and R. van Nuffelen were responsible for scanning the images not already available as digital files. Valuable contributions by Ms. N. Meier, C. Maissen, and M. Husarik are also very much appreciated. Mr. M. Wittwer provided important information regarding cost calculations. Finally, we thank all our clinical colleagues who have sent us interesting patients to evaluate and the colleagues from the Department of Medical Radiology at our institution who have given us invaluable advice and comments on the clinical image material.

This book is sponsored by an unrestricted educational grant from GE Medical Systems.

PART I

Basic Aspects of Clinical PET Imaging

1

Introduction

Gustav K. von Schulthess

GENERAL CONSIDERATIONS

Positron emission tomography (PET) imaging has been around for more than 20 years and has had an interesting history of development. Because of its expense, it has been in the hands of a few high-level scientific investigators for a long time. These investigators have carried out a multitude of sophisticated quantitative analyses of normal volunteers and patients with various disease conditions using a multitude of radioisotopes. These studies have shed much light on biochemical processes, *in vivo* brain function, and other aspects of human physiology and pathophysiology. However, the findings often have had little clinical impact, or the methodology developed has been so sophisticated that its use is impractical in clinical routine studies. Thus, clinical applications of PET have been in the doldrums for a long time, except at a few centers. These centers are large academic institutions that have had sufficient funds to operate an expensive PET system without regard to reimbursement issues.

By 1990, there were a few PET centers worldwide with predominant research interests and few budget limitations, run by scientists and physicians who were mainly interested in the research aspects of PET, while smaller institutions were unable even to consider installing a PET system. The data on the clinical use of PET originating from these research institutions were quite limited, and thus the medical community at large only slowly took notice of the fact that PET methodology could potentially provide important and clinically relevant information. As the installation and running of a PET center are considerably more complex than with a magnetic resonance (MR) imager, PET could not take off as quickly as MR. Cost issues and the fact that fewer clinical applications were obvious in PET than in MR made its widespread clinical introduction difficult. As a result, the introduction of clinically relevant PET has been occurring only since the early 1990s. Unfortunately, the 1990s were also the first years characterized by previously much less important cost pressures and negative feelings about high-tech medicine. Hence, PET imaging must be introduced into the clinical environment in a very adverse climate for an expensive new methodology.

G. K. von Schulthess: Nuclear Medicine, University Hospital, CH-8091 Zurich, Switzerland.

At the beginning of the 1990s, the medical community started to notice that interesting clinical data could be acquired with this method. The method in itself was very costly for several reasons:

1. Maintaining production capabilities in the industry for a few scanners rather than 100 or more per year resulted in a high price tag.
2. Building a full detector ring camera with a large axial field of view (15 cm) required a large amount of expensive detector material.
3. The production of radioisotopes was very costly because an expensive cyclotron and radiopharmacy laboratory were needed.
4. The logistics of providing radioisotope in a PET center or for a satellite PET camera was formidable.

At this point, the manufacturers started to rethink the design of PET scanners by realizing that an axial field of view on the order of 15 cm was necessary for efficient imaging. With this field of view, the brain and heart can be imaged in one acquisition, and by optimization of detector efficiency, short data acquisitions of five minutes or so permitted obtaining whole-body PET scans which could cover transaxial fields of view of 180 cm within 1 hour. These cameras were thus the first technically able to provide detector systems so efficient that clinically relevant imaging beyond the brain and the heart could be performed; "clinically relevant" is defined as an examination that requires 1 hour or less of imaging time. In parallel, small relatively cost-effective cyclotrons were built, and automated radiopharmaceutical synthesis systems came on the market, making it possible for a PET center to begin to produce fluorodeoxyglucose (FDG) at an acceptable cost in the range of $400 to $500 per patient and provide fluorine 18 radiopharmaceuticals to several satellite PETs with travel distances of around 3 hours or less from the cyclotron, a range that is still compatible with the half-life of 110 minutes.

Thus, in contrast to the early 1990s, in the late 1990s the necessary PET equipment existed to produce clinical whole-body examinations. As tumor staging appears to be the most relevant clinical indication for PET imaging, this is extremely important. It is now fully upon us, the clinical users, to generate the prospective data that will prove the relevance of clinical PET.

In most settings, PET data have to be viewed together with data from other imaging techniques, mainly computed tomography (CT) and MR imaging, that have attained a high level of clinical relevance: It is not possible to isolate PET from those examinations, and this is one of the themes of this text. This book aims at helping new users of PET in designing proper imaging protocols. It also provides the necessary information so that the medical imaging community and clinical users not running PET themselves understand that the method offers a vast array of clinically relevant data that may in fact be acquired cost-effectively.

This book draws on experience gleaned from roughly 3,500 clinical PET scans, of which approximately 60% were whole- or partial-body scans for tumor or infection detection and staging, 30% were scans for the evaluation of cerebral diseases, and 10% for cardiac studies. Except in cardiac studies, it is obvious that whenever PET shows pathology, its interpretation mandates close correlation with morphologic cross-sectional imaging data from CT or MR imaging. This has to do with the fact that in the brain it is sometimes difficult to distinguish hypermetabolic tumorous structures from normally metabolizing cortical areas, and that in the body FDG PET offers so few anatomic landmarks. Sometimes, electronic image fusion is necessary to provide optimum results. A hospitalwide network based on the DICOM 3.0 standard allows fusion of all modalities with each other within the PET software environment. Therefore, in many settings PET and the morphologic cross-sectional imaging modalities are complementary. PET provides the sensitivity for lesion detection, and the morphologic modalities the anatomic context. Thus, the tenets under which Nuclear Medicine at the University Hospital in Zurich operates and under which this book was written are the following:

1. Unless it can be quickly and convincingly demonstrated that PET is clinically relevant in some major applications, it will die before it ever starts to really live.

2. Running a clinical and cost-effective PET operation requires high patient throughput and minimized costs for radiopharmaceuticals.

3. Clinically relevant data have to be obtainable during an examination with a duration acceptable to patients. Imaging for much over 1 hour is unacceptable.

4. Tumor staging is the major clinical application of PET in most centers, and the application on which all discussions about cost effectiveness must be based.

5. In most applications, PET provides high sensitivity but inadequate morphologic information if lesions are found. Viewing data in conjunction with morphologic cross-sectional data is therefore mandatory. Image fusion is sometimes relevant and one even may consider combining a PET scanner with a morphologic imaging modality.

6. PET may be very relevant in assessing the effects of therapy, thus obviating lengthy regimens using expensive therapeutic agents.

7. Close collaboration of nuclear physicians and radiologists is mandatory. An integrated approach to image interpretation must be taken. A very strict separation between radiology and nuclear medicine may be particularly detrimental to the introduction of clinically useful PET, and thus antagonism between these related disciplines should be minimized.

As a result, this book contains a limited amount of technical information and information on radiopharmaceuticals and ancillary technology. The emphasis is on educating clinicians who are not interested in the intricacies of reconstruction algorithms and other "horrors." Since clinical applications in the brain and the heart, staging of tumors, and possibly the search for infectious foci are currently the most clinically relevant endeavors in clinical PET, these applications are discussed. Probably, at this point the most relevant clinical application of PET in most institutions is tumor staging. This is not surprising. The accumulation of FDG in malignant tumors is strong in most instances, while with the exceptions of the brain, the heart, and the urinary collecting system, little FDG is taken up by normal body structures. As a result, the signal-to-noise ratio for detecting a pathologic lesion is extremely high. This makes PET a wonderfully effective tumor staging method. In contrast to morphologic cross-sectional imaging, where the radiologist must carefully evaluate the numerous morphologic structures seen on equally numerous cross-sectional images, pathologic foci light up on PET like light bulbs. In essence, the "clever" radiopharmaceuticals do part of the work for the nuclear physician interpreting PET scans, while the contrast media used by the radiologist are unable to do so. This fact can be illustrated quite well using a page of one of the famous children's books by Richard Scarry, where the child is asked to identify "Lowly the Worm." This creature can be likened to the pathologic lymph node to be identified in tumor staging. Morphologic examinations present a vast amount of information, much of which is irrelevant to the task of staging, very much as in Fig. 1-1, where most of the structures are irrelevant for finding Lowly the Worm. The task of tumor staging with FDG is more adequately represented by Fig. 1-2, in which all irrelevant structures are blurred and only Lowly the Worm is seen in his apple car. Because PET provides little anatomic information, correlation with morphologic cross-sectional images is relevant whenever a lesion is seen.

CONSENSUS CLASSIFICATION OF USEFULNESS AND REIMBURSEMENT STATUS

During the past decade, a simple classification scheme has been devised to indicate whether or not a method is clinically useful. The classification has three broad groups, which are defined below. This book gives the most recent classifications according to this scheme obtained at several consensus conferences in Germany, as well as some other information on reimbursement status. This is useful information because if PET has been classified as useful or is reimbursed for a certain indication, this is a good sign that an objective panel has critically reviewed the existing literature and come to the conclusion that PET indeed has clinical relevance for the indication cited.

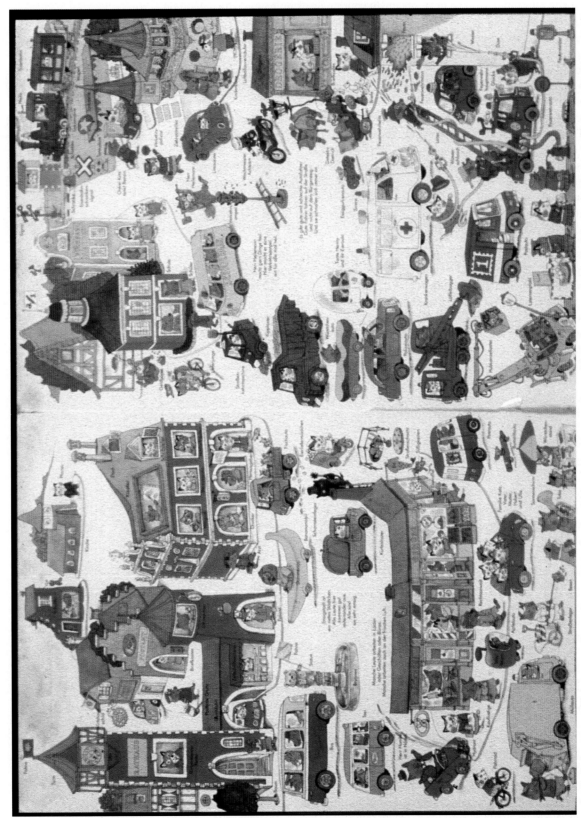

Figure 1-1. A page of a Richard Scarry children's book, which is full of information. Finding "Lowly the Worm" is quite a task, which is like finding a single lymph node metastasis.

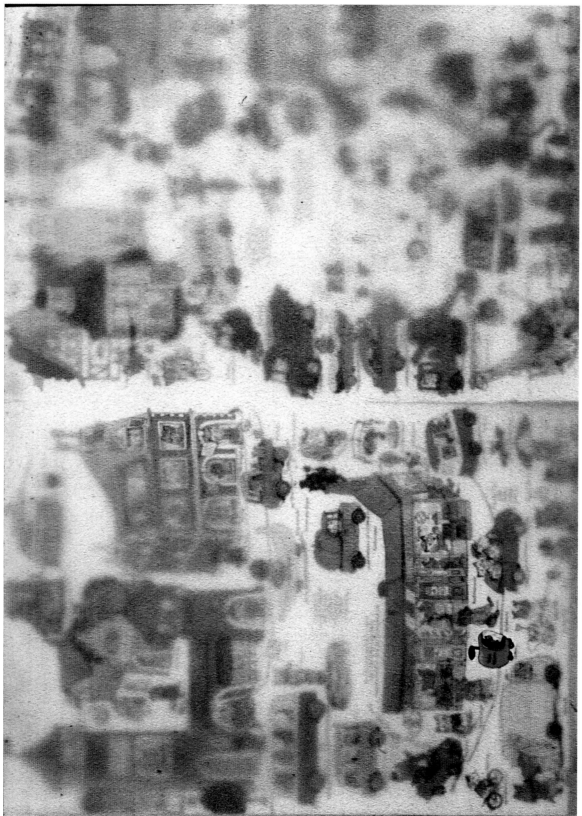

Figure 1-2. The same page blurred with chalk paper superimposed onto the picture. The area where "Lowly the Worm" is found is cut out. Thus, very much as in a FDG PET scan, the essential finding is enhanced, while the normal structures are barely seen.

The classification scheme used is as follows:

1a: appropriate and clinically useful;
1b: acceptable, predominantly clinically useful;
2a: helpful, only preliminary results on clinical benefits available;
2b: no evaluation possible, as not enough data available;
3: in general without benefit.

Furthermore, all indications discussed are classified according to a scheme from 0 to 4, summarizing the assessment of PET's usefulness, appraising the potential of PET to replace existing techniques, and giving the reimbursement status in Switzerland and the United States. It should be noted that while the reimbursed indications in Switzerland are relatively numerous, new Swiss medical law permits limiting the number of parties having the right to be reimbursed when a technology such as PET is classified as an expensive procedure. Currently, for a population of 7 million, there are only two PET sites having the right to be reimbursed.

The classification scheme devised by us is as follows:

0: useless—no replacement potential;
1: may show relevant information—may yield information to suggest another study;
2: relevant but inferior to other imaging—may obviate other study if PET is already available;
3: good, at least equivalent to other imaging-usually obviates other study;
4: clearly superior to other imaging modalities—other study usually adds no information.

2

Physical Principles and Practical Aspects of Clinical PET Imaging

Cyrill Burger and Thomas Berthold

The basic principle of positron emission tomography (PET) is simple: A PET tracer is administered to a patient and takes part in physiologic processes. First, the tracer is distributed in the body by the vascular system. If it is not a strictly intravascular tracer, some fraction of it is extracted into tissue during capillary passage. Depending on the tracer molecule, it may then undergo metabolic transformations or be bound at specific binding sites, and may eventually be washed out again. As the exchange and conversion processes are inherently dynamic, the concentration of tracer in the different forms and locations is instantaneously changing. Only for a few tracers, such as fluorine 18 (^{18}F)-labeled fluorodeoxyglucose (FDG), is an equilibrium situation reached in which concentrations are relatively stable.

The PET scanner continuously detects signals from the tracer in its field of view. It is able to localize these signals, but it can not attribute them to a specific form of the tracer if there are several. So the result of a PET scan is the total tracer concentration in each image pixel averaged over the acquisition duration. In experimental protocols, a series of sequential scans is initiated after tracer administration to monitor tracer uptake. In clinical PET, however, only a single scan is usually acquired at a certain time after tracer administration. The appropriate acquisition timing depends on the kinetic behavior of the tracer and on the half-life of the radionuclide used for labeling. With FDG, for example, a waiting period of 40 minutes must be observed between FDG injection and the PET scan.

The resulting PET images show functional information related to the processes in which the tracer is involved. It is important to note that without additional image processing, the information obtained is not purely quantitative. For instance, the images from a oxygen 15 ($H_2{}^{15}O$) water scan are "perfusion-weighted," rather than representing absolute perfusion in milliliters per minute per milliliter of tissue, or images of a FDG PET scan show "glucose uptake" rather than glucose turnover in milligrams per minute per 100 mL of tissue.

C. Burger and T. Berthold: Nuclear Medicine, University Hospital, CH-8091 Zurich, Switzerland.

PET is essentially a volumetric imaging technique. Data are simultaneously acquired in the entire field of view and represented as a stack of adjacent transaxial slice images. In some cases, however, different views of the data are helpful in finding the final diagnosis. This is no problem with PET images: As the axial resolution is about equal to the in-plane resolution, the data set may readily be resliced to generate coronal, sagittal, or even oblique slices without introducing disturbing effects.

The next section briefly explains the operation principle and the design of a PET scanner. How accurate PET images can be obtained is then outlined. Besides an appropriate data acquisition, this requires several calibrations and corrections. The chapter ends with a section dedicated to practical considerations on how to perform PET scans.

PRINCIPLES OF THE PET SCANNER

Basic Physical Effect: Positron Decay

PET tracers are labeled with positron-emitting radionuclides. These nuclides are proton-rich and hence unstable. They tend to reach a more stable state by positron decay, that is, by converting an excess proton into a neutron, a neutrino, and a positron, as sketched in Fig. 2-1. The positron—a positively charged electron—is emitted from the nucleus. It is slowed down by interactions and finally interacts with an electron, its antiparticle. This reaction is called *annihilation*: The masses of the positron and the electron are converted into energy, namely, into two photons of 511 keV each. These photons are emitted from the site of annihilation and travel in opposite directions, enclosing a 180-degree angle.

Detection of Annihilation Photons: Single Events

The PET scanner can detect the photon pair arriving from an annihilation event. To this end, it is equipped with scintillator crystals and subsequent processing devices, as outlined in Fig. 2-2. When a photon enters such a crystal, it is slowed by interactions with crystal atoms until it stops. By this time, it has transferred all its energy to the crystal atoms, whereby they become excited. When returning to the ground state, these atoms emit visible light photons. The number of light photons released by the crystal is proportional to the energy of the incident photon. This property can be used to discriminate between the 511 keV photons from annihilation events and photons from other sources. Adjacent to the crystal is an amplification device, a photomultiplier, that converts the light input into a current and feeds it into a processing device. If the energy calculated indicates arrival of a 511-keV photon, a single-event "511-keV photon entering crystal x at time t" is recorded.

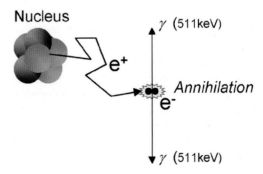

Figure 2-1. Physical effect used in PET imaging. A positron is emitted from the nucleus, is slowed down, and finally interacts with an electron in an annihilation process. The masses are converted in two 511-keV photons that travel in opposite directions.

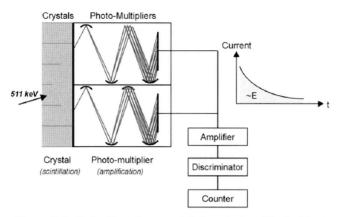

Figure 2-2. Detection of an annihilation photon. The incident photon produces a light flash in the detector crystal, causing photoelectrons to be released from the light-sensitive surface of the photomultiplier. The electrons are amplified to a current that is proportional to the energy of the entering photon. If the energy is in the acceptance range, the single-event counter is incremented.

Localization of the Annihilation: Coincidence Events

Relevant to the formation of a PET image is the location where the positron was emitted, namely, the nucleus of the radionuclide, which marks the presence of a tracer molecule. This location, however, cannot accurately be determined. Only annihilation photons can be detected and used to reconstruct the site of annihilation (Fig. 2-3). Annihilation photons can be detected with scintillation detectors. But how can the origin of the arriving photons be determined? The answer is that there is not enough information to locate it precisely. A PET detection system can only find a line along which a photon must have been traveling and hence on which the annihilation must have taken place. Two properties of the annihilation photon pair help find this line: The two photons are emitted in opposite directions along one common line, and they are traveling at the speed of light. Therefore, they must hit two opposing detectors at practically the same time. Put conversely: if two detectors register a single event at the same time, an annihilation must have happened on the line between the two crystals involved. In this case, the PET system records a *coincidence event* on a *line of response* (LOR). To account for the various delays in the detection of single events, coinci-

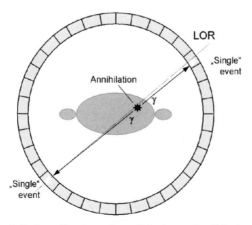

Figure 2-3. Localization of annihilations. Annihilation photons always occur in pairs, traveling at light-speed into opposite directions. Simultaneous detection of two 511-keV photons therefore signals an annihilation on the line between the two detectors involved.

Detector Rings

1   2   3   4   .....

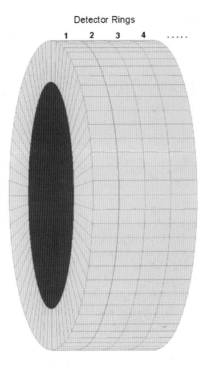

Figure 2-4. Full-ring PET scanner. A cylindrical field of view is enclosed by rings of detectors that stop and record the annihilation photons.

dence is weakened to events occurring within a short time interval (*coincidence window*) in real PET scanners. Usually, coincidence windows of 10 to 20 ns are applied (1).

Full-ring PET Scanner Design

The PET tracer distributed in the body radiates equally into all directions in space. To record as many coincidences as possible, the organ of interest should ideally be enclosed by detectors. Therefore, PET scanners are equipped with many detectors, usually assembled as a cylindrical arrangement of detector rings (Fig. 2-4). The body part to be examined is positioned within the rings. Modern PET scanners operate in two- (2D) or three-dimensional (3D) mode, as shown in Fig. 2-5. The preferred mode for quantitative acquisitions is the 2D mode, whereby coincidences are only accepted between crystals within transaxial rings. To prevent obliquely traveling photons from reaching detectors and saturating the scanner electronics, the rings are shielded from each other by tungsten septa that absorb the

A) 2D Mode   B) 3D Mode

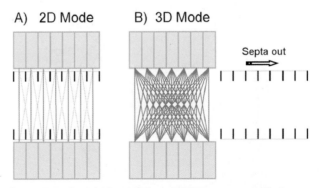

Septa out

Figure 2-5. Acquisition modes of PET scanners with ring geometry. **A:** LORs in a 2D acquisition. Tungsten septa stop photons traveling at inclined angles. To increase sensitivity, coincidences between neighboring rings may also be allowed as indicated by the *dashed lines*. **B:** In 3D acquisition mode, the septa are removed, and coincidences allowed at large axial angles.

undesired photons. The septa are removed for 3D acquisitions, and coincidences are allowed for crystals pertaining to different rings. With this, the solid angle and hence the scanner sensitivity are significantly improved. On the other hand, distortion effects are introduced, and correcting them is much more difficult than in 2D mode.

Reconstruction of a PET Image from Coincidence Events

During an acquisition, the PET scanner continually records coincidence events. At the end, it has the information available on how many annihilations happened on any allowed LOR between two detectors. These data are usually organized into raw data sinograms. To ascertain the nature of the PET raw data, all events on parallel LORs are sorted out, as illustrated in Fig. 2-6. For each ring, a row of count numbers is obtained. A count number represents the number of annihilations that took place in the slab, which defines the LOR, and sent the two 511-keV photons along the direction considered. Obviously, the more tracer is contained within the slab, the higher is the number of recorded counts. This means that the row of counts represents a projection of the spatial tracer concentration in the slice along the direction of the LORs. In a full-ring PET scanner, there are LORs at all directions

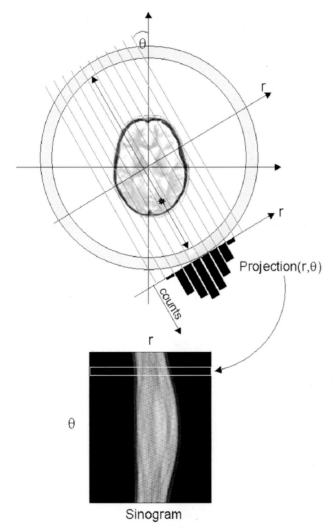

Figure 2-6. Geometry for obtaining PET raw data in 2D. Each coincidence belongs to a LOR that covers a slab in a transaxial slice and is given by its angulation (θ) and by its distance (r) from the center. The numbers of counts in all parallel LORs form a projection of the tracer distribution that is entered as a row into the sinogram data structure.

around 360 degrees. As events on all LORs are simultaneously recorded, projections through the tracer distribution are available at all angles after an acquisition. The data obtained are comparable to computed tomography (CT) scanning, although in that case the projections are sequentially measured by rotating an x-ray tube about the body. From the set of PET projection data, the underlying distribution must be calculated. There are several (approximate) solutions for this reconstruction-from-projections problem. Traditionally, a process called *filtered back-projection* has been applied because it is fast and robust. However, it suffers from artefacts around sharp discontinuities of the tracer distribution, as shown in Fig. 2-7. Therefore, *iterative reconstructions* are becoming the new standard, producing more accurate images in such problematic cases. The PET reconstruction delivers images that represent the tracer concentration in transaxial slices.

Alternative PET Scanner Designs

The full-ring PET scanner represents the current state-of-the-art with respect to sensitivity and resolution. Such devices, however, are expensive due to the large number of detectors employed (up to 28,000) which contain costly bismuth germanate (BGO) scintillation crystals. To make PET more affordable, two alternative designs have been implemented in commercial scanners.

A system developed by UGM Medical Systems (Philadelphia, Pennsylvania) reduces costs in two ways: Less expensive scintillation crystals from sodium iodine are used instead of BGO, and only a few large detectors instead of many small ones are employed. Six rectangular crystals are hexagonally arranged as illustrated in Fig. 2-8. The back of each crystal is covered by an array of square photomultipliers. Upon interaction of a photon in a crystal, the different amounts of light seen by the photomultipliers are used for the calculation of the photon entry point. The system always operates in 3D mode and accepts coincidences over a large axial acceptance angle. The spatial resolution of this system is about 6 mm and hence almost as good as that of full-ring systems operating in 3D mode. Sensitivity, however, is less by a factor of 3 (2). The system has recently been improved by replacement of the plain crystals by curved ones and is now marketed as CPET by ADAC Medical Systems (Milpitas, California).

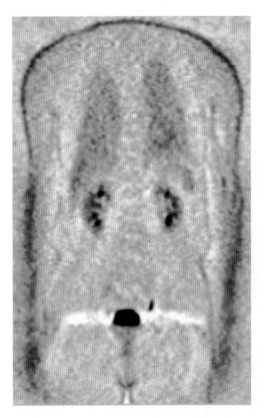

Figure 2-7. Typical artefact of PET image reconstruction by the filtered back-projection algorithm. The high accumulated dose in the bladder causes a ring effect that completely distorts the image around it.

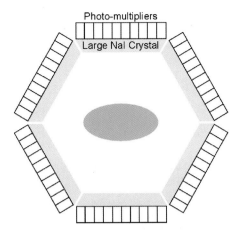

Figure 2-8. Alternative PET scanner design (UGM Medical Systems). It consists of six large sodium iodine scintillation crystals arranged as a hexagon and inherently operates in 3D to increase sensitivity.

The other alternative system, the ECAT ART marketed by CTI PET Systems (Knoxville, Tennessee) is based on the BGO multiring design. Instead of the full 360 degrees, only two 60-degree arcs are covered by two rotating detector buckets (Fig. 2-9). Only one-third the number of the detectors is thus required, resulting in substantial cost savings. To counterbalance the loss in sensitivity, the ART system always operates in 3D acquisition mode. The detectors rotate at 30 revolutions per minute, limiting the minimal acquisition duration to 2 seconds. The resolution is slightly worse than that of the CPET system, and the sensitivity is about 40% less (2).

CORRECTION STEPS FOR THE GENERATION OF PET IMAGES

PET scanners can produce images showing the absolute concentration of tracer throughout the field of view. However, ending up with correct concentrations requires a rigorous scheme of corrections and quality-control procedures.

Corrections for System Limitations during Detection

What must first be ensured is that only unscattered 511-keV photons from annihilations are detected and that their incidence is attributed to the correct crystal. The difficulties are that each crystal has a different light output and amplification differs among photomultipliers. These properties are assessed in quality-control procedures involving lengthy phantom acquisitions and transformed into appropriate correction maps.

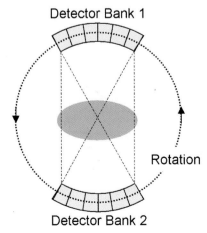

Figure 2-9. Alternative PET scanner design (ECAT ART). The full rings have been replaced by two rotating BGO detector buckets that cover 60 degrees each.

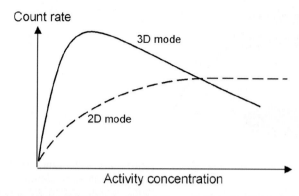

Figure 2-10. Relation between the activity in the field of view and the measured count rate. In 3D mode, the optimal performance is achieved with low activity concentrations. PET systems become saturated at high activity levels.

On the next level, it must be ensured that none of the arriving photons is missed. As misses cannot be avoided, they must at least be compensated for. A miss occurs when two (unrelated) photons arrive almost simultaneously at the same detector block. One such situation is *pulse pile-up*: The two photons are so close in time that their light flashes overlap. Therefore, the energy calculated from the light output is greater than 511 keV, and the event is discarded, so that both photons are lost. Another loss situation is *system dead-time*: The second photon arrives after the first has been accepted but while the processing unit is still busy handling its signal. In this case, only the second photon is lost. The frequency of single-event losses depends on the design of the detector system and increases with the rate of arriving photons. The characteristic is that of a saturating system, as shown in Fig. 2-10: At low activities, a further increase in activity results in a proportional increase in the detected count rate. However, as the activity is raised more and more, the system becomes flooded with events that it cannot handle any more, and after flattening, the count rate even begins to drop. This means that care must be taken to administer an appropriate tracer dose so that the system runs well below saturation. In this case, there are procedures to estimate the losses and compensate for them (Fig. 2-11).

Corrections for Interactions of Photons with Matter

Not all emitted photons are able to follow the initial direction until they hit the detector. Some are deflected, so they may not be used any more for determining the line where the annihilation took place. Others are absorbed in body tissue. This *attenuation* effect is so se-

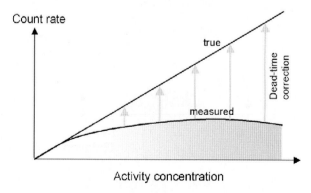

Figure 2-11. Dead-time correction. The characteristic response of the PET system to different activity levels is measured in phantom scans. Count rates recorded in patient scans are corrected accordingly.

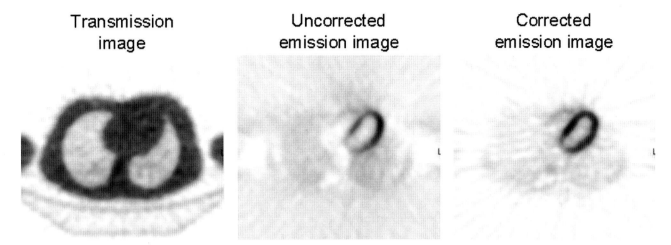

| Transmission image | Uncorrected emission image | Corrected emission image |

Figure 2-12. Effect of attenuation correction. The transmission image (20-minute acquisition time using two germanium 68 line sources) represents the linear absorption coefficient, which differs among body tissues. Without correction for photon attenuation, septal activity appears reduced in a FDG heart scan (20-minute acquisition time in 2D mode). The artefact disappears with attenuation correction.

vere that the number of detected photons is reduced by a factor up to 20. As the reduction depends on the amount of body tissue to be passed and hence on the anatomic location, attenuation must be compensated for to obtain any quantitative images. The attenuation correction is relatively easy for PET. The reason is that PET requires the detection of both annihilation photons to record a coincidence. The chance that one or both of the photons becomes attenuated depends on the total path length of tissue that must be penetrated. Hence, it is independent of the position on the line where the photons started their travel, meaning that attenuation is constant on a LOR. With an additional *transmission scan,* this attenuation can be measured and transformed into a map of *attenuation correction factors* (ACFs). Compensation for attenuation is then very easy: The number of detected coincidences on each LOR can simply be multiplied by the corresponding ACF. Figure 2-12 shows the effect of attenuation in the example of a FDG heart scan.

Scattering of photons manifests itself as a reduction of correctly detected coincidences. Some photons are deflected in a way that they miss the detectors, and others lose enough energy that they can be identified as scattered photons and discarded, but some are still accepted and cause misregistered coincidences (Fig. 2-13). The fraction of such scattered co-

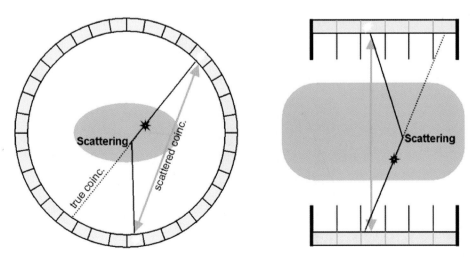

Figure 2-13. Misregistered events due to scattering. Some fraction of the deflected photons does not lose enough energy to be identifiable as being scattered. If they are detected by coincident crystals, a coincidence is counted on a wrong LOR.

incidences is high, ranging up to 20% for 2D acquisition mode and 70% for 3D mode. Clearly, then, scatter must be corrected for. While there is no accurate solution for the problem, heuristic correction schemes are routinely applied. They work well for 2D acquisitions but are problematic for 3D acquisitions when the activity is not well concentrated within the field of view.

There is an additional source of wrong coincidences. Two unrelated photons may be detected within a coincidence window and registered as a "random" coincidence (Fig. 2-14). Prerequisite for such a situation is that the other two photons belonging to the two annihilations are lost either by missing the field of view or by being absorbed. The correction for random coincidences is not problematic, as their rate can be measured and accurately be compensated for by the detection system.

Absolute Calibration

Even if all the above corrections have been performed, the reconstructed images still represent counts rather than activity concentrations. The problem is that the sensitivity of the scanner differs over the field of view. This means that the same activity produces different count numbers when placed at different locations, depending on the scanner design and the actual acquisition mode. In 3D mode, for instance, sensitivity increases tremendously toward the central slices, as they are covered by many axially inclined LORs. However, this behavior can be assessed in calibration scans with a homogeneous phantom of a known activity concentration, and appropriate translation tables can be derived.

Limits of PET Systems

The spatial resolution that can be attained with a PET scanner is limited by two phenomena (3). First, the positron travels some distance before it is annihilated. The maximum path length depends on the positron emitter, ranging from 2.4 mm for ^{18}F up to 20 mm for rubidium 82. However, as the positron's path is not straight, the resolution loss is much smaller, ranging from 0.2 to 2.6 mm. Second, the direction of the two annihilation photons may slightly deviate from 180 degrees due to a residual momentum. This noncollinearity causes a resolution loss of about 2 mm for a whole-body scanner. Put together, the fundamental resolution limit of PET is about 3 mm. In practice, commercial scanners provide resolutions of 4 mm and upward, depending on the scanner design and the location in the field of view.

Temporal resolution is related to many factors such as tracer dose, system sensitivity, and

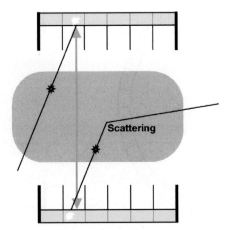

Figure 2-14. Random coincidence. Two unrelated photons arriving simultaneously at the two detectors of a LOR are erroneously interpreted as a coincidence.

signal-to-noise ratio required in the final image. System sensitivity depends on the scanner design, as well as the acquisition mode. For instance, at most, 3% of annihilation events can be detected in 2D mode. In 3D mode, sensitivity increases by a factor of 5 to 8. The shortest acquisition times are employed in experimental protocols to sample the initial phase of tracer uptake, and range down to 2 seconds. For clinical acquisitions, however, acquisition times typically range from 5 to 20 minutes.

PET SCANNING AND IMAGE PROCESSING

A brain investigation using FDG PET will serve as an overview of PET scanning. Early in the morning, a blank scan is performed to recalibrate the scanner, and FDG is prepared in the radiopharmacy laboratory. When the patient, who has fasted for at least 4 hours, arrives at the PET center, he or she is brought to an uptake room and asked to lie on a bed and relax. The FDG tracer is injected, and the patient rests for 40 minutes, during which time the labeled glucose is distributed throughout the body and metabolically trapped. The patient is then transferred to the table of the PET scanner (Fig. 2-15). The organ of interest is positioned within the scanner's field of view, and the acquisition is started. Emission counts are collected for 20 minutes; then a 10-minute transmission scan is initiated. After this, the patient is discharged, and the images are reconstructed for reviewing and archived (Table 2-1).

Study Protocol

The above sequence of events reflects the underlying protocol of a FDG PET study. Other types of PET studies are conducted according to similar protocols, which ensure that optimal images are obtained. A study protocol contains the information listed in Table 2-1: As study protocols specify the timing of the different steps, they allow stream-

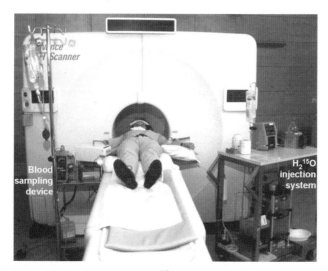

Figure 2-15. Setup for a H$_2$^{15}O PET brain study. The patient's head is positioned within the field of view of the PET scanner. Located on the right is an injection device that can be remotely controlled to reduce technicians' radioactive exposure. This device administers the tracer as a fast bolus. On the left is an automatic blood sampler that continually withdraws blood from the artery, measuring the contained radioactivity. These data are only required for quantitative procedures.

TABLE 2-1. *Protocol items for PET scanning and image processing*

Protocol item	Comment
Patient information	Due to the radioactive decay of tracers, it is essential for patients to arrive at the scheduled time and in adequate physical condition. With FDG studies, for example, the patient must have fasted and avoided exercise before the examination because the muscles would show an increased uptake
Patient preparation	Preparation depends on the actual study. For FDG studies, the following issues must be observed: During the uptake phase, the patient must be as relaxed as possible both physically and mentally. Therefore, rest in a dark, silent room on a comfortable bed is advised. A high dose often accumulates in the bladder during the waiting time. As severe reconstruction artefacts appear around extreme activity concentrations (see Fig. 2-7), the bladder should be cleared before any acquisition near the abdomen. Further preparation steps include blood sampling, medication (rest/stress studies), and proper positioning of the organ to be investigated in the field of view
Tracer dose administered	Two important issues must be considered. The activity accumulated in the field of view of the scanner should not be too small, as the images would get noisy, and should not be too large to avoid system saturation. Furthermore, the dose should be small enough if the tracer has a pharmacologic effect
Waiting time between administration and acquisition	Most tracers do not require a significant waiting time after tracer administration. In the case of $H_2{}^{15}O$ water studies, for instance, it is even essential to scan during tracer uptake
Scanning mode	Most scanners support different scanning modes, which must be selected according to the requirements of the study
Duration of emission scan	The duration should be as short as possible to avoid motion artefacts, yet long enough that the signal-to-noise ratio of the resulting images is sufficient
Transmission scan	The transmission scan is required for nonuniform attenuation correction. Duration in the same order as the emission scan is preferable but may be reduced due to time constraints
Reconstruction parameters	Images are reconstructed from projection data. Filters can be applied in this process for reducing noise, although at a loss of resolution, and the images can be zoomed
Image presentation	The reconstructed images can be transformed into various representations, such as coronal or sagittal views or bull's-eye plots for heart studies
Archival	There are two options for digitally archiving the data: saving the entire raw data set or just the reconstructed images. The former allows redoing reconstructions at a later time with different reconstruction parameters or algorithms, but requires huge amounts of storage capacity

lining of the PET center work flow with respect to tracer production and patient throughput. The most important steps of PET scanning are discussed further in the sections that follow.

Blank Scan

The blank scan is a daily quality-assurance procedure. It is routinely performed in the morning, before the first patient arrives. The blank scan is essentially a transmission scan without a body in the scanner field of view (Fig. 2-16A). Its purpose is to measure the gain of detectors in the system, which may drift over time, and to calculate correction maps. The information obtained is presented to the operator as a set of sinogram images, within which defective detector blocks appear as dark strikes (Fig. 2-16B).

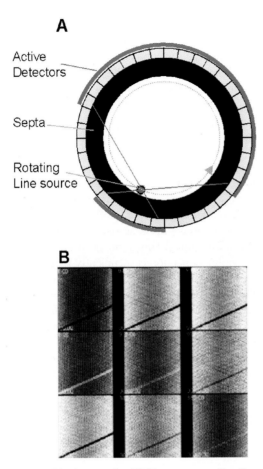

Figure 2-16. Blank scan for PET scanner calibration. **A:** A weak radioactive source is rotated around the empty field of view, and the coincidences are measured. **B:** The acquired counts are presented as sinograms, one for each slice. A black strike signals a detector problem.

Transmission Scan

A transmission scan is the counterpart of an emission scan. It uses photons that are emitted from an external source and pass the body, rather than photons emitted from a radioactively labeled tracer within body tissue. The most common experimental setup is sketched in Fig. 2-17. While the patient is positioned in the field of view, a robot pulls a radioactive

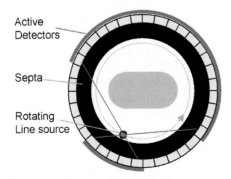

Figure 2-17. Transmission scan for obtaining ACFs. A line source is rotated about the body. A simple relation between the number of emitted (expected) photons and the number of detected ones allows calculation of the ACFs as well as CT images do.

line source out of a shielding container. It then rotates it about the body for some acquisition duration. Photons are continually emitted from the source at a known rate. Some of them may pass the body and reach an opposing detector; others are attenuated. After enough transmission counts have been detected, the line source is pushed back into its container. From the blank scan, it is already known how many photons would have been detected without obstructing tissue in the field of view. Thus, the two count numbers—transmission and blank scan—can be directly related with each other to derive the attenuation coefficient of the penetrated tissue. Furthermore, they allow the derivation of ACFs, which must be multiplied with the emission counts to compensate for attenuation. Because attenuation is constant on every LOR, the ACFs are directly obtained by dividing the blank scan counts by the transmission counts (4).

There is an important issue to observe with transmission scans: Wrong attenuation coefficients introduce severe artefacts into the final emission images. Therefore, it is essential that the patient does not move between the emission and the transmission scans. Furthermore, the transmission image must be accurate enough, meaning that the duration of transmission photon collection is sufficiently long, usually on the order of the duration of the emission scan. However, a recent approach promises to shorten the transmission scan while at the same time improving the accuracy of the attenuation maps. The principle is based on the observation that there is only a small number of tissue types with respect to attenuation, such as lung, soft tissue, and bone. Each of these tissue types has a known linear attenuation coefficient. The task to perform is a *segmentation* of the transmission image: Each pixel in the image must be classified, and the measured pixel value must be replaced by the ideal attenuation coefficient of that tissue type. The artificial attenuation coefficients obtained are then employed during attenuation correction. Several segmentation procedures have been implemented and are being introduced into clinical packages.

Emission Scan

The ultimate aim of PET scanning is to assess the spatial distribution of the PET tracer. It manifests itself by radiations—emitted annihilation photons—collected during the emission scan as emission counts. The emission scan is performed in one of several scanning modes. These modes can be categorized according to the detector configuration and acquisition type.

A multiring PET scanner can be operated using a 2D or a 3D configuration of the detectors (see Fig. 2-5). Most modern machines have septa that automatically slide into place if the operator selects a 2D acquisition, and are retracted if the mode is switched to 3D acquisition. Upon retraction of the septa, the number of LORs increases by a factor of 8 to 12. This increase has the advantage of improving system sensitivity, although it also complicates many issues (5): The data sets become exceedingly large and require reconstruction times of about 10 minutes per field of view. The scatter fraction increases from about 10% to 15% to 30% to 40%, so that accurate scatter correction becomes absolutely essential. Furthermore, attenuation correction and system calibration become much more complex. As a consequence, 3D acquisitions have mainly been used in brain-mapping studies, where relative blood flow changes are sufficient for the localization of activation sites, and only to a limited extent in neuroreceptor studies. The validation of the 3D methodology for studies in the chest (myocardial blood flow, tumor uptake) and the abdomen (tumor uptake) is not yet completed. Hence, current opinion is that 2D acquisition represents the "gold standard" and is usually accurate to within 5%.

In clinical studies, the data are usually acquired as one static scan: All counts between the start of the acquisition and its end are collected, and the average is calculated over the acquisition duration. Such an acquisition is usually termed a *frame.* If the dynamic distribution of the tracer within the body is to be assessed, a sequence of short consecutive frames is initiated at the time of tracer administration. The result of such a dynamic scan is a set of volume images showing the activity concentration at different times. These images cannot be directly interpreted by visual inspection. Rather, they must be further processed

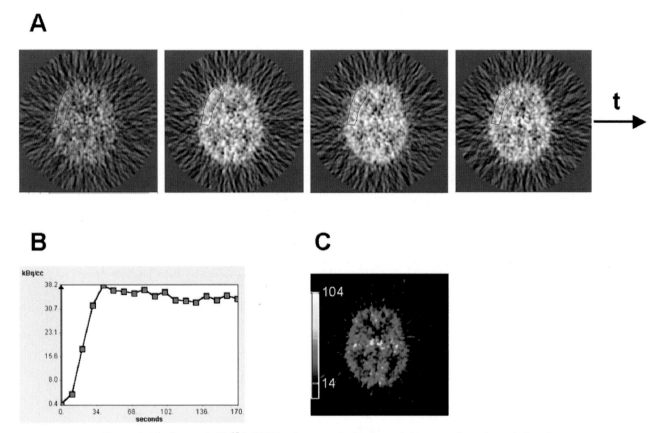

Figure 2-18. Dynamic $H_2^{15}O$ PET brain scan. **A:** Some early images of a selected slice during a sequence of 10-second frames that measure the uptake of water into tissue during the passage of the bolus. **B:** Curve shows the instantaneous tracer concentration within the region of interest shown in **A** at increasing times. **C:** Functional map shows absolute perfusion in milliliters per minute per 100 mL tissue, as calculated by a time-weighted integral approach (6) from the dynamic sequence.

to extract functional information, as shown in Fig. 2-18 for a $H_2^{15}O$ PET perfusion scan. Often, in oncologic studies, large parts of the body must be investigated to find metastases. As the axial field of view is typically only about 15 cm (25 cm at most), several adjacent static scans must be performed to cover the entire volume of interest. Current PET scanners support such whole-body scans in that their control software is able to incrementally adjust the table position by exactly the required offset and the reconstruction software combines the resulting images into one 3D data set (see Fig. 2-7). A rarely used acquisition type is the gated scan, which allows synchronization of the acquisition with beating of the heart. Triggered by the electrocardiogram, the collected counts are continuously sorted into a set of bins corresponding to different heart phases. These bins are separately reconstructed and allow resolution of heart motion as opposed to static heart scans, which only provide averaged images.

Image Presentation

PET has the advantage of being a volumetric technique with nearly isotropic resolution. Therefore, the image volume obtained can be resliced along arbitrary directions without introducing artefacts. This property is very helpful in different contexts: Long- and short-axis views can be readily generated for heart scans. Coronal and sagittal images can be displayed for whole-body scans to quickly get an overview of large parts of the body. Specifically, it allows easy fusion of PET data with images from anatomic studies such as magnetic resonance imaging. PET data can be reoriented without loss of information and resliced so that the calculated PET slices are congruent with the anatomic slices. Then, the anatomic images and the functional PET images can be presented as fused images (see Chapter 6: Image Fusion).

REFERENCES

1. Daube-Witherspoon ME. Positron emission tomography (PET): operational guidlines. In: Wagner HN, Szabo Z, Buchanan JW, eds. *Principles of nuclear medicine,* 2nd ed. Philadelphia: WB Saunders, 1995.
2. Townsend DW, Isoardi RA, Bendriem B. Volume imaging tomographs. In: Bendriem B, Townsend DW, eds. *The theory and practice of 3D PET, vol 32: developments in nuclear medicine.* Dordrecht/Boston/London: Kluwer Academic Publishers, 1998:111–133.
3. Muehllehner G, Karp JS. Positron emission tomography imaging—technical considerations, *Semin Nucl Med* 1986;16:35–50.
4. Bailey DL. Transmission scanning in emission tomography. *Eur J Nucl Med* 1998;25:774–787.
5. Townsend DW, Bendriem B. Introduction to 3D PET. In: Bendriem B, Townsend DW, eds. *The theory and practice of 3D PET, vol 32: developments in nuclear medicine.* Dordrecht/Boston/London: Kluwer Academic Publishers, 1998:1–10.
6. Alpert NM, Eriksson L, Chang JY, et al. Strategy for the measurement of regional cerebral blood flow using short-lived tracers and emission tomography. *J Cereb Blood Flow Metab* 1984;4:28–34.

3

Clinical Radiopharmacy

Gerrit Westera and P. August Schubiger

The specifics of clinical radiopharmacy in positron emission tomography (PET) stem from the (ultra)short half-lives of positron-emitting isotopes and the fairly high energy (511 keV) of the annihilation gamma rays. This means on-the-spot production of large amounts of radioisotopes (but see below) and synthetic chemistry that must proceed quickly behind a fair amount of shielding, using remotely controlled, automated equipment (Table 3-1).

PET RADIONUCLIDES

A self-sufficient PET center is equipped with an in-house cyclotron (Fig. 3-1) to produce the common positron emitters: carbon 11 (^{11}C), nitrogen 13 (^{13}N), oxygen 15 (^{15}O), and fluorine 18 (^{18}F) (Table 3-1). Today's compact cyclotrons are the negative-ion type: Hydrogen or deuterium is accelerated as negative ions, and the negatively charged electrons are stripped off by passing the beam through a carbon foil, which also diverts the particles to the targets. These cyclotrons fit into a small vault or are self-shielding and are highly automated, permitting operation by laboratory technicians. A special case in this respect is the [^{15}O]oxygen generator (1). It is a small, low-energy deuterium accelerator that is self-shielded and fits into any small corner up to 50 m removed from the PET camera.

Satellite PET centers can operate on ^{18}F products supplied by a cyclotron that is not too far away, as well as gallium (^{68}Ga) and rubidium 82 (^{82}Rb) generator products, eventually supplemented with a [^{15}O]oxygen generator.

PET RADIOPHARMACEUTICALS

The inherent beauty of ^{11}C, ^{13}N, ^{15}O is the occurrence of their stable counterparts in biomolecules, enabling the probing of biochemical processes in living human beings. ^{18}F

G. Westera: Nuclear Medicine, University Hospital, CH-8091 Zurich, Switzerland.

P. A. Schubiger: Joint Center for Radiopharmaceutical Sciences of the Paul Scherrer Institute, Villigen, Swiss Federal Institute for Technology and University Hospital, CH-8091 Zurich, Switzerland.

TABLE 3-1. *PET radionuclides*

| Radionuclide | Half-life (min) | Nuclear reaction | Specific activity (Ci/μmole) | | Max β^+ energy, (MeV) | Max range in H$_2$O (mm) |
			Theoretical	In practice		
^{11}C	20.3	^{14}N (p,α) ^{11}C	9×10^3	2–50	0.97	5.4
^{13}N	10.0	^{16}O (p,α) ^{13}N	19×10^3		1.2	5.4
^{15}O	2.0	^{14}N (d,n) ^{15}O	90×10^3		1.72	8.2
		^{15}N (p,n) ^{15}O				
^{18}F	109.6	^{18}O (p,n) ^{18}F	1.7×10^3	5–100 F$^-$	0.64	2.4
		^{20}Ne (d,α) ^{18}F		<0.080 F2		
^{68}Ga	68	^{68}Ge-generator, $T_{1/2}$= 271 d	—		—	—
^{82}Rb	1.3	^{82}Sr-generator, $T_{1/2}$ = 25 d	—		—	—

can often replace hydrogen or hydroxyl groups without modifying essential biologic activity. With automated synthesis under optimized reaction conditions (Fig. 3-2), production time can be limited, and ^{18}F's almost 2-hour half-life is sufficient for regional distribution.

The synthetic strategies are different for isotopes with ultrashort half-lives. Whereas complicated ^{11}C products can still be produced batchwise for in-house use, the use of ^{13}N and ^{15}O is practically restricted to simple molecules. ^{15}O is best produced continuously and in-line converted to the desired radiopharmaceutical (e.g., [^{15}O]water), which may then be applied as needed.

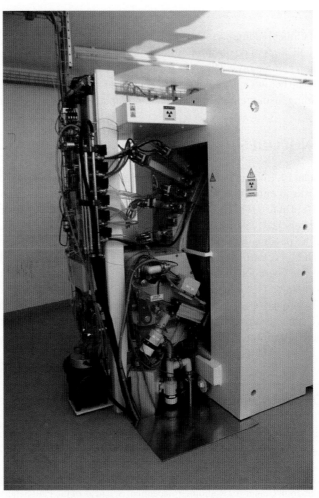

Figure 3-1. Cyclotron with targetry.

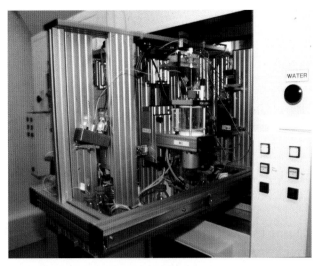

Figure 3-2. Versatile automatic production apparatus.

Currently, only a few compounds are generally being used in clinical routine (Table 3-2). However, other compounds have locally acquired similar status in particular institutions.

[^{18}F]FDG

2-[^{18}F]fluoro-2-deoxy-d-glucose ([^{18}F]FDG) represents a good example of the technical conditions needed for radiopharmaceutical production. It is produced according to scheme 1 in Fig. 3-3. The basic chemistry is long known (2), but recent refinements and optimization now allow commercial production of curie amounts of injectable [^{18}F]FDG of pharmaceutical quality (3,4). The synthesis time, including purification, packaging, and quality control, of curie amounts of [^{18}F]FDG can be less than 40 minutes after the end of bombardment.

[^{11}C]methionine

Methionine tagged with ^{11}C ([^{11}C]methionine) is the ^{11}C compound that comes closest to a routine clinical radiopharmaceutical. It is made according to scheme 2 in Fig. 3-3 by methylation of the demethylated substrate (5,6). Analogously, many ^{11}C radiopharmaceuticals of high specific activity can be made in quantities allowing one or two injections (with deterioration of the specific activity between applications).

It takes about 1 hour to prepare and check the quality of an ^{11}C product, which explains why the starting activity needs to be an order of magnitude more than the amount required for the application. This schedule is common, and depending on the overall yield of the reactions, further optimization is often hardly worthwhile because with imaging times of 1 hour per injection, a third injection six half-lives after the end of synthesis would need a prohibitively large amount of ^{11}C.

TABLE 3-2. *Routine PET radiopharmaceuticals*

Radiopharmaceutical	Application
[^{13}N]ammonia	Blood flow (cardiology)
[^{15}O]water	Blood flow
[^{18}F]FDG	Glucose metabolism
[^{11}C]methionine	Amino acid metabolism and transport

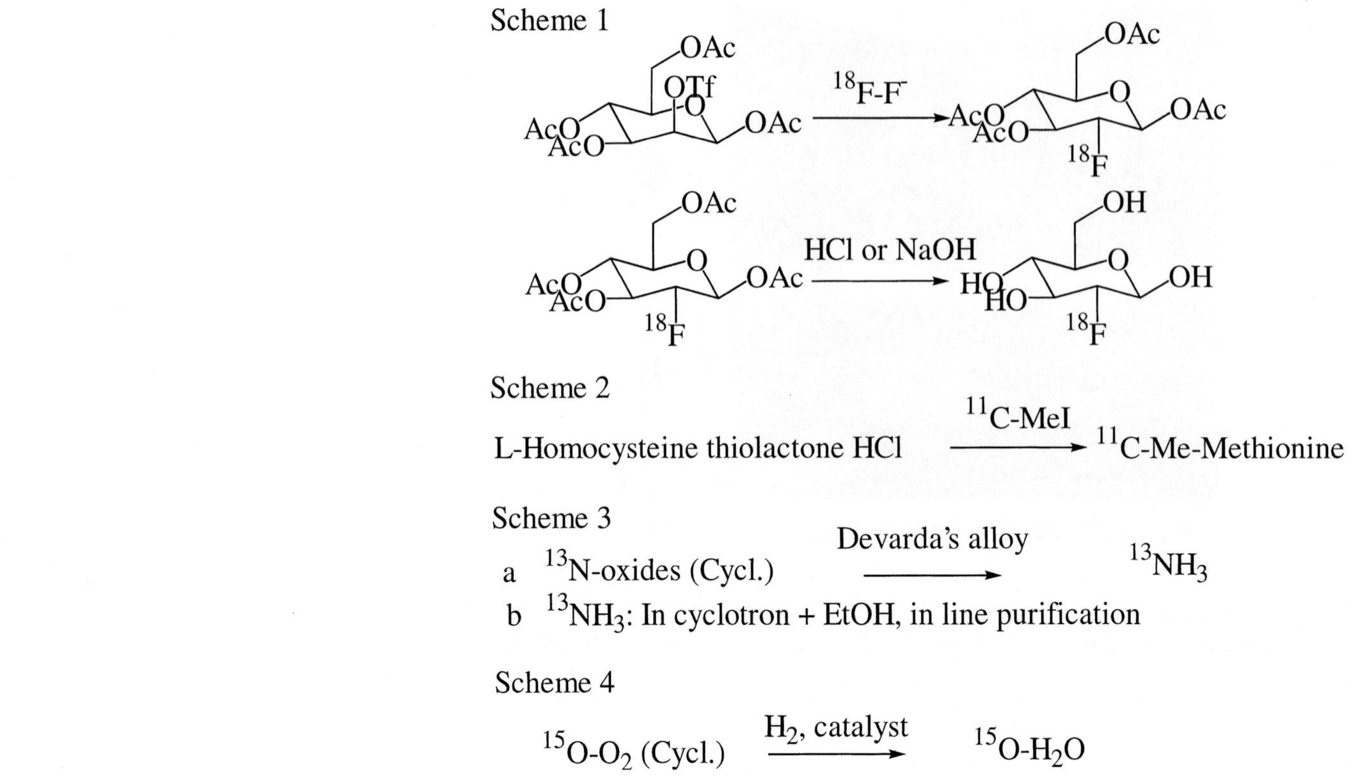

Scheme 1

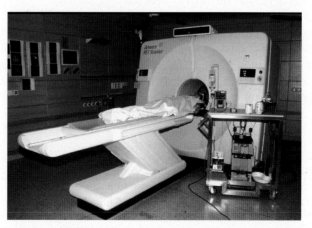

Scheme 2

L-Homocysteine thiolactone HCl $\xrightarrow{^{11}\text{C-MeI}}$ ^{11}C-Me-Methionine

Scheme 3

a ^{13}N-oxides (Cycl.) $\xrightarrow{\text{Devarda's alloy}}$ ^{13}NH$_3$

b ^{13}NH$_3$: In cyclotron + EtOH, in line purification

Scheme 4

^{15}O-O$_2$ (Cycl.) $\xrightarrow{\text{H}_2,\ \text{catalyst}}$ ^{15}O-H$_2$O

Figure 3-3. Reaction schemes.

[^{13}N]ammonia

Although nitrogen is part of peptides and many biologically important macromolecules, the short half-life of ^{13}N makes ammonia the only ^{13}N product in clinical routine. Two useful production methods are shown in scheme 3 in Fig. 3-3 (7,8). Batch productions sufficient for two consecutive injections are feasible.

[^{15}O]water

Several simple [^{15}O] compounds—with oxygen, carbon dioxide, carbon monoxide, or water—can be produced continuously in line with a continuous cyclotron bombardment.

Figure 3-4. Bedside water infusor.

TABLE 3-3. *Classification of air quality*

Class	Maximum amount of particles/m^3 > 0.5 µm	> 5 µm	Maximum number of microorganisms
A	3,500	0	< 1
B	3,500	0	< 5
C	350,000	2000	100
D	3,500,000	20,000	500

[^{15}O]water is the radiopharmaceutical that is generally used clinically; it is made according to scheme 4 in Fig. 3-3. An infusor has been developed that allows multiple injections at 4- to 5-minute intervals (9,10) (Fig. 3-4).

PHARMACEUTICAL ASPECTS

Chemical and radiochemical quality control is integrated into the production process. The pharmaceutical aspects can only be checked after application of the radiopharmaceutical. Sterility and apyrogenicity are assured by performing the syntheses according to rigorous standard operating procedures and checking representative samples afterward. The syntheses must be performed in a closed apparatus with terminal sterilization.

The requirements for the laboratories (air quality and building requirements to prevent dust accumulation) and for the documentation should be defined according to international conventions in agreement with the local authorities (see Nordic Council on Medicines, 1998 (11); Pharmaceutical Inspection Convention, 1989 (12); U.S. Department of Health and Human Services, 1997) (13,14). There seems to be a trend to accept the following guidelines:

If the product is distributed, the air in the laboratories must be of purity class D; manipulations in open equipment must be performed in class A laminar flow hoods, surrounded by class B air (Table 3-3).

If the product is used only in house, the requirements may be less stringently implemented.

OUTLOOK

Synthetic methods have been developed that allow routine production of some short-lived clinical PET radiopharmaceuticals. The development of more flexible automation will eventually allow other, more complicated syntheses of new in-house products to be performed. All production facilities will have to be improved to fulfill pharmaceutical standards of good manufacturing practice. This will also permit production of more ^{18}F compounds for regional distribution to satellite PET centers. Emerging candidates are F-dopa and fluorinated tyrosine.

REFERENCES

1. Clark JC, Morelle J-L. An oxygen-15 generator. In: Targetry 91: proceedings of the IVth international workshop on targetry and target chemistry, PSI Villigen, Switzerland, September 1991:34–35.
2. Hamacher K, Coenen HH, Stöcklin G. Efficient stereospecific synthesis of no-carrier-added 2-[^{18}F]-fluoro-2-deoxy-d-glucose using aminopolyether-supported nucleophilic substitution. *J Nucl Med* 1986;27:235–238.
3. Moerlein SM, Bockhorst JL, Gaehle GG, Lechner KL, Siegel BA, Welch MJ. Preparation of fluorodeoxyglucose F-18 injection via the GE microlab device: the Washington University experience. *J Labelled Compounds Radiopharmaceut* 1995;37:653–654.
4. Zijlstra S, Medema J, Elzinga PH, Notohamiprodjo G, Vaalburg W. Optimisation of ^{18}F-FDG production using commercially available SPE-cartridges. *J Labelled Compounds Radiopharmaceut* 1997;40:229–231.
5. Comar D, Cartron J-C, Mazière M, Marazano C. Labelling and metabolism of methionine-methyl-[^{11}C]. *Eur J Nucl Med* 1976;1:11–16.

6. Mizuno K-I, Yamazaki S, Iwata R, Pascali C, Ido T. Improved preparation of l-[methyl-^{11}C]methionine by on-line [^{11}C]methylation. *Appl Radiat Isot* 1993;44:788–790.
7. Vaalburg W, Kamphuis JAA, Beerling-vander Molen HD, Reiffers S, Rijskamp A, Woldring MG. An improved method for the cyclotron production of ^{13}N-labelled ammonia. *Int J Appl Radiat Isot* 1975;26:316–317.
8. Korsakov MV, Krasikova RN, Fedorova OS. Production of high-yield [^{13}N]ammonia by proton irradiation from pressurized aqueous solutions. *J Radioanalyt Nucl Chem* 1996;204:231–239.
9. Tochon-Danguy HJ, Clark JC, Janus A, Sachinidis JI. Technical performance and operating procedure of a bedside [^{15}O]water infusor. *J Labelled Compounds Radiopharmaceut* 1995;37:662–664.
10. Westera G, Schubiger PA. A versatile [^{15}O]water infusor. Presented at the seventh international workshop on targetry and target chemistry, Heidelberg, June 1997.
11. Nordic Council on Medicines. *Short-lived radionuclides for positron emission tomography: application of the EC guidelines for radiopharmaceuticals.* NLH Publication 1998, No. 46.
12. Pharmaceutical Inspection Convention. *Guide to good manufacturing practice for pharmaceutical products.* 1989.
13. U.S. Department of Health and Human Services, Food and Drug Administration, Center for Drug Evaluation and Research. *Guidance for industry: current good manufacturing practices for positron emission tomographic (PET) drug products.* 1997.
14. Meyer G-J, Waters SL, Coenen HH, Luxen A, Mazière B, Langström B. PET radiopharmaceuticals in Europe: current use and data relevant for the formulation of summaries of product characteristics (SPCs). *Eur J Nucl Med* 1995;22:1420–1432.

4

Radiation Doses and Radiation Protection

Stefan Kneifel

In a nuclear medicine examination and in general, it is good practice to adhere to the ALARA (As Low As Reasonably Achievable) rule and identify all steps that can reduce radiation exposures to patients and personnel. This chapter summarizes some radiation issues relevant for individuals involved in PET imaging.

PATIENT RADIATION DOSES

Generally, the absorbed dose for any radiopharmaceutical depends on several factors:

Type of decay;
γ-Ray energy;
β^+ ray energy;
Distribution, kinetics, and metabolism in the body;
Radionuclide half-life (physical half-life);
Clearance from the body (biologic half-life).

For all PET radiopharmaceuticals, the first two factors are constant. They all emit positrons that annihilate with an electron, resulting in two γ-rays of 511-keV energy each. Thus, the dose absorbed by a patient during a PET examination depends on the distribution of the radiopharmaceutical and its physical and biologic half-lives (see Table 4-1).

$$T_{eff} = T_{phys} \times T_{biol}/(T_{phys} + T_{biol}).$$

When using radionuclides with a short physical half-life such as oxygen 15 (^{15}O) or nitrogen 13 (^{13}N), the biologic half-life is of minor relevance for the radiation dose obtained by the patient because the effective half-life relevant for the radiation dose is very close to the shorter of the two half-lives, provided that either the physical or biologic half-life is very different. In radionuclides with a longer physical half-life such as fluorine–18 (^{18}F), the clearance becomes more relevant for the dose. ^{18}F-labeled fluorodeoxyglucose ([^{18}F]FDG), the most widely used in clinical PET, is taken up by the brain and excreted via the kidneys into the bladder. Thus, the organs with the greatest radiation exposure in a [^{18}F]FDG study are the kidneys, the bladder wall, and the brain because of this radiopharmaceuticals high activity accumulation.

S. Kneifel: Nuclear Medicine, University Hospital, CH-8091 Zurich, Switzerland.

TABLE 4-1. *Single-organ absorbed doses in PET studies*

Target organ	[^{18}F]FDG (μGy/MBq)	H$_2$[^{15}O]water (μGy/MBq)
Brain	37	0.71
Heart	16	0.67
Kidneys	28	0.95
Liver	19	0.75
Bone marrow	5	1.49
Lungs	18	0.57
Breast	9	1.16
Stomach	12	1.21
Small intestine	14	1.05
Upper large intestine	14	1.26
Lower large intestine	14	1.54
Spleen	14	1.19
Testes	14	1.11
Ovaries	15	1.79
Thyroid	13	1.11

Calculated for 70-kg body weight.

The calculation of single-organ doses (measured in gray [Gy]; 1 Gy = 1 J/kg) and whole-body effective dose (measured in sievert [Sv]; 1 Sv = 1 J/kg, multiplied by a weighting factor for different decay types) is sophisticated and based on complex calculation models that take the uptake values for different organs and their spatial neighborhood into account. Tables 4-1 to 4-3 show single-organ doses and whole-body effective doses for the most frequently used PET tracers: [^{18}F]FDG (1), ^{15}O water ([H$_2$^{15}O]water) (2), and ammonia tagged with ^{13}N ([^{13}N]ammonia) (whole-body doses only) (3). They are calculated for an average body weight of 70 kg.

In newborns, the brain uptake of [^{18}F]FDG is higher and its extraction into the urine is less than in adults. The radiation exposure of most organs with the exception of the bladder wall is therefore higher, resulting in an increased whole-body effective dose. For newborns, the effective dose is about 430 μSv/MBq, which is 14 times higher than in adults (4).

RADIATION PROTECTION FOR PET SCANNER PERSONNEL

As in any environment with ionizing radiation, the three principles of radiation protection apply: exposure time, shielding, and distance. (In German, these are the three A's, respectively, *Aufenthaltsdauer, Abschirmung,* and *Abstand.*)

TABLE 4–2. *Whole-body effective doses of radiopharmaceutical for PET studies*

	[^{13}N]ammonia	[^{18}F]FDG	[H$_2$^{15}O]water
μSv/MBq	2.0	29	1.16

Calculated for 70-kg body weight.

Table 4–3. *Whole-body effective doses for some routine PET examinations*

Examination	Tracer	Activity (MBq)	Whole-body dose (mSv)
Whole-body FDG PET	[^{18}F]FDG	400	11.6
Myocardial viability	[^{18}F]FDG	250	7.2
Brain FDG PET	[^{18}F]FDG	200	5.8
Myocardial perfusion	[^{13}N]ammonia	2 × 800 = 1600 (rest/stress)	3.2
Brain perfusion	[H$_2$^{15}O]water	2 × 800 = 1600 (baseline/diamox)	1.8

Calculated for 70-kg body weight.

TABLE 4–4. *Gamma energy: 2 × 511 keV*

Shielding material	Half-value layer (cm)
Concrete (2.35 g/cm^3)	5
Lead	0.42

Exposure Time

Work time close to patients receiving radiopharmaceuticals and to unshielded radiation sources, such as syringes, can be minimized through optimal planning of the work to be done.

Shielding

Due to the high gamma energy, effective shielding becomes very thick and therefore shields are heavy (Table 4-4). Therefore, radiation protection considerations must be taken into account when construction of the examination and radionuclide application rooms are being planned. Mobile shields must be mounted onto wheels and are too heavy to be carried around in most instances. If patients are injected by hand, the radiation dose to the fingers by positrons must be taken into consideration. Adequate protection can be achieved with Plexiglas shielding, as this material is light, stops positrons, and increases the distance between the radiation source and the fingers.

Distance

As with single photon emitters, increasing the distance between radiation sources and personnel is a cheap and efficient radiation protection measure (Table 4-5).

Guidelines

Injection of the radionuclides should always occur through an intravenous line placed prior to radionuclide application. If possible, an automated injector system should be used. If it is necessary to draw repeated blood samples or to take repeated blood pressure measurements, these should be performed using automated systems.

Dosimetry

It is not enough to monitor only the whole-body dose of personnel. High partial-body radiation burdens occur, particularly in the fingers, during preparation of syringes containing the radiopharmaceuticals and during injection. This radiation burden should be monitored with finger dosimeters (thermoluminescence dosimeters). To check potential contamination, hand–foot monitors and monitors checking contamination of clothes must be avail-

TABLE 4–5. *Comparison of radiation doses of ^{18}F and ^{99m}Tc*

	h10 (mSv/h)/GBq distance 1 m	h0.07 (mSv/h)/GBq distance 10 cm
^{99m}Tc	0.022	300
^{18}F	0.16	2000

^{99m}Tc, technetium 99m.

able. Incorporation of positron emitters during PET examinations is rare. Because of the short half-life of the standard PET radionuclides, they can barely be measured.

REFERENCES

1. Deloar HM, Fujiwara T, Shidahara M, et al. Estimation of absorbed dose for ^{18}FDG using whole-body PET and MRI. *Eur J Nucl Med* 1998;25:565–574.
2. Brihaye C, Depresseux JC, Comar D. Radiation dosimetry for bolus administration of H_2^{15}O. *J Nucl Med* 1995;36:651–656.
3. Johansson L, Mattsson S, Nosslin B, Leide-Svegborn S. Effective dose from radiopharmaceuticals. *Eur J Nucl Med* 1992;19:933–938.
4. Ruotsalainen U, Suhonen-Polvi H, Eronen E, et al. Estimated radiation dose to the newborn in ^{18}FDG-PET studies. *J Nucl Med* 1996;37:387–393.

5

Financial Considerations

Gustav K. von Schulthess

Positron emission tomography (PET) is a costly business, and this is a key reason why this excellent imaging modality has not yet found widespread introduction into clinical practice. Running a financially successful PET operation obviously depends on the level of reimbursement for an examination. In this chapter, the cost side of running a PET operation is analyzed, and the analysis assumes income per scan as reimbursed in Switzerland. Although reimbursement for PET in Switzerland is relatively low, this has the advantage of truly optimizing PET scanning with regard to cost. As PET involves not only the scanning itself but also production or purchase of the necessary radiopharmaceuticals, both aspects must be considered. On the scanner side, the logistics of performing a large number of PET scans during the short time when the radiopharmaceuticals are available is important. This applies for both a PET center (an operation that includes one or more scanners and a cyclotron) and a PET satellite, where there is only a scanner. On the cyclotron/radiopharmacy side, the issue is to provide the radiopharmaceuticals as cheaply, as quickly, and as plentifully as possible.

GENERAL CONSIDERATIONS

Currently, the only clinically useful and potentially widely available radiopharmaceutical is fluorodeoxyglucose tagged with fluorine-18 ($[^{18}F]FDG$); the ^{18}F isotope has a half-life of approximately 110 minutes. It can be efficiently produced in automated systems in large batches and activities in the range of 200 to 1,000 mCi. Table 5-1 delineates how much $[^{18}F]FDG$ (or any other ^{18}F-containing compound or ^{18}F itself) is available after various intervals of waiting time. This is important because $[^{18}F]FDG$ is typically delivered to the scanner in a vial at the beginning of the day, and appropriate patient doses are taken from the vial into the syringe used for application as time goes by. This is very similar to technetium-labeled bone scanning agents. The first column in the table gives the times at which the activity is measured after an initial time point of deliv-

G. K. von Schulthess: Nuclear Medicine, University Hospital, CH-8091 Zurich, Switzerland.

TABLE 5-1. *Availability of [^{18}F]FDG after various time intervals*

Time elapsed (min)	Multiplication factor	Remaining activity (starting at 100 mCi)	Initial activity required for injected dose	
			5　mCi	10　mCi
0	1	100	5	10
55	0.71	71	7.0	14.1
110 (1 h 50)	0.5	50	10	20
165 (2 h 45)	0.35	35	14.3	28.6
220 (3 h 40)	0.25	25	20	40
275 (4 h 35)	0.177	17.7	28.2	56.4
330 (5 h 30)	0.125	12.5	40	80
385 (6 h 25)	0.088	8.8	56.8	112.6
440 (7 h 20)	0.068	6.8	80	160
495 (8 h 15)	0.044	4.4	113.6	227.2
550 (9 h 10)	0.031	3.1	160	320

The half-life of [18F]FDG is 110 minutes.

ery. The multiplication factor permits calculation of how much remains of a given dose of [^{18}F]FDG after the time indicated in column 1. If one wants to calculate how much [^{18}F]FDG remains 275 minutes after initial delivery of 50 mCi for injection, one takes the dose and multiplies it by the multiplication factor, which in this example yields approximately 9 mCi. This is tabulated in the third column for a starting activity of 100 mCi. Usually, one wants to find out how much activity one needs to deliver initially, so that at a certain time after delivery, a dose of 5 mCi or 10 mCi can be injected. The computations for this setting are provided in the last two columns. When one plans a scanning day during which five patients will be examined with 10 mCi of [^{18}F]FDG (the first at 0 minutes, the second at 55 minutes, the third at 110 minutes, the fourth at 220 minutes, and the fifth at 330 minutes), one must add the respective values in the last column, that is, 10 + 14.1 + 20 + 40 + 80 = 164.1 mCi. Thus, very high initial doses of [^{18}F]FDG are needed for the last patient, and with a single [^{18}F]FDG delivery of around 300 mCi, six to eight patients can easily be scanned in a day, given an efficient scanner. Table 5-1 is important, as it documents how prohibitive it becomes to perform a PET scan using [^{18}F]FDG produced 7 hours or more before injection because of the huge required dose to be prepared at time 0 minutes.

More accurate calculations, which in practice are rarely needed, can be obtained by using the half-life formula:

$$A = A_0 \exp (-t \ln2/t_{1/2}) \text{ or}$$

$$A_0 = A/[\exp (-t \ln2/t_{1/2})]$$

Where A is the activity needed, A_0 is the initial activity delivered, t is the delivery time, and $t_{1/2}$ corresponds to the half-life, which is 110 minutes for ^{18}F (when calculations are made for other positron emitters, the appropriate half-life would replace this value). ln2 equals 0.693, and for ^{18}F, $t_{1/2}$. ln2 equals 158.7 minutes. As one is usually interested in computing how much initial activity is needed to yield a dose A after a time t, the second formula is required.

COST CONSIDERATIONS IN PET SCANNING

Let us look at the scanner side of things first. For a 10-mCi dose of [^{18}F]FDG injected roughly 7 hours after delivery from the radiopharmacy laboratory, one requires 160 mCi rather than just 10 mCi. Assume a scanner is receiving a [^{18}F]FDG shipment once a day and one wants to run it for 8 hours, with the last injection taking place after 7 hours. Based on these premises and the assumption that the average examination lasts for 1 hour (or 55 minutes to make calculations simple), the total amount of [^{18}F]FDG needed is 183 mCi for 5-mCi injections and 366 mCi for 10-mCi injections, as computed by using Table 5-1. A 1-hour clinical scan time for a whole-body PET (WB PET) can be achieved with present-day top-of-the-line PET scanners. Thus, with production of approximately 400 mCi and tight scheduling, eight patients obtaining a FDG PET can be imaged on a high-throughput scanner; however, a more realistic figure would probably be six or seven patients.

In Switzerland, a simple reimbursement scheme has been established, whereby 1 hour of a top-of-the-line scanner costs SFr 800 ($540). A brain PET is charged 0.75 hour, an additional absorption correction 0.25 hour, and a scan with an additional isotope also 0.25 hour. WB PET is charged 1 hour of scan time, and so is a partial-body PET with an absorption correction. If four WB PET scans and three brain PET scans are performed with [^{18}F]FDG during 250 working days per year, the number of scans performed is 1,750, and the revenue per day is SFr 5,400 ($3,600), or SFr 1.35 million ($911,000) per year. In addition, performing one study with ammonia tagged with nitrogen 13 ([^{13}N]ammonia) or one water study per day adds 250 examinations and revenues of 250 × SFr 200 ($135) or 250 × SFr 600 ($400), or SFr 50,000 ($34,000) or SFr 150,000 ($101,000), respectively, depending on whether or not the study is an add-on. Table 5-2 shows that with these numbers, a full-ring detector PET camera can be run to cover costs even in a satellite setting. However, an adequate [^{18}F]FDG source is mandatory. Cheaper cameras will have lower patient throughput, in the range of five or six in an 8-hour working day. This generates decreased revenue, assuming two brain and three WB FDG PET scans (3 × SFr 800 + 2 × SFr 600 = SFr 3,600 × 250 = SFr 900,000 or $607,000), and the radiopharmaceutical cost is higher because of less efficient use of the delivered dose. However, this is offset by the lower price of the PET equipment.

The numbers relating to this information in Table 5-2 are given in column 2 for a high-end scanner and in column 3 for a low-end scanner. They are self-explanatory. Personnel costs, as well as building costs, may vary substantially from country to country, while capital costs are currently in the range given above in a wide range of countries. In addition, the numbers of personnel have been estimated at a low level, as efficiency of working personnel is increasingly demanded.

TABLE 5-2. *Summary of costs involved in PET center operations*

Item	High-end scanner ($)	Low-end scanner ($)	Cyclotron/radiopharmacy L ($)
Equipment cost	2,200,000	1,000,000	3,500,000
Per year	275,000 (8 yr)	125,000 (8 yr)	220,000 (16 yr)
Capital cost (5%)	110,000	50,000	175,000
Service contract	100,000	60,000	150,000
Upgrading	100,000	60,000	150,000
Supplies	—	—	50,000–100,000
Personnel	250,000[a]	200,000[a]	350,000[b]
Subtotal	835,000	495,000	1,100,000
Building	1,000,000	1,000,000	3,000,000
Capital cost	40,000	40,000	120,000
Depreciation (40 years)	25,000	25,000	75,000
Maintenance, including power	25,000	25,000	75,000
Total Expenditures	925,000	585,000	1,370,000
Revenues			
In house [^{18}F]FDG use	900,000–1,000,000	600,000	700,000
In house [H$_2$^{15}O] water, [^{13}N] ammonia use	—	—	125,000
			575,000
[^{18}F]FDG sale (0.25 of mCi) charged	—	—	575,000
Total revenues	900,000–1.000.000	600,000	1,400,000

[a] $^1/_2$ MD and two technicians/administrators for high-end scanner, $^1/_2$ MD and 1$^1/_2$ technicians/administrators for low-end scanner.
[b] 1 PhD and 2$^1/_2$ lab technicians/administrators.

COST CONSIDERATIONS IN A PET RADIOPHARMACY LABORATORY

With regard to the cyclotron/radiopharmacy (CRP) side of things, a CRP unit needs to deliver 200 to 400 mCi of [^{18}F]FDG per day to run a scanner at the above rate. The Swiss scheme reimburses SFr 650 ($440) for [^{18}F]FDG and SFr 340 ($230) for [^{13}N]ammonia and oxygen 15 water ([H$_2$^{15}O]water). Six [^{18}F]FDG injections thus generate an income of about SFr 4,000 ($2,600) per day, or SFr 1,000,000 ($675,000) per year (250 days). Assuming that the PET center can also handle two [^{13}N]ammonia or two [H$_2$^{15}O]water scans (or one of each) on top of the [^{18}F]FDG examinations and these can be performed either before or after all [^{18}F]FDG patients have been scanned, the daily income at the reimbursement rate of SFr 350 ($240) per injection is an additional SFr 700 ($470) per day, or SFr 175,000 ($118,000) per year. Thus, the net income from radiopharmaceuticals dispensed for one scanner at a PET center can be reasonably expected to amount to SFr 1.125 million ($760,000).

Table 5-2 presents cost calculations representing the approximate cost for the system at the University Hospital in Zurich. While PET scanning with a single scanner can and must be run cost-effectively, the CRP operation requires additional income. This can be generated by installing a second scanner if the patient load permits this, by selling [^{18}F]FDG to satellite PET installations, or both. Producing a total of 800 mCi will support two scanners operating at the level discussed above, doubling the revenue to more than $1,520,000, which covers cost. Alternatively, it permits the CRP operation to sell 400 mCi. If calibration is delayed by one (or two) half-lives, approximately 200 (or 100) mCi can be charged for. At our institution, 1 mCi sells for SFr 35 ($25); thus, an additional daily revenue of SFr 7,000 (or SFr 3,500), or SFr 1,750,000 (or SFr 875,000) per year, can be generated, which corresponds to approximately $1,180,000 (or $590,000). Hence, selling [^{18}F]FDG is important, and, if properly organized, a CRP operation can become cost-effective when delivering to satellite PET installations. As [^{18}F]FDG can readily be produced twice a day if the corresponding systems for synthesis are available, a CRP operation can cover its cost and may even generate some income. In fact, when on average 200 mCi of [^{18}F]FDG can be charged per day, the revenue will be more than $1,000,000, which should make cost coverage readily attainable. What is important is that the numbers suggest that the price for [^{18}F]FDG can potentially be lowered substantially if a CRP unit can supply several satellites and produce [^{18}F]FDG efficiently. Hence, once PET becomes more widespread, not only equipment costs, but [^{18}F]FDG costs may also go down, making PET imaging even less costly than the current examination cost of SFr 1,200 to SFr 1,500 ($800 to $1,000).

RADIOPHARMACEUTICAL COSTS FOR A SATELLITE PET

When a PET satellite installation purchases a total dose of 200 mCi of [^{18}F]FDG calibrated to the arrival time at the satellite, the radiopharmaceutical costs are SFr 6,000 (SFr 30/mCi) ($4,000). For a site around 110 minutes away, the CRP has to produce 400 mCi because typically one half-life of 110 minutes is lost with handling and delivery. The revenue from scanning five to seven patients is approximately SFr 3,200 to SFr 4,500 ($2,200 to $3,000) in the Swiss reimbursement scheme, where an [^{18}F]FDG injection costs SFr 650 ($440) assuming a 5- to 10-mCi dose. This reimbursement was requested for two reasons: First, it makes sense to have radiopharmaceutical costs that are in the range of currently available radiopharmaceuticals; second, their cost should not be an order of magnitude larger than magnetic resonance (MR) and computed tomography (CT) contrast media, which are priced in the range of SFr 100 to SFr 200 ($68 to $135). Hence, covering the radiopharmaceutical costs in a satellite PET environment heavily depends on the calibration time of the dose, which can be negotiated with the CRP. Indeed, if calibration occurs at time of delivery, cost coverage is not possible, as the numbers above indicate. Calibration to one half-life (110 minutes) after arrival of the radiopharmaceutical at the satellite halves the cost and makes cost coverage possible. Hence, costs of SFr 3,000 ($2,000) are offset by revenues of SFr 3,200 to SFr 4,500 ($2,200 to $3,000). Transport of the radiopharmaceutical is in the range of SFr 150 to SFr 300 ($100 to $200). This calculation demonstrates that one of the most essential aspects of running cost-covering PET imaging in a satellite setting is the requirement of having [^{18}F]FDG available as cheaply as possible. Developments in CRP technology and radiopharmaceutical production suggest that this is indeed a realistic scenario, and the calculations for a CRP delineated in the previous section demonstrate that charging 100 mCi for every 400 mCi produced is still cost-covering if at least 400 mCi can be sold daily.

CONCLUSION

Thus, it appears possible to run a cost-effective PET center or satellite at reimbursement rates comparable to those for MR imaging (higher if only one body region is imaged or comparable if multiple body regions are imaged, as CT and MR imaging are typically charged per region imaged). Adequate patient throughput of seven to nine (five to six) patients must be achieved on the cameras, and the CRP unit must supply more than a single camera with [^{18}F]FDG. The cost of [^{18}F]FDG is approximately four times the cost of nonionic x-ray contrast agents and MR contrast agents, with considerable potential for cost reduction when properly produced by an efficient CRP with several satellite clients or two cameras. Further, it should be noted that quite a number of radiopharmaceuticals, such as metaiodobenzylguanidine and octreotide, cost twice as much as [^{18}F]FDG. Thus, an FDG PET scan is comparable in cost even by the standards of sophisticated nuclear medicine examinations.

It may be argued that the numbers used above are overly optimistic. These figures can be attained with proper planning and organization, although it requires a substantial effort. The key notion, however, is that unless clinical PET scanners are run in a similar fashion to how the morphologic cross-sectional imaging modalities are run, a PET examination will price itself right out of the market, and this would definitely be the demise of this very effective and promising technique. Physicians running PET scanners must be aware that tinkering with PET is not affordable for most sites in a decade when cost constraints are key. Few centers around the world can do this. The law of numbers, illustrated by the concept that increasing production of [^{18}F]FDG will lower costs, also applies to the scanner side. If the demand for PET scanners increases, manufacturers will eventually be able to produce highly efficient scanners at a substantially lower cost. So it is upon the physicians running PET to make the technology fly.

6

Image Fusion

Cyrill Burger and Thomas Berthold

Positron emission tomography (PET) is inherently a functional modality. Its aim is to provide images that quantitatively portray a specific function of the tissue under investigation. Therefore, tracers are designed so that they selectively label the process of interest. As a result, PET imaging is highly sensitive: Tissues with disturbed function become evident. On the other hand, tissues from different organs often behave similarly with respect to tracer uptake, such that organ boundaries are not clearly visible. This means that the presence and extent of a lesion might well be found in PET images but that it is sometimes difficult to exactly interpret the finding in the anatomic context. In this situation, it is helpful to correlate the relatively coarse PET images to high-resolution anatomic images acquired by magnetic resonance (MR) imaging or computed tomography.

In the paradigmatic example of brain tumor grading, state-of-the-art technique is to perform a needle biopsy under control of an interventional MR scanner. With this technique, MR images are continually acquired, showing the brain tissue and the location of the needle. The problem is that tumor tissue is often highly heterogeneous. Hence, the most malignant part of the tumor must be sampled to grade the tumor correctly. Information about the tumor proliferation rate, however, is not contained in MR images. It must therefore be borrowed from an appropriate functional image, for example, from a previous fluorine 18–tagged fluorodeoxyglucose ($[^{18}F]FDG$) PET scan, as illustrated in Fig. 6-1. With the combined (fused) anatomic and functional information, the target can clearly be identified and subsequently sampled with the needle.

This example illustrates how image fusion techniques allow obtaining the maximal information out of imaging studies covering a common anatomic extent. Generally, two successive steps are involved. First, the two image sets must be brought into geometric alignment, meaning that the position and the orientation of organs are identical. Several solutions exist for this image-registration task, and these are outlined in the next section. After the image sets have been registered, each image pixel of one study is related to the corresponding pixel in the other study. As a consequence, congruent slice images can eas-

C. Burger and T. Berthold: Nuclear Medicine, University Hospital, CH-8091 Zurich, Switzerland.

MR   FDG-PET

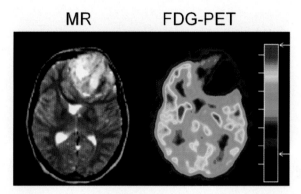

Figure 6-1. Tumor grading with needle biopsy. The MR image allows tumor extent to be assessed at a high resolution but gives no indication as to which part of the tissue is most malignant. The PET image gives less anatomic information. However, it shows [^{18}F]FDG uptake related to the tumor proliferation rate, allowing definition of the tissue that should be sampled for accurate tumor grading. This location can be transferred to the MR image and used to guide the intervention.

ily be generated and presented to the physician in the classic side-by-side manner. With computer-assisted image-fusion tools, however, the joint information can be explored in a dynamic way to better assess the extent and severity of lesions.

IMAGE REGISTRATION

Initially, two image sets from different studies are available, covering about the same extent of a patient's body, although the overlap need not be perfect. The images have been acquired with specific scan parameters and within the given geometry of the scanners. In the resulting images, the organs are therefore shown at different locations, are cut at different angles, and are potentially represented by image elements (pixels) of different size. The aim of image registration is to compensate for all differences in acquisition geometry and thus put the organs from both imaging studies into a common frame of reference. In practice, one study is regarded as the *reference* study and stays fixed, while only the other study, the *reslice* study, is transformed. The three components of a registration method include the following:

1. **Transformation**: A model must be defined as to how the objects in the reslice study are related to those in the model study. In clinical studies, it is generally assumed that the body is a rigid object, and instrumental distortions are neglected. In this case, a rigid transformation is sought that accounts for two effects: The body may be (a) rotated in space and (b) placed differently within the field of view of the scanners. The rigid-body transformation is described by six parameters, namely, one rotation angle and one offset distance for each of the three spatial dimensions. The assumption of rigidity is very reasonable for brain studies, as long as the skull remains closed, but is problematic for all other studies. Nonrigid transformations have been described, attempting to compensate for organ distortions such as shearing or even for smooth elastic deformations. However, the integrity of such transformations is difficult to ensure. Therefore, image registration is rarely used for studies outside the brain. In prospective investigations of the chest, attempts have been made to improve the situation by special support systems to provide data suitable for registration. An example is shown in Fig. 6-2, whereby the patient's body is kept in as constant a position as possible for successive scans on different scanners with the support a vacuum mattress.

2. **Matching criterion**: The aim of an image-registration method is to calculate those transformation parameters that result in an optimal geometric alignment, when applied to the reslice study. Every automatic method to determine these optimal parameters requires a formal criterion for measuring the quality of the alignment, that is, a formula that can be evaluated for any parameter set. Such a matching criterion can only be formed if there is enough common information detectable in both studies. Basically, there are two different approaches: Either the pixel values themselves (gray value–based registration) or some derived high-level information (feature-based registration) can be used. The latter requires a preprocessing step to find the information feature, such as the localization of anatomic landmarks or the delineation of an organ surface.

3. **Optimization method**: After the matching criterion has been established, a procedure is required to actually calculate the optimal values for the transformation parameters. In the ideal case, a closed-form solution can be derived that immediately delivers the optimal parameter set. Such a solution, however, does not exist for most types of transformations and matching criteria, and iterative optimization strategies must then be employed. They start from an initial set of transformation parameters. Then, the reslice study is transformed accordingly, the matching criterion is evaluated, and the parameters are updated such that a better alignment is expected. This cycle is repeated until the matching criterion can not be further improved.

Some popular registration methods are outlined in the rest of this section. All assume that the investigated body part is rigid. Their applicability mainly depends on the type of studies that are to be registered. As the methods are based on the alignment of anatomic information, it is sometimes helpful if transmission images are available from PET studies. These images show the attenuation coefficient of tissue and hence allow precise localization of the body surface, as well as bony structures. The registration can then be done between the PET transmission study and an anatomic study, and the obtained transformation parameters applied to the PET emission study.

Interactive Registration

Interactive registration is the most robust of all methods, as it is driven by the pattern-matching capabilities of a professional user who is familiar with the anatomy of the investigated organs and understands the characteristics of the presented images. Three components form an interactive registration tool: (a) a user interface for entering trial transformation parameters, (b) an algorithm that transforms the reslice study accordingly, and (c) image correlation tools that allow controlling the accuracy of matching. An exam-

A

B

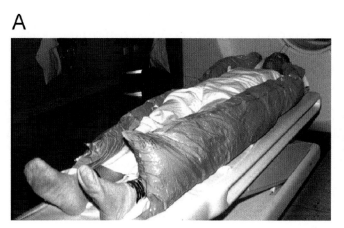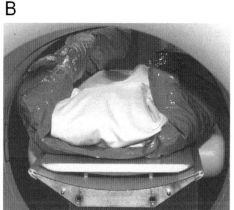

Figure 6-2. Fixation aid for examinations of the thorax. **A:** The patient is embedded into a mattress that, when evacuated, fits itself to the body contours. The shape is maintained throughout successive scans, efficiently limiting patient motion. **B:** To prevent errors from bending on different tables, an equalization board is used for each scanner.

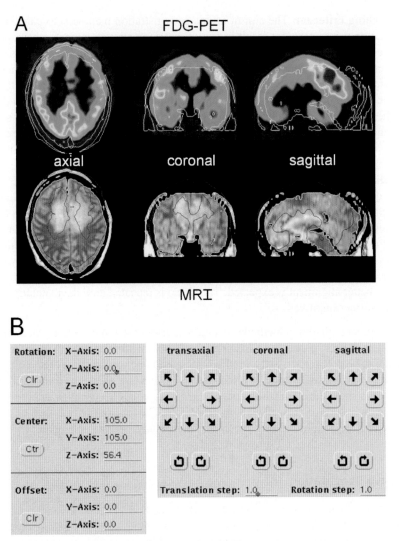

Figure 6-3. Interactive image registration of a [^{18}F]FDG PET study to a T1-weighted MR study in the same patient using the MPITool. **A:** Images of orthogonal slices through the PET and the MR data sets are shown in the first and the second row, respectively. The two studies are not yet aligned as indicated by the mismatch of the exchanged contour lines. **B:** User interface elements for the operator to modify the transformation parameters, namely, three rotation angles and three spatial offsets.

ple of such a tool—the MPITool (Advanced Tomo Vision GmbH, Erftstadt, Germany) — is given in Fig. 6-3. Three orthogonal slices of the studies to be matched are shown in parallel, interpolated to the same display resolution. The user must specify the six parameter values of the rigid transformation (three offsets, three rotation angles). When one parameter is modified, the reslice study is immediately transformed, and the orthogonal slices are recalculated and redisplayed. Contours are exchanged between the studies and serve as visual indicators of the matching accuracy. The user incrementally modifies the transformation until satisfied with the match, that is, until the exchanged contours closely follow the organ structures. At this point, corresponding slices are shown in the orthogonal sections of the two studies.

Interactive registration is applicable for a broad range of studies, as long as they contain sufficient anatomic information. Due to the manual-matching procedure, the result is prone to some subjectivity. However, systematic studies have shown that the variability is not significant, as long as standard processing guidelines are followed (1). Reproducibility and accuracy are reported to be comparable to or even better than those of other registration methods in a large variety of registration tasks.

Surface Matching

The concept of the surface-matching method is straightforward. It requires that the boundaries of an object be visible in both studies. From these boundaries, a three-dimensional (3D) surface of the object is generated, which according to the assumption of rigidity must be identical in the two studies. An iterative optimization algorithm is applied to find those parameters that bring the two surfaces into optimal alignment, and the entire reslice study is transformed accordingly.

The main difficulty with this approach is the initial segmentation step to find the organ boundaries. They are always represented with limited resolution and are often not clearly identifiable in functional images. Therefore, fully automatic segmentations only succeed in well controlled environments where the image contrast is predictable and the tissue coverage is predetermined. These conditions are difficult to ensure in a clinical setting, so manual or computer-aided segmentations must usually be applied. Surface matching was developed and has mostly been applied for registration of studies in the head, using the brain surface, which is relatively easy to segment for most modalities (2).

Automatic Image Registration

The popular automatic image registration (AIR) method was developed by Woods et al. (3). It directly uses the pixel values, assuming that the images to be registered show essentially the same pattern. More precisely, AIR assumes that each pixel value in the reslice study equals the value of the corresponding pixel in the reference study multiplied by a global factor F. So if the two studies were aligned, the pixelwise division of reslice/reference study would result in factor F's being everywhere. In practice, of course, this idealization will not precisely hold due to effects such as noise or sampling differences, as well as to physiologic differences. Therefore, the assumption is relaxed to the criterion that an optimal match is reflected by a minimal variance of the reslice-to-reference ratio over the images. As the ratio deteriorates outside the extent of body tissue, it must be limited to the common tissue overlap of the two studies by applying masks. An iterative optimization procedure adjusts the transformation parameters until the ratio image gets as flat as possible. The only input to the algorithm is a threshold value for defining the tissue mask. This value can be empirically determined and fixed for each study type. Everything else runs fully automatically.

The AIR method is best suited for the registration of images from studies replicated on a single modality. In this case, highly accurate results are obtained. It can be extended for cross-modality registration, although preprocessing steps are then involved.

IMAGE FUSION

The registration of two studies establishes a transform that allows bringing two image sets into a common coordinate system. In practice, one of the two studies is transformed into the coordinate space of the other, resulting in a new aligned image set. It is advisable to reslice that study which has more isotropic resolution because otherwise disturbing interpolation effects might occur (Fig. 6-4). In a wide sense, image fusion includes all techniques that allow the integration of the information of two or more aligned image studies. There are two interactive approaches that are simple yet helpful and accurate:

1. Contours can be defined and exchanged between the studies.
2. A coupled cursor can be moved about the images. It simultaneously marks the same anatomic position in both studies. The coupled cursor is especially useful if it is combined with an interactive 3D cursor that allows rapid updating of the display with orthogonal slices through a new point of interest.

There are also several methods to generate images within which the information of two studies is explicitly fused. To this end, congruent slice images with the same resolution are

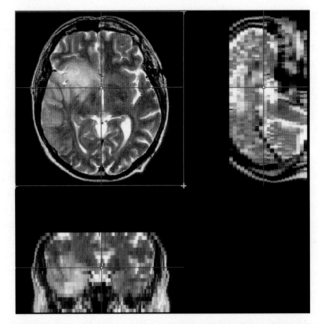

Figure 6-4. Effects of anisotropic resolution. The T2-weighted MR data set shown has a 512×512×23 matrix with 0.39×0.39×4mm pixel size, meaning that the slice thickness is ten times larger than the in-plane pixel resolution. Therefore, disturbing interpolation artefacts appear in the coronal and sagittal views, as well as in any oblique planes.

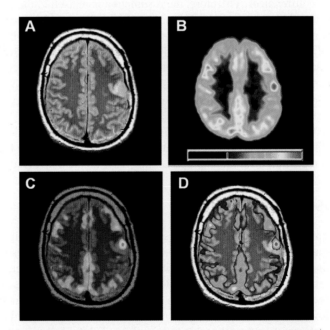

Figure 6-5. Generation of explicitly fused images. **A:** T2-weighted MR image. **B:** [18F]FDG PET resliced and interpolated to the MR resolution. **C:** Fused image formed by alternating the MR and the PET pixel values. **D:** Fused image formed by displaying all PET pixels above a threshold and MR pixels elsewhere. Note that the lower level of the PET color table has been increased relative to that in **B**.

calculated for both studies. Then, one of the following approaches may be applied to generate the fused images, as illustrated in Fig. 6-5:

1. The pixels in the fused image are alternatingly taken from either of the two studies, forming a checkerboard-like pattern. The original pixel colors are retained and can be adjusted separately for the two pixel types.
2. A threshold can be defined for one of the studies—the *lesion* study. All pixels with values above the threshold are taken from this lesion study, while the remaining pixels are filled with values from the other study. This approach allows retaining the full resolution of the two information components in specific regions. It is particularly powerful when the threshold is interactively moved, whereby the information content of the fused images is shifted toward one or the other of the studies.

Image fusion represents an improvement over the classic way of correlative image reading. No longer are physicians given only a set of static slice or projection images and asked to integrate the information in their mind. They now have a set of tools that allow exploring the information interactively and with different methods, until the situation has been clarified. Even more sophisticated fusion methods are just around the corner. Figure 6-6 shows an example that represents two fused studies in the form of a virtual reality scene.

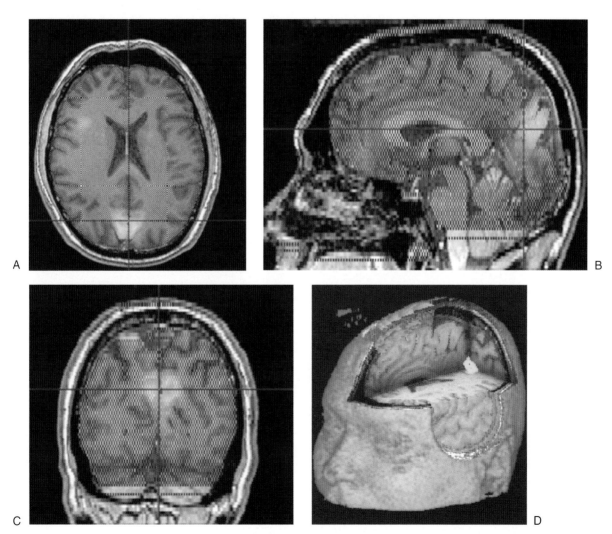

Figure 6-6. Image fusion as a virtual reality scene. Activation images of a visual stimulation experiment acquired with [$H_2{}^{15}O$]water PET are projected onto anatomic MR images. **A–C:** The fused images of three orthogonal slices that intersect at the visual cortex. **D:** After segmentation of the skin and the brain surface in the MR images, the data set can be rendered as a 3D scene. The PET information is painted onto the MR surface, whereby the color has been leveled so that only the strongest activation is shown. Software tools allow punching through the skull at arbitrary locations or cutting away planar sections of the brain.

REFERENCES

1. Pietrzyk U, Herholz K, Fink G, et al. An interactive technique for three-dimensional image registration: validation for PET, SPECT, MRI and CT brain studies. *J Nucl Med* 1994;35:2011–2018.
2. Pelizzari CA, Chen GT, Spelbring DR, Weichselbaum RR, Chen CT. Accurate three-dimensional registration of CT, PET, and/or MR images of the brain. *J Comput Assist Tomogr* 1989;13:20–26.
3. Woods RP, Cherry SR, Mazziotta JC. Rapid automated algorithm for aligning and reslicing PET images. *J Comput Assist Tomogr* 1992;16:620–633.

7

The Normal PET Scan

Gustav K. von Schulthess, Georg Kacl, and Katrin D. M. Stumpe

Depending on the indication, positron emission tomography (PET) is performed in a limited body region only, or extended fields of view are scanned. The former is the case in PET imaging of brain and heart disease, while the latter is mainly used to evaluate patients with tumors for staging purposes. However, PET may also become an important method to search for infectious foci, a setting where extensive body regions may have to be scanned, as well. There is an ongoing debate on whether scans with transmission correction should be used exclusively, or whether "emission only" scans are suitable in some instances. Partly, the issue is one of appropriate software. At the University Hospital in Zurich, we use partial-body transmission-corrected scans, for example, when staging bronchial carcinoma, but whole-body emission-only scans when staging patients with malignant melanoma. In general, we find uncorrected scans preferable when quantification is not necessary, and this is the case in most instances of tumor staging.

There are good clinical reasons for using emission-only scans. The preconditions are that no lesions are missed compared to transmission-corrected scans, and that quantification is not needed. In our experience, lesions are not missed in emission-only scans, but it is well known that their shape may be altered (1). Emission-only scans require only one-half the acquisition time, compared to scans where emission and transmission data are acquired, because both are typically run equally long. There have been software developments where emission and transmission data are acquired simultaneously (2–4). When a whole-body scan with 10 or more cradle positions is performed, the time penalty is huge when a transmission scan is acquired. Then, a whole-body staging scan may take 2 hours rather than 1 hour, which certainly is not pleasant for the patient and results in inadequate patient throughput, making PET too expensive. In addition, corrected scans are computed from noisy emission and transmission data, so that the quality of the transmission-corrected scans is often far inferior to that of emission-only scans, particularly when the data reconstruction does not use iterative reconstruction algorithms.

G. K. von Schulthess and K. D. M. Stumpe: Nuclear Medicine, University Hospital, CH-8091 Zurich, Switzerland.

G. Kacl: Department of Diagnostic Radiology and Nuclear Medicine, Spital Limmattal, CH-8902 Urdorf, Switzerland.

Many organs, organ systems, and body structures can show uptake of fluorodeoxyglu-cose tagged with fluorine 18 ([^{18}F]FDG), and it is important to recognize such uptake as normal in order to distinguish it from pathologic accumulations. The uptake patterns described in this chapter are semiquantitatively graded into five levels ranging from 0 to 4, with an additional "overrange" of uptake, which can be called grade >4 or grade 5 and is stronger than brain uptake. The definitions of these grades of uptake patterns are as follows:

Grade 0: no uptake, comparable to the background and that found with compact bone;
Grade 1: little uptake;
Grade 2: moderate uptake;
Grade 3: strong uptake;
Grade 4: very strong uptake, comparable to brain uptake;
Grade >4 or 5: uptake stronger than brain uptake.

An example showing some uptake and relative associated grades is shown in Fig. 7-1. In this chapter, uptake into the various organs, organ systems, and body structures is discussed systematically and irrespectively of whether transmission-corrected or uncorrected scans are involved. Illustrations are mostly of uncorrected scans because of their better quality. At the

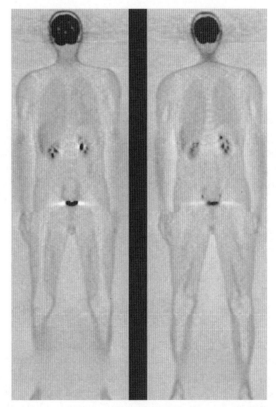

Figure 7-1. Coronal section of a normal whole-body PET scan shows variable organ uptake of [^{18}F]FDG. By definition, brain activity would be graded as 4. Grade 4 activity is also seen in the bladder and the renal calices, with some spot-like activities in the distal ureters. Much of the inhomogeneous abdominal and thoracic uptake would be graded as 1. The liver in the regions close to the surface attain grade 2. There is some intravascular activity of grade 2 in the superficial femoral/popliteal vessels. The uptake in the compact bone of the femora and tibiae is grade 0, with some grade 1 uptake into the bone marrow mainly in the vertebral bodies. Image misregistration occurring at the floor of the pelvis is due to acquisition in the upper body first and then turning of the patient for acquisition of the lower extremities.

end of this chapter, issues specific to transmission-corrected and uncorrected scans will be discussed. It should also be noted that the appearance of various organs depends on the reconstruction algorithms used and thus can vary somewhat. The images shown were all acquired with a GE PET Advance scanner (GE Medical Systems, Waukesha, Wisconsin).

[^{18}F]FDG ACTIVITY IN THE BRAIN

The clinically most relevant radiopharmaceuticals in PET brain imaging are [^{18}F]FDG and, in some sites, water labeled with oxygen 15 ([^{15}O]water).

Cerebral [^{18}F]FDG uptake is consistently strong because the brain's sole energy source is glucose; hence [^{18}F]FDG uptake in the brain of an alive, conscious person is essentially constant from individual to individual. As a result, brain uptake can be used as a semiquantitative reference to which the uptake of lesions can be compared, and it is useful to window and level whole- or partial-body PET scans so that brain activity falls into the top range of the window. Using this approach to represent the scans will thus permit application of the uptake grading scheme, with the brain showing an uptake of grade 4.

Strong uptake (grade 4) is seen in the cerebral cortex, the caudate nucleus, the thalamus, and the cerebellar structures. The white matter uptake is lower (grade 3). Obviously, the cerebral ventricular system containing fluid shows little uptake (Fig. 7-2). Due to partial-volume artefacts, this is not necessarily obvious in patients with normal ventricles, but when a patient exhibits enlarged intra- or extracerebral fluid spaces, the corresponding regions not taking up [^{18}F]FDG stand out. There is some normal variation in cortical [^{18}F]FDG uptake, related partly to extrinsic stimuli that the patient is subject to during the [^{18}F]FDG uptake phase in the first 10 to 20 minutes after intravenous injection of the radiopharmaceutical. This can be minimized by keeping the patient in a dark room during this phase, although for tumor staging the physiologically induced variations in cerebral [^{18}F]FDG uptake are irrelevant. Slightly lower [^{18}F]FDG uptake in the parietal regions relative to the frontal cortical regions is considered normal and probably due to a somewhat lower gyration of cortex in the parietal areas (5). Asymmetries in the posterior cerebral poles are also normal findings, often noted on morphologic imaging.

The uptake patterns of [^{15}O]water scans are similar to those found with [^{18}F]FDG (Fig. 7-3).

HEART AND CARDIOVASCULAR

[^{18}F]FDG Activity in the Heart

The heart and vascular system show variable uptake. The heart can be consistently visualized only when the patient is not in a fasting state. When fasting, 80% or more of individuals show no myocardial [^{18}F]FDG uptake. Hence, cardiac PET studies with [^{18}F]FDG require that the patient receive a glucose load before scanning, typically 50 g of sugar (6). In contrast, the patients scanned for tumor staging or infection-focus search are kept on nothing-by-mouth status (7).

The appearance of the heart is influenced by the time elapsed between the [^{18}F]FDG injection and the scanning. Since [^{18}F]FDG uptake is relatively slow, occurring over 20 to 60 minutes, substantial intraventricular activity is noted in the early phases, up to around 20 minutes (Fig 7-4). As time progresses, the ventricular wall activity becomes dominant and intraventricular activity recedes. After the typical uptake time of 30 to 40 minutes, intraventricular activity is minimal. Uptake in the walls is homogeneous with a typically slightly lower uptake at the apex of the left ventricle (thought to be due to the increased motility of the heart in this region and therefore to physiologic partial-volume averaging when scanning is not gated to the cardiac cycle) (Fig. 7-5). Transmission correction is always applied

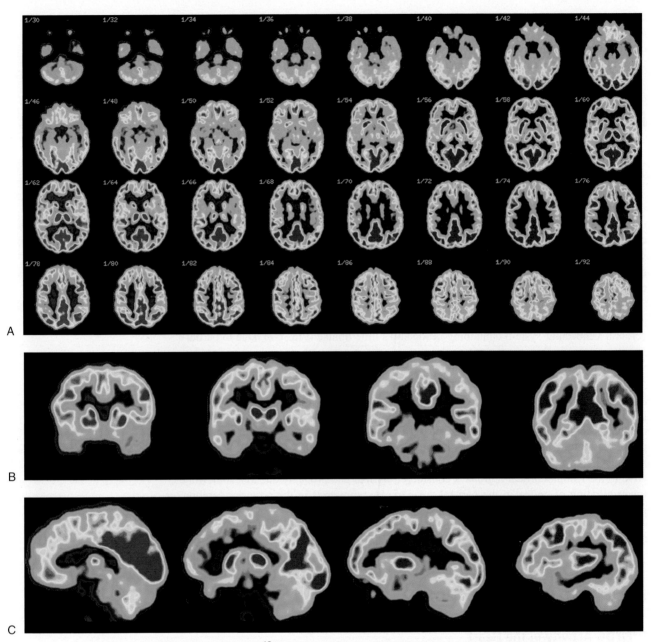

Figure 7-2. A: Normal uptake of [^{18}F]FDG. In a series of axial brain scans, activity is prominent in the cortex, the basal ganglia, the thalamus, and the cerebellum. Note the increased activity in the region of the eye sockets corresponding to the orbital musculature. Coronal **(B)** and sagittal **(C)** sections cover the left hemisphere from lateral to midline.

for proper heart scanning to correct for decreased photon penetration from the inferoposterior and lateral walls. Strongly inhomogeneous uptake can be noted in diabetic patients. This is a result of inadequate insulin blood levels. It can be so detrimental to image quality that PET scans in diabetes become uninterpretable, unless the patient is examined under a glucose clamp (8). The right ventricular wall is frequently not seen and, if seen, usually indicates right ventricular overload leading to concomitant increased glucose utilization. When the heart shows [^{18}F]FDG uptake in tumor staging, the appearance is similar to that described above, even in scans uncorrected for absorption.

Because there is a sizable blood pool present in the field of view during cardiac scanning, quantitative uptake measurements can be done by using the arterial input function from a region of interest taken from the left intraventricular region (9,10). Only a venous sample is needed for quantification of data in this case.

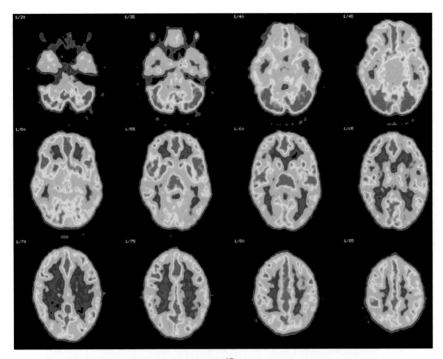

Figure 7-3. Normal uptake of [^{15}O]water in a series of axial brain scans. Note that the distribution pattern is similar to that of [^{18}F]FDG in Fig. 7-2, with the notable exception of the ocular muscles, which do not appear in the water scan. The image quality is somewhat inferior because of the short half-life of water and thus the reduced data acquisition time.

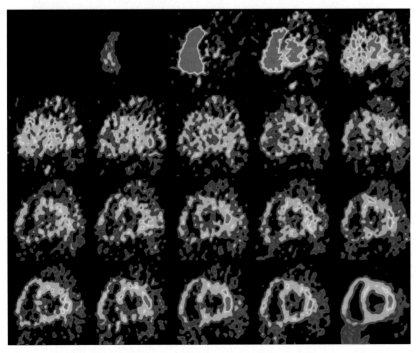

Figure 7-4. Dynamic short-axis heart series showing uptake of [^{18}F]FDG. Data acquisition for the first eight frames was 10 minutes, for the next six frames 15 minutes, for the next three 20 minutes, and then two for 30 minutes; the last is a static image acquired during 15 minutes.

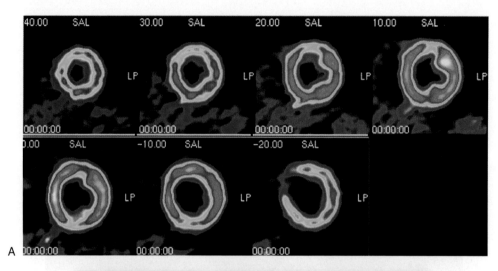

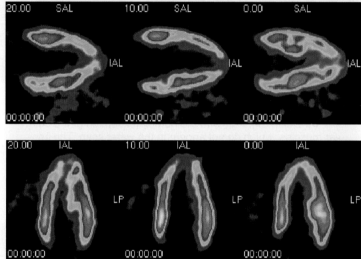

Figure 7-5. Normal uptake pattern of [^{18}F]FDG into the heart, late phase at 40 to 60 minutes. **A:** Cuts vertical to the long axis of the left ventricle starting at the apex; **B:** the first three images show vertical cuts parallel to the long axis, and the second three sections horizontal cuts parallel to the long axis. Note the absence of [^{18}F]FDG uptake into the septum membranaceum (**top right**, section closest to the cardiac base) and the very weak accumulation of [^{18}F]FDG in the right ventricle. Furthermore, there is decreased [^{18}F]FDG uptake at the apex of the left ventricle, which is frequently noted and normal.

Ammonia Activity in the Heart

The normal myocardial uptake pattern for PET using ammonia tagged with nitrogen 13 ([^{13}N]ammonia) is comparable to that using [^{18}F]FDG (Fig 7-6). However, it is obviously independent of the fasting state of the patient.

[^{18}F]FDG Activity in the Vascular System

Vascular [^{18}F]FDG activity depends on the time elapsed between injection and scanning, with intravascular [^{18}F]FDG decreasing and eventually disappearing into the intracellular compartments as uptake progresses and into the urinary system, through which it is excreted. In scans not corrected for transmission, vascular activity in the thighs and the pelvis localizable to the large vessels can be noted relatively frequently (80% of all patients) (Fig. 7-7). Sometimes, such activity is also seen in the neck and the upper extremities.

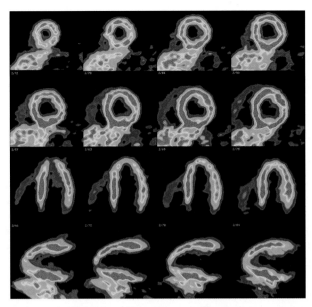

Figure 7-6. Normal uptake pattern of [^{13}N]ammonia scans of the heart. **Top two rows:** Eight short-axis scans starting at the apex and ending at the base; **third and fourth rows:** four horizontal and vertical long-axis cuts, respectively. Note the lower activity in the thinner right ventricular wall. Liver accumulation of [^{13}N]ammonia is prominent.

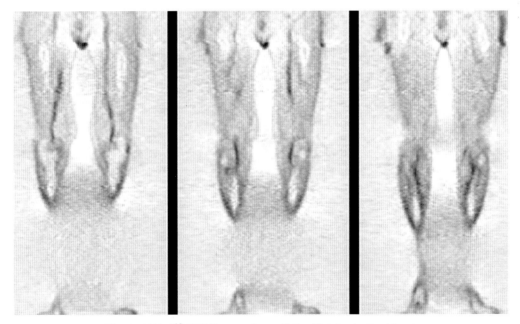

Figure 7-7. [^{18}F]FDG vascular activity. Uptake in the blood vessels of the thighs probably represents the superficial femoral/popliteal arteries and femoral veins jointly.

[^{18}F]FDG ACTIVITY IN KIDNEYS AND URINE COLLECTING SYSTEM

[^{18}F]FDG is excreted through the kidney, as it is not quantitatively recuperated by the kidneys as glucose is. Hence, clearance of glucose from the vascular compartment occurs prominently through the kidneys, and activity appears in the renal collecting system, the ureters, the bladder, and the urethra (see Fig. 7-1). This can lead to potential urinary contamination and thus unwanted activity in the groin area. As tomographic scans are acquired, this is less of a potential problem in image interpretation as in bone scanning, where planar images are acquired. By the time PET scans are acquired, the renal parenchyma no longer contains noticeable amounts of activity and is usually not noticed. However, the renal calices contain prominent activity in most patients, and the more prominent this activity is, the more likely the patient has ectatic renal calices. The activity of urine is most often of grade 5 (in overrange), when the brain is windowed to be at the upper window level with grade 4. The ureters also contain activity. Due to their peristaltic activity, they usually do not appear in their entire length, even when coronal scans are paged through. Their appearance can even be spot-like but is usually filament-like (Fig. 7-8). This occasionally causes a problem when tumor staging involves the identification of abdominal, paraaortic, or iliac lymph nodes that lie in proximity to the ureters (11). Cine-mode viewing of whole-body PET data in the coronal plane can be helpful in this setting, as the longitudinal course of the ureters is well appreciated in this way.

The bladder obviously also exhibits the intensity of urine activity. As this activity is usually very high, it can lead to severe deterioration of the image quality of pelvic data that affects the transaxially acquired data containing the bladder. It is therefore good practice when whole- or partial-body scans involving the bladder region are acquired that the pa-

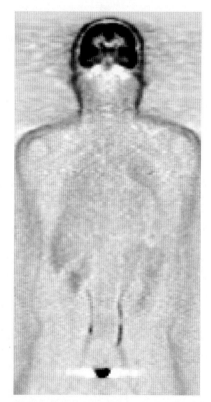

Figure 7-8. [^{18}F]FDG activity in the mid- and distal portions of both ureters and the bladder. This coronal PET scan is normal and also shows slight activity from the right anterior parts of the kidney. Normal liver uptake is enhanced in the surface aspects (emission scan uncorrected for transmission).

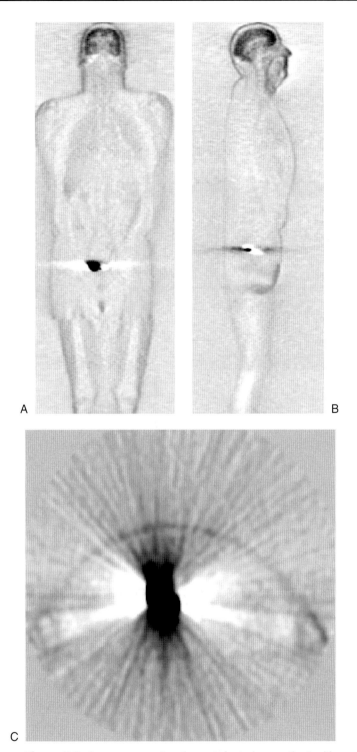

Figure 7-9. Image reconstruction artefacts in a patient with relatively high bladder activity.

tient is sent to void before the scan and that data acquisition is started in the pelvic area containing the bladder. This obviously is to no avail in patients with urinary retention. In diagnostically critical situations, it may be necessary to install a bladder catheter and permanently rinse the bladder during scanning. Some groups use iterative reconstruction of data in this region, which substantially improves the quality of scans containing significant bladder activity (Fig. 7-9). Occasionally, activity is noted in the urethra and obviously in the bladder neck in patients after transuretheral resection of benign prostatic hypertrophy.

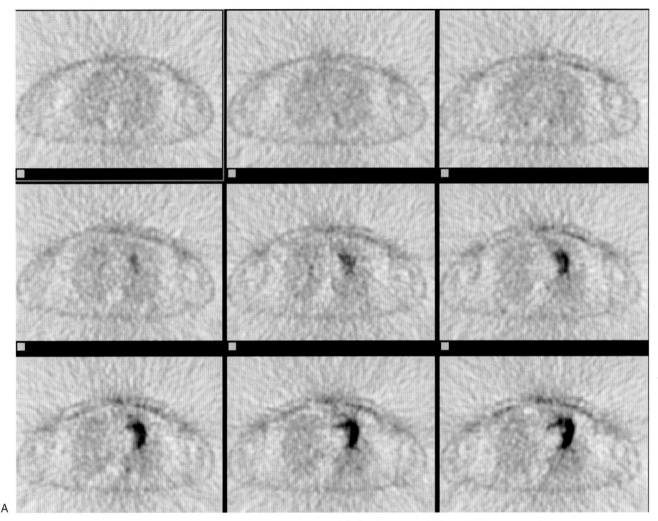

A

Figure 7-10. Normal transaxial PET scans of the lung at the upper border of the heart. **A:** Uncorrected scan shows very weak outlines of the lung.

[^{18}F]FDG ACTIVITY IN THE CHEST AND MEDIASTINUM

In scans not corrected for transmission, slight lung uptake is noted that is never higher than grade 1 in normal individuals; with reconstruction these scans may show some slightly stronger activity peripherally. In such scans, the lungs have clearly more activity than the surrounding soft tissues. Whether this is due to some remaining circulating [^{18}F]FDG, uptake of [^{18}F]FDG into lung macrophages, or both is not clear (see Fig. 7-1). Activity in the mediastinum is typically less than in the lungs on uncorrected images, but greater on corrected scans (Fig. 7-10).

[^{18}F]FDG ACTIVITY IN LIVER, SPLEEN, BONE MARROW, AND THYMUS

Liver uptake on uncorrected scans is similar to uptake in the lungs (grade 1), also with some peripheral increase. There is no activity in the gallbladder, as [^{18}F]FDG is excreted strictly by the kidneys. It is therefore possible to recognize liver metastases relatively easily, as their activity level is grade 3 to 4. The same is true for the spleen. Bone marrow and thymus are organs harboring many white cells, which are known to take up [^{18}F]FDG; however, uptake is only strong when these cells are activated (12) (see Chapter 20: Clinical PET Imaging of Inflammatory Diseases). The thymus is seen in normal children and young adults (Fig. 7-11), and hematopoietic bone marrow is seen through adulthood. They both

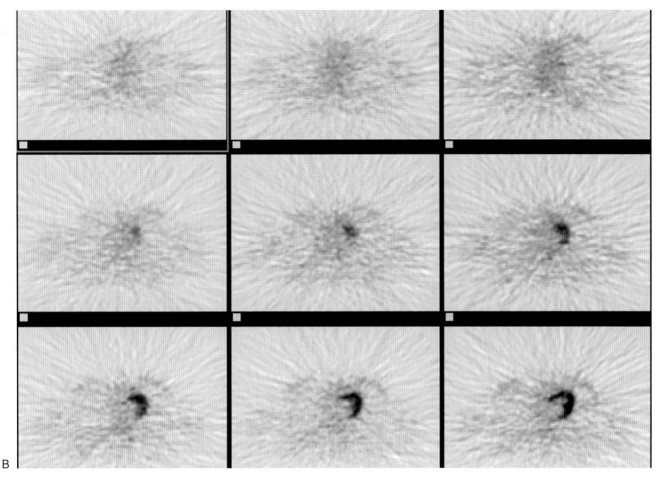

Figure 7-10. *(continued)* **B:** In contrast, a scan corrected for absorption shows how prominent image degradation in uncorrected scans can be.

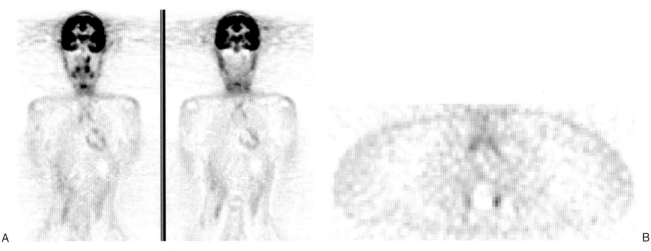

Figure 7-11. [^{18}F]FDG activity in the thymus. Coronal **(A)** and transaxial **(B)** sections show grade 2 activity, together with activity in the pharyngeal lymph nodes and some sublingual activity in a 16-year-old patient. On the transaxial section, the thymus exhibits the typical V-shaped appearance known from morphologic images.

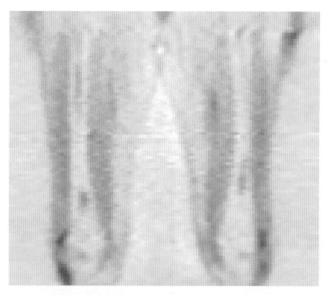

Figure 7-12. [^{18}F]FDG activity in bone marrow. Normal but relatively strong activity is seen in the marrow cavities of the femora when there is some expansion of hematopoietic bone marrow.

have activity levels of grade 1 or 2, and hematopoietic bone marrow in the vertebral bodies is seen in most patients. Weak bone marrow activity is also seen in the femora in approximately 50% of patients, in the pelvis in 20%, and in the ribs in approximately 10% (Fig. 7-12). Increased bone marrow activity is seen in patients with acute infection, probably reflecting increased production of white cells, as evidenced by the left-shift observed in blood samples and in patients undergoing chemotherapy in settings where the bone marrow is recovering (13) (Fig. 7-13).

[^{18}F]FDG ACTIVITY IN THE DIGESTIVE SYSTEM

The digestive system shows activity in various parts. As [^{18}F]FDG is accumulated and excreted by the salivary glands, the glands, as well as saliva, can contain substantial amounts of activity, producing foci that occasionally even reach grade 4 level but are typically grade 2 to 3 (see Fig. 7-11). These accumulations must be carefully evaluated, particularly in patients with head and neck pathology, as they can be mistaken for pathology (14,15) (Fig 7-14). In fact, they represent a major pitfall in interpreting PET scans in that region. It is very important that scans be viewed in all orientations and that the reader of the scans can superimpose a mental image of the underlying anatomy. Activity deposits are seen typically down to the level of the larynx, sometimes localized in the region of the valleculae, while activity in the esophagus and the stomach is not noted in normal individuals.

Activity in the small and the large intestines is seen relatively frequently, and is grade 1 but can reach grade 2. The cause of this activity is not known but may be related to slight regional inflammation or to smooth muscle activity during peristalsis. On occasion, there is activity arousing suspicion that there may be some underlying pathology present. As [^{18}F]FDG accumulates strongly in inflammatory foci and can be used to detect sites of acute infection (see Chapter 20), the suspicion is that the patient is suffering from an unrecognized inflammatory condition of the bowel. Clarification of the meaning of such accumulations is awaiting further investigation. Hence, finding activity up to grade 2 is a normal finding (Fig. 7-15). More prominent activity of grade 3 or higher should raise suspicion that some inflammatory process of unclear clinical significance may be present in the bowel, and should trigger a report alerting the clinician to undertake further studies to clarify the underlying reason for such activity. Increased uptake in patients with ulcerative col-

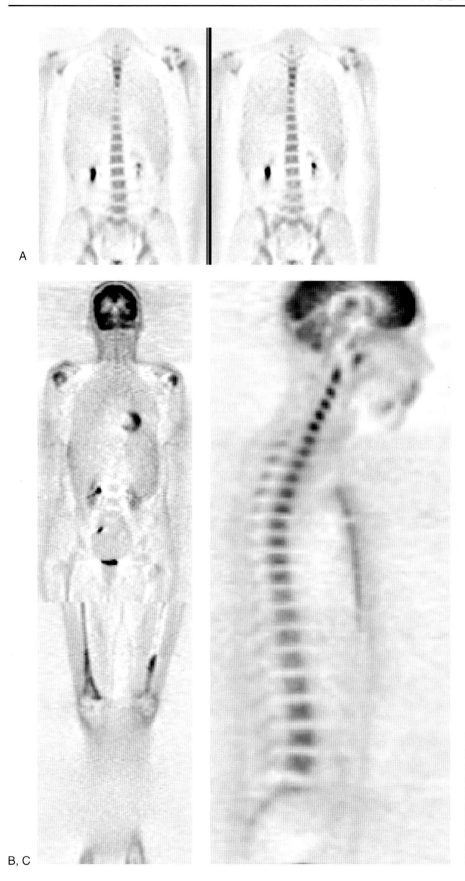

A

B, C

Figure 7-13. Recovering normal hematopoietic bone marrow. The coronal **(A,B)** and sagittal **(C)** scans in a patient who received high-dose hematotoxic chemotherapy for lymphoma show intense bone marrow uptake (grade 3 to 4) in the entire axial skeleton, the pelvis, the sternum, and the proximal appendicular skeleton.

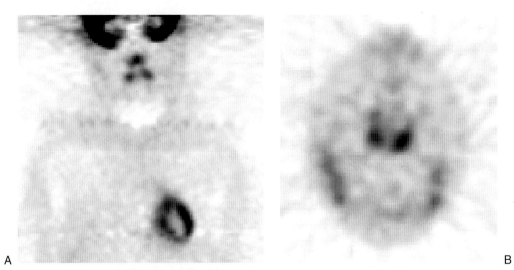

A   B

Figure 7-14. [^{18}F]FDG activity in pharyngeal lymph nodes. Coronal **(A)** and transaxial **(B)** scans show intense lymph node uptake. Cardiac activity in the coronal scan is also strong.

itis and Crohn's disease has been demonstrated (16,17), and incidental focal uptake suggesting diverticulitis has also been noted in our clinical material.

[^{18}F]FDG ACTIVITY IN THE MUSCULOSKELETAL SYSTEM

[^{18}F]FDG activity in the musculoskeletal system is common. While normal activity in bony structures is related to uptake of the radiopharmaceutical into hematopoietic bone marrow (see above), uptake into muscles and joints is the focus of this discussion.

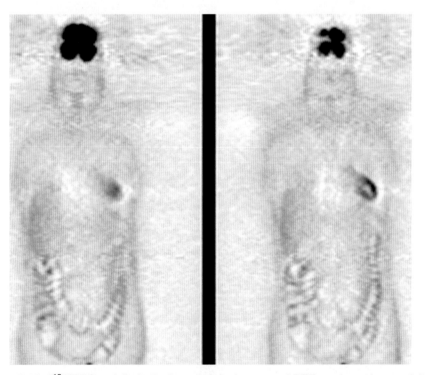

Figure 7-15. [^{18}F]FDG activity in the bowel. Anterior coronal PET sections show activity of grade 2 to 3 in the entire colon. While this can be seen relatively frequently and is considered normal, it cannot be excluded that the bowel shown here exhibits inflammatory changes.

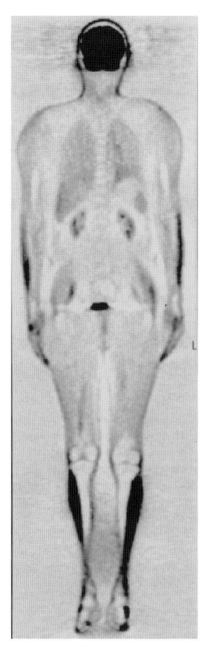

Figure 7-16. Increased [^{18}F]FDG activity in the calf and fore-arm muscles.

Muscles use glucose when they are exercised, and it is therefore not surprising to find moderate to prominent [^{18}F]FDG uptake in patients who for some reason have increased muscular activity in parts of their skeletal musculature. This increased activity can have several causes. The most frequent is probably a patient's hurrying to a late appointment that results in increased activity in the leg musculature, mainly the hamstrings (Fig. 7-16). Quite frequently, activity is also noted in the muscles of the neck, which are apparently prone to some spasticity (Fig. 7-17). This is usually unknown to the patient, although we have seen patients with torticollis showing very strong activity (grade 4) in the affected musculature. Muscular uptake, when present, is typically strong (grade 3 to 4). Suggesting to patients that they relax during the injection and making sure that they are lying comfortably, are important measures in reducing the frequency with which muscular activity in the scans is noted; however, these measures will not completely suppress it. This

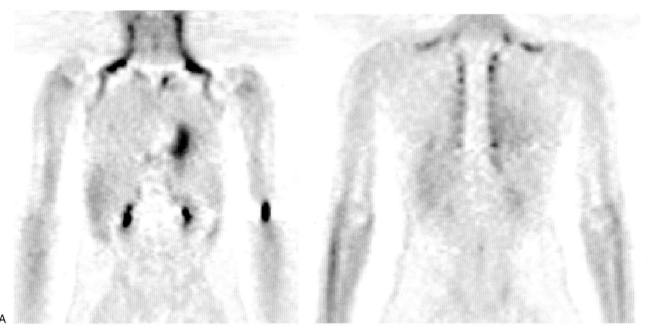

A   B

Figure 7-17. Increased [^{18}F]FDG muscular activity. **A:** The trapezius muscles in the neck region. **B:** The thoracic spinal musculature.

is understandable because [^{18}F]FDG accumulates in muscles that have been exercised prior to the injection, and it is difficult to get control over this. In addition, many patients probably have localized muscular spasticity, unknown to them, that can result even in decreased [^{18}F]FDG uptake on dynamic scans in the lumbar muscles (18). Other reasons for increased muscular activity can be the occasional patient who feels cold and is shivering. This can result in generalized increased muscular [^{18}F]FDG uptake. Ocular muscular activity is very frequently noted, as these muscles are constantly activated physiologically (see Fig. 7-2), and parabuccal activity has also been noted by us in a large series of over 300 PET scans recently reviewed to better understand sites of normal [^{18}F]FDG accumulation (Fig. 7-18). Parabuccal activity is probably physiologic, resulting from speaking activity prior to [^{18}F]FDG injection or motions of the mouth muscles unrelated to speaking activity (19,20).

Identifying muscular uptake in the head and neck region is relevant and is the second major pitfall that can affect the specificity of evaluating tumors in this region. As with pharyngeal activity, viewing coronal sections of a study in cine mode can be most helpful. This is so because muscles are always longish structures that accumulate [^{18}F]FDG along their entire length. Thus, a focal spot of uptake noticed on a single section will be identified on cine-mode viewing as activity in a muscle running obliquely to the scan plane. Most frequently, the sternocleidomastoid muscles are involved.

Accumulation of [^{18}F]FDG in joints also appears to be quite frequent. Often, activity of grade 1 and occasionally grade 2 is noted. The joints of the foot are seen in more than 40% of studies and the knee joints in more than 50%; the hips are also frequently noted (>35%). Surprisingly, accumulation in the shoulder is seen in about 80% of patients, with very frequent (45%) visualization of the acromioclavicular joints (Fig. 7-19). The clinical significance of these findings is again not clear. Presumably, accumulation of [^{18}F]FDG is an expression of slight regional inflammatory reactions (see Chapter 20), but the activity noted could also be an expression of normal synovial activity resulting from joint use.

In summary, muscular and joint activities are frequently noted, and the former can be a pitfall in head and neck tumor staging. The accumulations are probably rarely of clinical

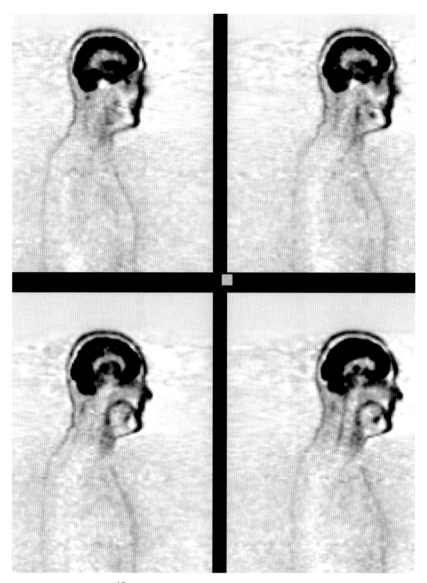

Figure 7-18. Parabuccal [^{18}F]FDG activity. Sagittal sections show activity that probably resides in the musculature. Furthermore, there is some salivary activity lining the tongue and the buccal cavity.

significance but should be noted in reports, as they could point to minor pathology that may eventually become relevant. While muscular activity is high-grade and typically grade 3 to 4, joint activity is grade 1 and occasionally grade 2. Stronger joint accumulations suggest that one is indeed dealing with relevant joint pathology.

OTHER ORGANS AND BODY STRUCTURES

Other organs occasionally showing prominent uptake that is presumably physiologic are the thyroid and the female breasts during the later phases of the menstrual cycle or during lactation.

[^{18}F]FDG Activity in the Thyroid

The thyroid shows prominent uptake of grade 2 to 4 in some patients, but on coronal scans this uptake is easily mistaken for uptake into the laryngeal musculature, which is seen

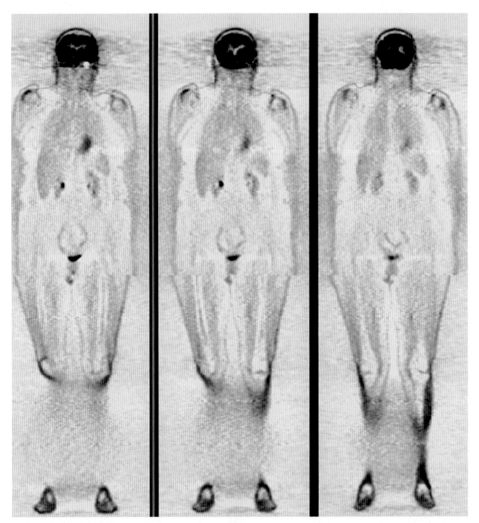

Figure 7-19. [^{18}F]FDG activity in the shoulder area. In addition to both shoulder joints, there is uptake of grade 2 to 3 in the acromioclavicular and glenohumoral joints, which is relatively unusual and can suggest active arthritis.

quite frequently and probably the result of patient phonation. Due to its position, the thyroid is easily noted and usually does not contribute to a potential pitfall situation (Fig. 7-20). If uptake occurs in the region of the thyroid and does not show the standard bilobar thyroidal anatomy, further investigation into potential underlying thyroid disease may be warranted (21–24).

[^{18}F]FDG Activity in the Breasts

The female breasts can show prominent [^{18}F]FDG accumulation (25). While the mamillae are frequently seen, the entire breast can accumulate [^{18}F]FDG in the later phases of the menstrual cycle, but the activity is low-grade, rarely exceeding grade 1. During lactation, however, the breasts take up substantial amounts of [^{18}F]FDG (Fig. 7-21), so that radiation protection measures for an infant are indicated after a PET is performed in a lactating woman (no breast-feeding for 24 hours afterward). As uptake is diffuse rather than focal, the danger of misinterpreting such uptake as pathologic is small. Although there is no clinical series of PET examinations available involving women with inflammatory breast disease, we have occasionally noted substantial uptake even in unsymptomatic women. Of note, breast implants may result in local uptake, possibly by

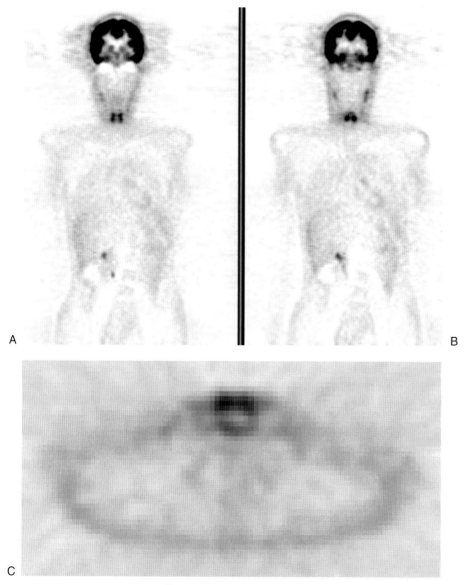

Figure 7-20. Thyroid uptake of [^{18}F]FDG. Axial-plane section shows the anterior location of the two thyroid lobes. If the activity is located farther posteriorly, it is then within the laryngeal muscles.

provoking a chronic inflammatory reaction that may be unknown to the patient, as in the case shown in Fig. 7-22.

NORMAL [^{18}F]FDG ACCUMULATIONS NOTED ON CORRECTED AND UNCORRECTED SCANS

Except in the setting of whole-body tumor staging, interpretation of brain scans that are not corrected for transmission is inadmissible. Probably, it is also necessary to do a transmission scan rather than correcting for absorption using a theoretical model, particularly if quantitative data must be acquired.

Transmission correction for cardiac scans, even if only analyzed qualitatively, is mandatory to correct for posterior and lateral wall absorption. In whole-body scans, no substantial issues have arisen in our experience, as long as no quantification of [^{18}F]FDG uptake

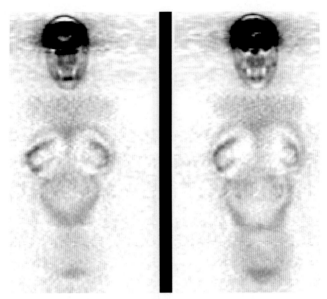

Figure 7-21. Normal uptake pattern of [^{18}F]FDG in the breasts of a lactating woman.

intensity is required. In most tumor staging, this is indeed not necessary. It may be necessary if [^{18}F]FDG uptake is determined for purposes of following up therapeutic success. However, this indication is rarely warranted at this stage in the development of clinical PET scanning.

In whole- or partial-body PET scans, some organs and organ structures can appear differently on corrected and uncorrected scans. This is particularly true for tissues exhibiting weak activity. As pointed out, the appearances of the lungs, the liver, and the spleen differ

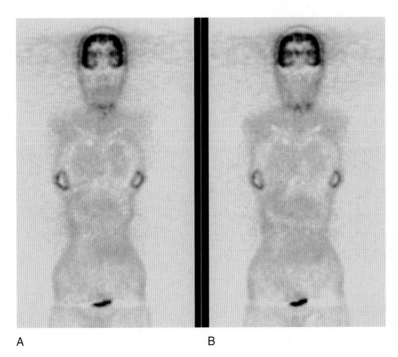

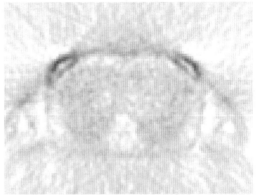

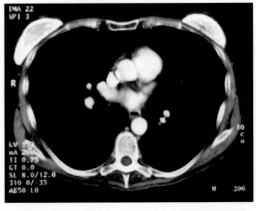

Figure 7-22. [^{18}F]FDG uptake in a patient with breast implants. Coronal **(A,B)** and axial **(C)** sections show uptake around the implants, which appear as photopenic regions. The axial section **(C)** was taken at the same level as a corresponding CT section **(D)**.

somewhat when viewed in corrected and uncorrected scans, but these differences do not interfere with proper evaluation of relevant pathology. Also noted on uncorrected scans is an artefactual increase of surface activity, located at the patient's skin, thus making the patient outlines somewhat more prominent. While this is easily noticeable, it can again be distinguished readily from physiologic and pathologic accumulations of [18F]FDG in the skin (see Fig. 7-10).

There is a set of other apparently abnormal accumulations or uptake deficiencies of [18F]FDG that are due to technical problems in the camera system or absorption due to metallic implants in patients such as dental work, pacemakers, and hip prostheses. Such accumulations or uptake deficiencies are readily identified and distinguished from pathologies. Therefore, commenting on them in this chapter has been largely suppressed. Overall, the normal PET scan shows little [18F]FDG accumulation, except in the brain, the heart, and the renal excretion system. As a result, pathology stands out prominently in most [18F]FDG PET scans. This represents a major strength of PET for tumor staging and possibly infectious-focus search.

REFERENCES

1. Bengel FM, Ziegler SI, Avril N, Weber W, Laubenbacher C, Schwaiger M. Whole-body positron emission tomography in clinical oncology: comparison between attenuation-corrected and uncorrected images. *Eur J Nucl Med* 1997;24:1091–1098.
2. Meikle SR, Bailey DL, Hooper PK, et al. Simultaneous emission and transmission measurements for attenuation correction in whole-body PET. *J Nucl Med* 1995;36:1680–1688.
3. Eberl S, Kanno I, Fulton RR, Ryan A, Hutton BF, Fulham MJ. Automated interstudy image registration technique for SPECT and PET. *J Nucl Med* 1996;37:137–145.
4. Ho-Shon K, Feng D, Hawkins RA, Meikle S, Fulham MJ, Li X. Optimized sampling and parameter estimation for quantification in whole-body PET. *IEEE Trans Biomed Eng* 1996;43:1021–1028.
5. Bicik I, Radanov BP, Schäfer N, et al. A PET with fluorodesoxyglucose and hexamethylpropylene amine oxime SPECT in late whiplash syndrome. *Neurology* 1998;51:345–350.
6. Kubota K, Kubota R, Yamada S, Tada M, Takahashi T, Iwata R. Re-evaluation of myocardial FDG uptake in hyperglycemia. *J Nucl Med* 1996;37:1713–1737.
7. Lindholm P, Minn H, Leskinen-Kallio S, Bergman J, Ruotsalainen U, Joensuu H. Influence of the blood glucose concentration on FDG uptake in cancer: a PET study. *J Nucl Med* 1993;34:1–6.
8. Locher JT, Frey LD, Seybold K, Jenzer H. Myocardial 18F-FDG-PET: experiences with the euglycemic hyperinsulinemic clamp technique. *Angiology* 1995;46:313–320.
9. Schwaiger M. Myocardial perfusion imaging with PET. *J Nucl Med* 1994;35:693–698.
10. Schwaiger M, Hutchins G. Quantification of regional myocardial perfusion by PET: rationale and first clinical results. *Eur Heart J* 1995;16(suppl):84–91.
11. Hoh CK, Seltzer MA, Franklin J, deKernion JB, Phelps ME, Belldegrun A. Positron emission tomography in urological oncology *J Urol* 1998;159:347–356.
12. Patel PM, Alibazoglu H, Ali A, Fordham E, LaMonica G. Normal thymic uptake of FDG on PET imaging. *Clin Nucl Med* 1996;21:772–775.
13. Sugawara Y, Fisher SJ, Zasadny KR, Kison PV, Baker LH, Wahl RL. Preclinical and clinical studies of bone marrow uptake of fluorine-18-fluorodeoxyglucose with or without granulocyte colony-stimulating factor during chemotherapy. *J Clin Oncol* 1998;16:173–180.
14. Kostakoglu L, Wong JC, Barrington SF, Cronin BF, Dynes AM, Maisey MN. Speech-related visualization of laryngeal muscles with fluorine-18-FDG. *J Nucl Med* 1996;37:1771–1773.
15. Segall GM. Normal glucose uptake by tongue and pharyngeal muscles in FDG-PET imaging *J Nucl Med* 1996;37:1918–1924.
16. Bicik I, Bauerfeind P, Breitbach T, von Schulthess GK, Fried M. Inflammatory bowel disease activity measured by positron-emission tomography. *Lancet* 1997;350:262.
17. Miraldi F, Vesselle H, Faulhaber P, Adler LP, Leisure GP. Elimination of artifactual accumulation of FDG in PET imaging of colorectal cancer. *Clin Nucl Med* 1998;23:3–7.
18. Frey LD, Locher JT, Hrycaj P, et al. Determination of regional rate of glucose metabolism in lumbar muscles in patients with generalized tendomyopathy using dynamic 18F-FDG PET. *Z Rheumatol* 1992;51:238–242.
19. Engel H, Steinert H, Buck A, Berthold T, Huch-Boni RA, von Schulthess GK. Whole-body PET: physiological and artifactual fluorodeoxyglucose accumulations. *J Nucl Med* 1996;37:441–446.
20. Barrington SF, Maisey MN. Skeletal muscle uptake of fluorine-18-FDG: effect of oral diazepam. *J Nucl Med* 1996;37:1127–1129.
21. Yasuda S, Shohtsu A, Ide M, et al. Chronic thyroiditis: diffuse uptake of FDG at PET. *Radiology* 1998;207:775–778.
22. Adler LP, Bloom AD. Positron emission tomography of thyroid masses. *Thyroid* 1993;3:195–200.
23. Bloom AD, Adler LP, Shuck JM. Determination of malignancy of thyroid nodules with positron emission tomography. *Surgery* 1993;114:728–734;discussion 734–735.
24. Conti PS, Durski JM, Singer PA, Austin T. Incidence of thyroid gland uptake of F-18 FDG in cancer patients. *Radiology* 1997;205(suppl):220.
25. Avril N, Bense S, Ziegler SI, et al. Breast imaging with F-18 FDG PET: quantitative image analysis. *J Nucl Med* 1997;38:1186–1191.

Clinical PET Imaging of the Brain

8

Brain Tumors and Inflammation

Ivette Engel-Bicik

The primary symptoms of patients harboring an intracerebral tumor include focal neurologic and neuropsychologic deficits such as convulsions, headache, or changes in personality. These symptoms depend on tumor localization and size and the resulting intracranial pressure. The initial diagnosis is made by clinical history and cross-sectional radiologic examinations such as computed tomography (CT), magnetic resonance (MR) imaging, MR angiography, and conventional angiography. The differential diagnosis is usually narrowed by patient age, localization of the tumor, and its imaging appearance, such as calcifications and pattern and intensity of contrast enhancement. Some information regarding the histopathologic grade may also be obtained. However, neither CT nor MR imaging provide biochemically based estimates of active tumor growth or malignancy grade.

In the past decade, positron emission tomography (PET) has been used with different radioisotopes for functional imaging of the brain. Because tumor cells have been known to metabolize glucose to a higher degree than normal cells (1), brain tumors have been successfully imaged with radioactive glucose. *In vivo* measurement of intracerebral glucose metabolism in humans was made accessible in 1979 by Reivich et al. (2). This method, using fluorine 18–tagged fluorodeoxyglucose ([^{18}F]FDG) and PET, made it possible to monitor the metabolic state of intracerebral tumors. For tumor grading, differential diagnosis between tumor recurrence and radiation therapy (RT-)induced changes, and prediction of patient survival, [^{18}F]FDG PET has proved to be a valuable imaging method (3–7). Clinically useful indications for a [^{18}F]FDG PET brain study are listed in Table 8-1.

IMAGING PROTOCOL

For imaging of brain tumors with [^{18}F]FDG PET, patients may not take anything by mouth for at last 4 hours to ensure a satisfactory [^{18}F]FDG uptake into tumor cells. No other patient preparation is needed. Data acquisition is performed with the patient lying supine

I. Engel-Bicik: Nuclear Medicine, University Hospital, CH-8091 Zurich, Switzerland.

TABLE 8-1. *Indications for [^{18}F] FDG PET in patients with brain lesions*

Grading (determination of degree of malignancy)
Determination of regional differences of [^{18}F]FDG uptake before biopsy
Establishing prognostic criteria
Therapy monitoring
Diagnosis of grade change (dedifferentiation from low to high grade)
Differential diagnosis between tumor recurrence and radiation necrosis

Data from refs. 3, 5, 7–13.

and the head resting in a supportive device to minimize motion artefacts. In general, ear plugs or eye pads are not necessary for brain tumor imaging. Data are acquired 30 minutes after intravenous injection of 180 to 370 MBq of [^{18}F]FDG for 20 minutes in three-dimensional mode, with a transmission scan being performed for absorption correction. Image reconstruction is carried out with a noniterative reconstruction method (128×128 matrix, 2.34×2.34×4.25 voxel size).

[^{18}F]FDG PET images can be evaluated both visually and quantitatively (11). The visual image analysis provides the information of an area with increased or decreased [^{18}F]FDG uptake corresponding to the lesion seen on a neuroradiologic examination such as CT or MR imaging. Quantitative image analysis measures the absolute metabolic rates for each tumor. However, quantitative analysis requires multiple blood samples, either by arterial or arterialized venous sampling. Although there might be some difficulties in the visual analysis of [^{18}F]FDG PET data, a substantial overlap has been reported regarding [^{18}F]FDG uptake into tumors in quantitative analysis between different tumor types (11). Therefore, other models for quantifying tumor metabolism have been developed. Ratios of tumor to white matter (t/wm) or tumor to contralateral cortex (t/ctx) have been shown to provide relatively valuable, additional information for the grading of intracerebral tumors (14,15). This is also true for the standardized uptake value (SUV), for which [^{18}F]FDG uptake in the lesion as measured by the PET scanner is divided by the activity injected and the body weight. However, controversial opinions regarding the usefulness of the SUV exist, because there are many factors affecting the SUV (16).

Image fusion with CT or MR images can be very helpful with very small tumors located close to the gray matter, because [^{18}F]FDG uptake in the tumor can be of the same intensity as the cortical activity and therefore indistinguishable (Fig. 8-1). In large, heterogeneous tumors, image fusion can help in localizing the tumor region of highest activity and therefore highest dedifferentiation, which is closely related to prognosis. Another valuable indication for image coregistration is differentiation of tumor recurrence from RT-induced changes. Here, the lesion of interest is often extensive with an inhomogeneous appearance on both morphologic and [^{18}F]FDG PET imaging. Therefore, image fusion is needed to separate necrotic areas from recurrent tumor tissue, which is often close to the border of a resection site.

ASTROCYTOMAS, OLIGODENDROGLIOMAS, AND GLIOBLASTOMAS

Astrocytomas, oligodendrogliomas, and glioblastomas are derived from intracerebral glial cells. For practical purposes, the histopathologic characteristics of all primary brain tumors are condensed into a grading scheme. The World Health Organization (WHO) classification distinguishes among four histopathologic grades (I to IV). For diffuse astrocytomas (17), the St. Anne/Mayo grading system is more widely in use (18). The differences between these two grading schemes are highlighted in Table 8-2.

The histopathologic grading of glial cell tumors has proven to be closely related to prognosis and survival. Other prognostic factors include the postsurgical amount of tumor tissue (19,20), patient age (21), responsiveness to RT (22), and detection and treatment of early tumor recurrence by the differential diagnosis of postinterventional changes (23).

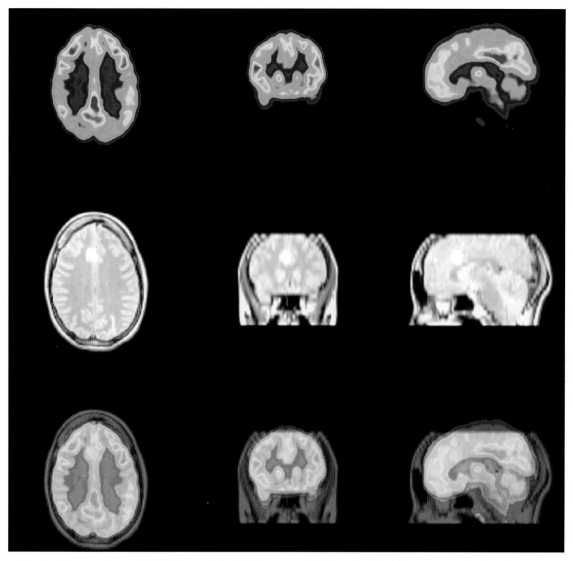

Figure 8-1. Image fusion of studies in a patient with a brain tumor. The fusion between [^{18}F]FDG PET **(top)** and MR imaging **(middle)** is displayed in three dimensions **(bottom)** using the MPITool (Advanced Tomo Vision GmbH, Erftstadt, Germany). (From ref. 83, with permission.)

Tumor Grading

Glioblastoma Multiforme and Anaplastic Astrocytoma (WHO Grades III to IV).

The diagnosis of a high-grade glioma, glioblastoma multiforme (GBM) in particular, can already be made with some confidence by considering a patient's age and the radiologic appearance of the lesion (24). GBM can occur in the posterior fossa or as a supraten-

TABLE 8-2. *Differences between the WHO classification and the St. Anne/Mayo grading system*

Grade	WHO	St. Anne/Mayo
I	Pilocytic astrocytoma	Astrocytoma grade 1
II	Astrocytoma (low-grade, diffuse)	Astrocytoma grade 2
III	Anaplastic astrocytoma	Astrocytoma grade 3
IV	Glioblastoma multiforme	Astrocytoma grade 4

Adapted from refs. 17, 18.

TABLE 8-3. *[¹⁸F]FDG uptake by visual analysis of different intracerebral lesions*

Lesion	PET [¹⁸F]FDG uptake	CT contrast enhancement	MR contrast enhancement	Necrosis	Edema
Glioblastoma multiforme	3–4	+	+	+	+
Anaplastic astrocytoma	3–4	+	+	−	+
Anaplastic oligodendroglioma	3–4	+	+	(+)	+
Mixed anaplastic astrocytoma	2–4	+	+	−	+
Grade II diffuse astrocytoma	1–2	−	−	−	(+)
Grade II oligodendroglioma	1–3	+/−	+/−	−	(+)
Grade II mixed astrocytoma	1–3	+/−	+/−	−	(+)
Pleomorphic xanthoastrocytoma	3	+	+	−	(+)
Juvenile pilocytic astrocytoma	3	+	+	−	(+)
Meningiomas	3–4	+	+	+/−	+
Primary CNS lymphomas	4	+	+	+/−	+
Radiation-induced necrosis	0–1	+	+	+	+/−
Brain metastases	3–4	+	+	+/−	+/−

0, [¹⁸F]FDG uptake equal to cerebrospinal fluid (at the level of the lateral ventricle); 1, uptake equal to white matter (at the level of the centrum semiovale); 2, uptake between white matter and contralateral gray matter; 3, uptake equal to contralateral gray matter; 4, uptake higher than that of contralateral gray matter; +, marked; −, absent; +/−, occasionally seen; (+), faint.

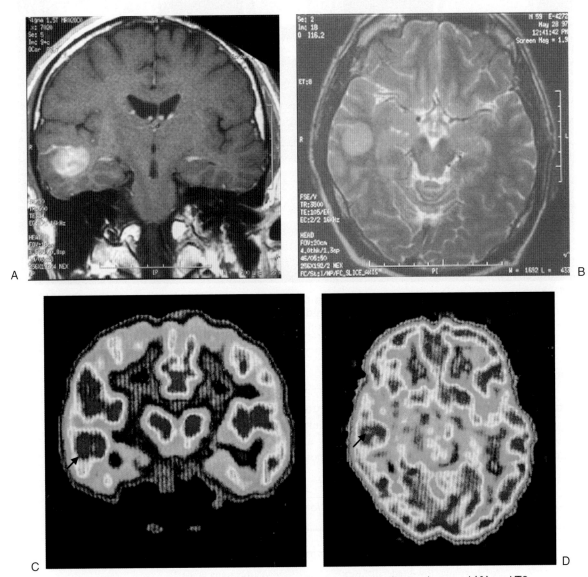

Figure 8-2. Right temporal lobe GBM. T1-weighted, contrast-enhanced coronal **(A)** and T2-weighted axial **(B)** MR sections demonstrate a small, round, contrast-enhanced lesion without mass effect. Coronal **(C)** and axial **(D)** [¹⁸F]FDG PET images show high tracer uptake by the tumor *(arrows)*.

torial mass. On neuroimaging examinations, the tumor most often presents with intratumoral necrosis, ring-like contrast enhancement, marked vasogenic edema, and mass effect. Contrast enhancement has been suggested to correlate with the degree of anaplastic change. However, studies have reported a lack of contrast enhancement on CT and MR imaging (25,26), making this diagnostic appearance unreliable for differentiating between high-grade and low-grade gliomas.

In general, untreated high-grade gliomas, such as GBM, can be separated by visual analysis from low-grade gliomas by their high [18F]FDG uptake on PET studies, the uptake usually being higher than that in the surrounding gray matter (6) (Table 8-3; Fig. 8-2). In most cases, the tumor can be readily differentiated from cortical tissue by peritumoral edema, which is more or less pronounced and shows a marked decrease in [18F]FDG uptake. Depending on tumor localization, a cerebellar diaschisis may also be seen. However, GBMs, anaplastic astrocytomas, and mixed gliomas can have a wide range of [18F]FDG uptake and may display a lower uptake than expected (Fig. 8-3). The amount of [18F]FDG uptake is

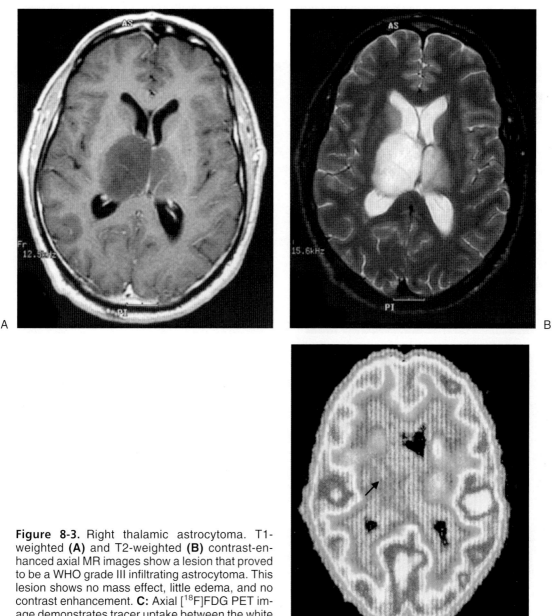

A

B

Figure 8-3. Right thalamic astrocytoma. T1-weighted **(A)** and T2-weighted **(B)** contrast-enhanced axial MR images show a lesion that proved to be a WHO grade III infiltrating astrocytoma. This lesion shows no mass effect, little edema, and no contrast enhancement. **C:** Axial [18F]FDG PET image demonstrates tracer uptake between the white and the gray matter *(arrow).*

C

mostly dependent on the amount of necrotic tissue and the proliferation rate of the tumor. Sometimes, the necrotic tissue of high-grade lesions can be very pronounced and the tumor rim very thin (Fig. 8-4). In these cases, differentiation from an infectious process can become a problem. Here, quantification by use of regions of interest and a t/wm or t/ctx ratio can help in differentiating between tumorous and nontumorous lesions. However, in quantitative image analysis, high standard deviations in [18F]FDG uptake for high-grade gliomas have been described (14).

The differential diagnosis between GBM and anaplastic glioma, as well as other intracerebral tumors with high [18F]FDG uptake such as lymphomas, meningiomas, or metastatic lesions, cannot be made with absolute certainty (see Table 8-3). Moreover, in GBM, multiple lesions occur in 4% to 6% of patients and therefore may be confused with metastatic disease or primary central nervous system (CNS) lymphoma. Thus, [18F]FDG PET studies must be read in conjunction with CT or MR imaging to improve diagnostic accuracy. This is also true for small tumors located close to the gray matter, which are still a problem. As the reconstructed in-plane resolution of currently available PET scanners is around 7 mm, image coregistration can offer additional information to discriminate between tumor tissue and normal cortical gray matter in tumors smaller than 1 cm in diameter (see Fig. 8-1).

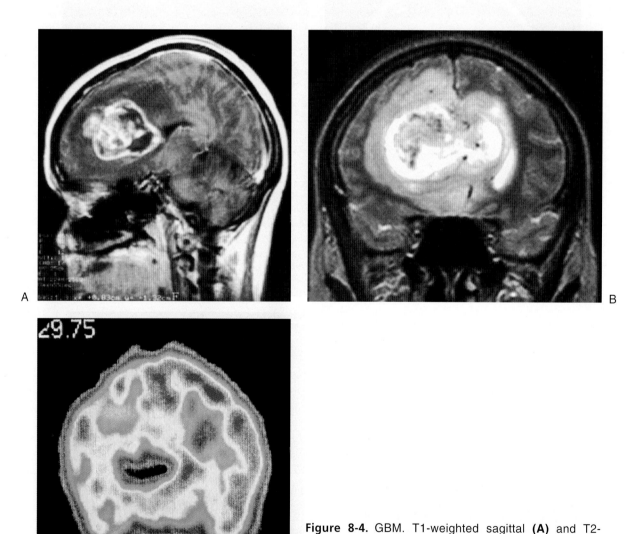

Figure 8-4. GBM. T1-weighted sagittal **(A)** and T2-weighted coronal **(B)** images with gadopentetic acid (Gd-DTPA) enhancement demonstrate avid contrast enhancement and edema. **C:** Coronal [18F]FDG PET image shows a central ametabolic lesion with a thin rim of high tracer uptake. The inner part of the tumor is therefore necrotic.

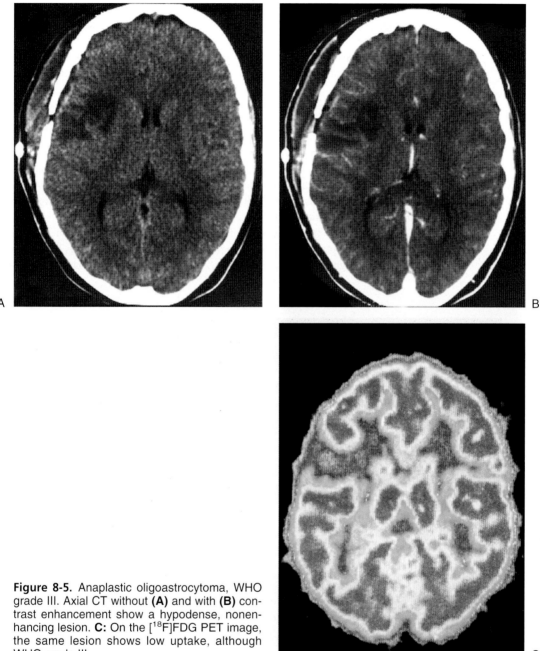

Figure 8-5. Anaplastic oligoastrocytoma, WHO grade III. Axial CT without **(A)** and with **(B)** contrast enhancement show a hypodense, nonenhancing lesion. **C:** On the [^{18}F]FDG PET image, the same lesion shows low uptake, although WHO grade III.

Although tumor grading with [^{18}F]FDG PET has been known to be very reliable in predicting prognosis (6,7), it must be closely related to tumor histology. Some difficulties in tumor grading are well known and are dependent on tumor location and histology, patient age, and the image resolution of the PET scanner. Oligodendrogliomas and mixed gliomas behave somewhat differently. [^{18}F]FDG PET grading of these tumors is known to be less reliable. Pure oligodendrogliomas have been described as having a higher [^{18}F]FDG uptake than astrocytomas or oligoastrocytomas (14), although they have a more favorable prognosis (Fig. 8-5). As a possible explanation for this behavior, specific metabolic properties and different cellular densities have been proposed (14).

Low-grade Gliomas (WHO Grade II). On CT, diffuse, low-grade astrocytomas most often present as ill-defined masses of low density without contrast enhancement. However, different degrees of enhancement also may be observed. On MR imaging, low-grade astrocytomas usually appear hypointense on T1-weighted images and hyperintense on T2-weighted images (Fig. 8-6A,B). Contrast enhancement is very seldom seen (27), generally appearing when progression to a more aggressive grade has taken place. Progression of low-grade astrocytomas to higher grades is known to have a genetic component (28) and occurs in about 75% to 80% of patients. Dedifferentiation into a GBM occurs in about 50% (24).

As glial cell tumors are derived from the white matter, low-grade gliomas present on [18F]FDG PET studies as lesions with low [18F]FDG uptake, generally lower than that of surrounding cortical gray matter (Fig. 8-6C,D; see Table 8-3). Differential diagnosis between low-grade gliomas and nontumorous lesions, such as infarction or infectious disease, is not possible by [18F]FDG PET. These pathologic entities have a glucose utilization rate close to that of white matter. The same is true for the differentiation between different types of grade II gliomas, such as diffuse astrocytoma, mixed grade II oligoastrocytoma, and grade II oligodendroglioma.

Pleomorphic xanthoastrocytoma (PXA), an astrocytic neoplasm occurring mostly in young adults, plays a somewhat special role. Although classified as WHO grade II, it shows clearly malignant histologic features (28). Progression to anaplastic PXA and even GBM

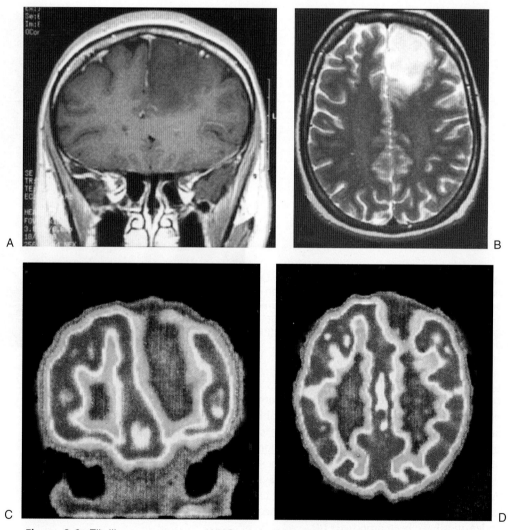

Figure 8-6. Fibrillary astrocytoma, WHO grade II. **A:** T1-weighted MR scan shows a left frontal lesion that is hypointense and nonenhancing. **B:** Axial T2-weighted MR image shows edema. On coronal **(C)** and axial **(D)** [18F]FDG PET sections, the lesion shows no tracer uptake, consistent with a low-grade glioma.

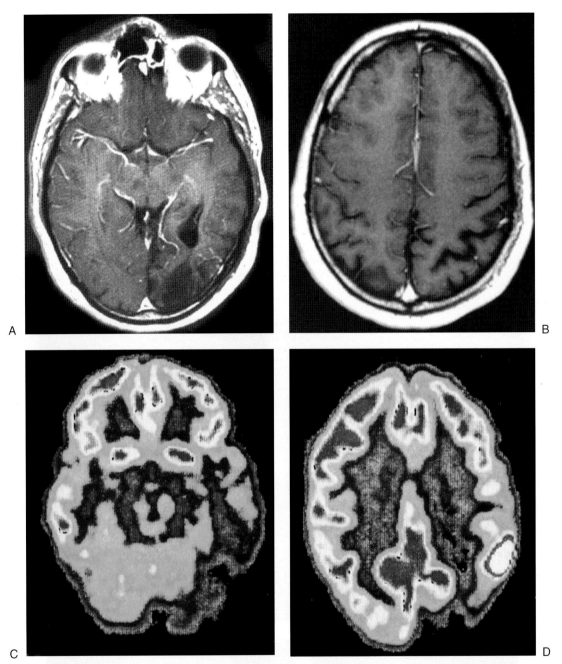

Figure 8-7. Epileptic disorder. **A,B:** T1-weighted axial MR images show a left occipital scar. **C:** On the [^{18}F]FDG PET image, a focus of high tracer uptake is evident at the anterior border of the scar, consistent with a subclinical seizure; this could be misinterpreted as a high-grade tumor. **D:** The scar itself presents as a lesion of low [^{18}F]FDG uptake.

has been described. Clinically, PXA usually behaves relatively benignly, although recurrences are often seen. On neuroimaging studies, the tumor is usually cystic in appearance with a small mural nodule, and enhances after contrast administration. On [^{18}F]FDG PET studies, the nuclear pleomorphism is reflected by high [^{18}F]FDG uptake in the mural nodule (29).

Special care should also be given to patients with a known convulsive disorder caused by the tumor. Subclinical seizures occurring during the [^{18}F]FDG-uptake phase (first 30 minutes) may light up as foci of high uptake and can be easily confused with a high-grade tumor (Fig. 8-7). Here, an electroencephalogram can be performed during the PET study to avoid misinterpretation.

Juvenile Pilocytic Astrocytoma (WHO Grade I). Pilocytic astrocytomas are circumscribed tumors occurring in children and young adults. They are slow-growing and clinically described as benign lesions; malignant dedifferentiation is rarely seen. On neuroimaging studies, juvenile pilocytic astrocytoma (JPA) often presents as a compact lesion with a cystic component; a mural nodule may be present. The cystic component and mural nodule strongly enhance after contrast administration.

Although these juvenile tumors are clinically described as benign, they are known to display a high [18F]FDG uptake in PET studies (14,30) (Fig. 8-8). The reason for this behavior may be their vascularity or a marked expression of the glucose transporter (30).

Determination of Regional [18F]FDG-uptake Differences. Stereotactic biopsies are widely used for diagnostic purposes to identify tumor type in current neurosurgical practice. Therapy management and patient survival are closely related to tumor grade and histology. Therefore, an attempt should be made to obtain the histologic diagnosis before a treatment plan is assigned. As tumors tend to be inhomogeneous and low-grade gliomas tend to dedifferentiate into higher grades, the most active tumor site must be biopsied to obtain the definitive diagnosis.

With [18F]FDG PET, regional metabolic differences in the tumor can be shown. When

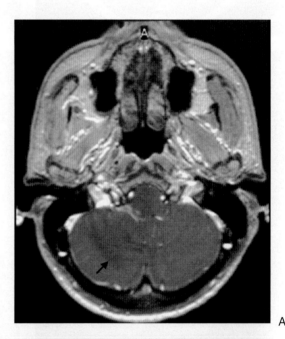

A

Figure 8-8. JPA, WHO grade I. **A:** T1-weighted, contrast-enhanced axial MR image shows a nonenhancing lesion of low intensity in the right cerebellar hemisphere *(arrow)*. **B,C:** [18F]FDG PET images show very high tracer uptake.

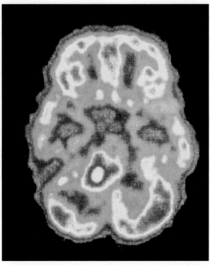

B

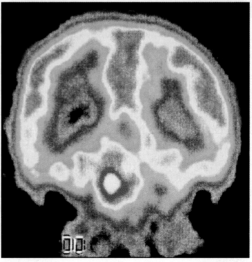

C

additional image coregistration between [^{18}F]FDG PET and CT or MR imaging is performed, the location of the most active tumor tissue can be marked for biopsy. This is particularly important in the diagnosis of large, heterogeneous lesions.

Establishing Prognostic Criteria and Therapy Monitoring

[^{18}F]FDG PET has also been used to establish prognostic criteria in patients with newly diagnosed intracerebral tumors (6,7,12,31). A major prognostic factor is the amount of [^{18}F]FDG uptake, which correlates with histologic grade. [^{18}F]FDG uptake has even been described as a more effective and reliable grading method than histology itself. Monitoring response to therapy with [^{18}F]FDG PET has proven to be of interest, as well (9,32), but larger studies need to be performed to obtain reliable data.

Diagnosis of Grade Change

Diffuse low-grade gliomas (WHO grade II) have a 75% to 80% chance of progressing to a higher grade (WHO grade III or IV). As there is still confusion whether low-grade gliomas should receive RT after surgical removal (33), the treatment plans are inconsistent. Some patients will not even receive total surgical removal, others will be treated by surgery alone, and still others will receive surgery and RT. In patients who have not had RT, close monitoring is necessary for detection of early progression to a WHO grade III or IV glioma.

With the morphologic imaging modalities of CT and MR imaging, only indirect signs can be used, such as tumor growth and new contrast enhancement, to detect changes in tumor grade. [^{18}F]FDG PET, however, has been shown to be reliable in diagnosing malignant degeneration of low-grade gliomas (34).

Differential Diagnosis between Tumor Recurrence and Postinterventional Changes

The diagnosis of tumor recurrence after surgery is initially made by clinical history and CT or MR imaging. If no additional therapy has been performed after the surgical procedure, recurrent tumor can be clearly visualized. However, if RT or chemotherapy has also been used, the differential diagnosis between tumor recurrence and postinterventional changes cannot be made with certainty with MR imaging or CT (35). Radiation necrosis can develop years after RT and can produce clinical symptoms similar to those of a recurrent brain tumor. On CT and MR imaging, radiation necrosis is hardly distinguishable from recurrent tumor, because new contrast-enhancing lesions, as well as edema and mass shift, can be seen in both radiation necrosis and tumor recurrence. In these cases, PET imaging has proven to be of substantial value (4,3,10,13,36).

Of special interest are high-grade gliomas, which are usually treated with surgery, RT, and sometimes even chemotherapy. As untreated high-grade tumors are known to have a high [^{18}F]FDG uptake, recurrent tumor is expected to display high [^{18}F]FDG uptake, as well. This is also true for clinically more benign tumors showing high [^{18}F]FDG uptake (JPA, PXA). Because low or even absent [^{18}F]FDG uptake is characteristic of radiation necrosis, differential diagnosis can readily be made by [^{18}F]FDG PET (Fig. 8-9; see Table 8-3).

However, high-grade tumors do not always recur in the form of a focus of high [^{18}F]FDG uptake. Other patterns of recurrence have also been described (37). At our own institution, two different growth patterns of recurrent brain tumors have been observed. One pattern is focal and the other diffuse in appearance. Focal recurrences occur at the rim of the surgical resection margin, often medial to or at the inferior or superior border. They display an increased glucose metabolism that is generally higher than that of the surrounding gray matter. This pattern was also described by Di Chiro et al. (5). If a recurrence appears in a focal manner with elevated [^{18}F]FDG uptake in the region of the previous tumor bed, there is

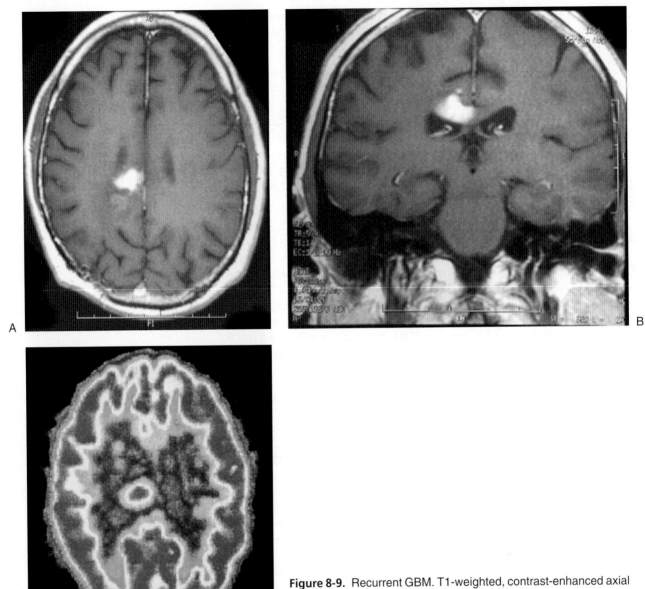

Figure 8-9. Recurrent GBM. T1-weighted, contrast-enhanced axial **(A)** and coronal **(B)** MR images show a small enhancing mass lesion above the right lateral ventricle. **C:** Axial [^{18}F]FDG PET image shows elevated tracer uptake, proving the lesion to be a recurrent high-grade glioma.

generally no difficulty in localizing the lesion. With a diffuse growth pattern, however, more difficulties are encountered. A diffuse growth pattern is generally accompanied by filling-in of the surgical cavity. This filling generally does not have an elevated [^{18}F]FDG uptake and is hardly distinguishable from surrounding cortical structures (Fig. 8-10).

Why tumor recurrence or progression shows a different growth pattern is not clear. It is known that [^{18}F]FDG uptake in neoplastic tissue is highly dependent on tissue oxygenation and regional blood flow (38). Both these factors are altered by RT. Another possible explanation may be that tumor cells receiving the full load of the RT dose change their biologic behavior (if they survive) and display a different [^{18}F]FDG-uptake mechanism from that of untreated tumor cells. One may speculate that this would lead, for example, to a decrease of [^{18}F]FDG uptake as observed in the diffuse growth pattern described above. In the other case, residual tumor cells would not have received the critical dose and therefore would not change their glucose metabolism (focal recurrences).

The differential diagnosis between recurrence of a low-grade glioma and RT-induced

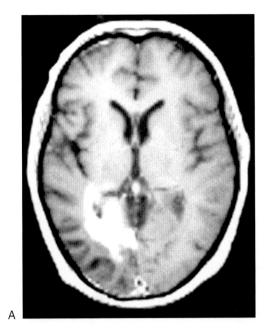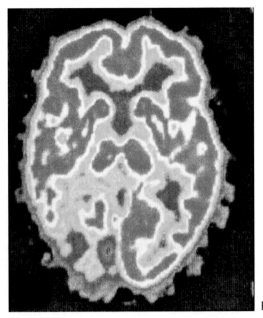

A   B

Figure 8-10. Recurrent GBM. **A:** T1-weighted axial MR image shows a right occipital, contrast-enhancing lesion, consistent with recurrent glioma. **B:** On an axial [^{18}F]FDG PET section, tracer uptake by the lesion is partly low and partly only slightly elevated.

changes cannot be obtained with [^{18}F]FDG PET. Both these entities display a low [^{18}F]FDG uptake. However, [^{18}F]FDG PET can be useful when there are indications that the recurrent tumor is also progressing to a higher grade.

MENINGIOMA

Meningiomas are the most common extraaxial neoplasms of the brain and constitute one-sixth of all intracranial neoplasms. They are derived from meningothelial (arachnoidal) cells and affect mostly middle-aged women, although they can occur in young children (papillary meningioma) and in adults of any age group. Some dependence on estrogen receptors has been implicated because in prepubertal meningiomas an equal sex distribution is seen and pregnancy has been reported to stimulate induction and growth of meningiomas.

As many meningiomas are very small, they often do not present with symptoms but are found incidentally on CT or MR scans performed for other reasons. Larger meningiomas are very slow-growing tumors and produce symptoms due to compression of adjacent brain structures, depending on tumor location. The most common location of CNS meningiomas is supratentorial, namely, in the parasagittal dura (25%), convexities (20%), sphenoid wing, cerebellopontine angle cistern, olfactory groove, and planum sphenoidale (24).

Meningiomas are known to be induced by radiation, with a latency period of 20 to 30 years. Radiation-induced meningiomas are more often atypical (WHO grade II) or anaplastic (WHO grade III), and multiple, and occur in younger age groups. Multiple meningiomas are also found in hereditary diseases, such as neurofibromatosis type 2 (NF2) or other familial non-NF2 diseases. Fewer than 10% of sporadic meningiomas are multiple.

Histopathologically, meningiomas are divided into a wide range of subtypes and are graded into WHO grades I to III. WHO grade I meningiomas, the most common, are considered benign and include frequent histopathologic subtypes such as meningothelial, fibrous, and transitional (mixed) meningiomas. In WHO grade II meningiomas (atypical meningiomas), cellularity and mitotic rate are increased, suggesting higher malignancy. This is also true for the very rare anaplastic (malignant) WHO grade III meningiomas, which show marked anaplasia, necrotic changes, and metastasis. However, histopathologic grading of meningiomas into higher grades (WHO grades II and III) seems to be very subjective because there is no consensus about specific histopathologic criteria (28).

Neuroimaging

The primary diagnosis of an intracerebral meningioma is often made by accident, and because of the tumor's location and neuroimaging appearance, the diagnosis is seldom questioned. Meningiomas are mostly sharply circumscribed, round or oval-shaped tumors with a smooth margin, appearing hyperdense on unenhanced CT imaging. In 20% to 25% of patients, calcifications can be seen. The amount of edema is variable and seems to depend on location and histopathologic subtype (28). Meningiomas enhance homogeneously and avidly after contrast administration on both CT and MR imaging, and may present with a necrotic center. Bony changes due to compression are found in approximately 20% of patients and may be osteolytic or hyperostotic.

On T1-weighted MR images, the tumor is mostly iso- to hyperintense relative to gray matter. A dural tail has been described as a typical feature of meningiomas. This is a linear enhancement of the dura, trailing off away from the lesion, and occurs in approximately 60% to 72% of patients. If angiography is performed, these tumors demonstrate high vascularity and a typical blush.

The most important entity to consider in the differential diagnosis of a CNS meningioma is a hemangiopericytoma, which does not calcify or produce hyperostosis and is usually irregularly shaped (Fig. 8-11). In the dorsum sellae, nonfunctioning pituitary adenoma and craniopharyngioma should be included in the differential diagnosis (see "Other Primary Tumors" below).

PET Imaging

In general, cellular proliferation increases from benign to atypical and anaplastic meningiomas, thus predicting a tumor's clinical behavior. Although many attempts have been made to characterize meningiomas, both CT and MR imaging are not able to predict tumor

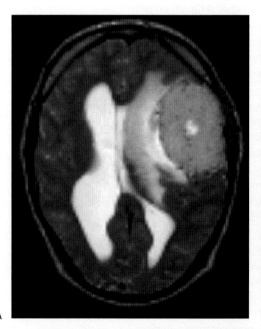
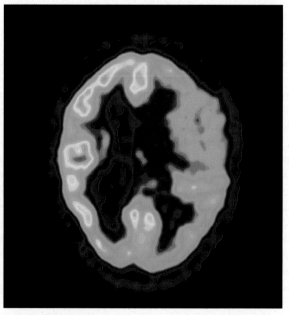

A   B

Figure 8-11. Hemangiopericytoma. **A:** T2-weighted axial MR image shows a circular mass in the left frontal lobe. **B:** On axial [^{18}F]FDG PET section, the lesion demonstrates intermediate tracer uptake, suggesting a WHO grade II to III tumor.

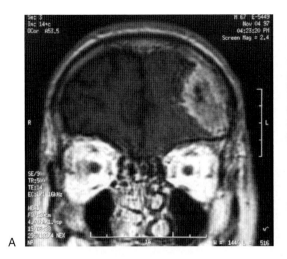
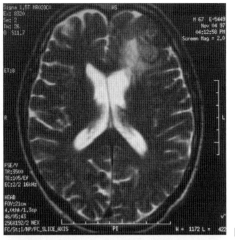

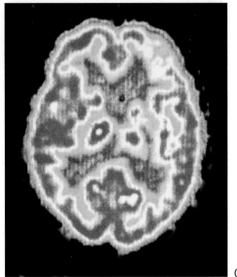

Figure 8-12. Meningioma. T1-weighted, contrast-enhanced coronal **(A)** and T2-weighted axial **(B)** MR images show a left frontal lesion consistent with meningioma. **C:** Axial [¹⁸F]FDG PET displays intermediate tracer uptake in the lesion, consistent with a WHO grade I tumor.

C

behavior (28), and therefore patient prognosis. On CT and MR imaging, the different histologic subtypes are not distinguishable. However, the major prognostic factors of patients harboring a meningioma are prediction of grade and recurrence. While benign meningiomas recur in approximately 7% to 20% and never change their histologic grade, atypical and anaplastic meningiomas have recurrence rates of 29% to 38% and 50% to 78%, respectively (28). Therefore, there is some need of a diagnostic method that can reliably predict tumor grading, tumor behavior, and recurrence rate.

[¹⁸F]FDG. Indications for [¹⁸F]FDG PET imaging in the management of patients with a meningioma are principally the same as for glial cell tumors. [¹⁸F]FDG PET can be used for histologic grading, prediction of tumor behavior, and diagnosis of recurrence. However, [¹⁸F]FDG PET has not been investigated to such a degree in meningiomas as in gliomas. Several studies were able to demonstrate that all meningiomas display a high [¹⁸F]FDG uptake, and WHO grade II and III meningiomas usually show higher activity than the surrounding cortical gray matter, thus putting meningioma in the same category for differential diagnosis as high-grade gliomas, lymphomas, and some metastases (Figs. 8-12 and 8-13; see Table 8-3).

[¹⁸F]FDG PET was investigated by Di Chiro et al. (39) and proven to be at least as reliable as the histologic classification for predicting the behavior and recurrence of meningiomas. The authors demonstrated that meningiomas displaying a relatively higher [¹⁸F]FDG uptake and higher histologic grade showed a faster and higher recurrence rate than those showing a lower [¹⁸F]FDG uptake. In more recent studies, Cremerius et al. (40)

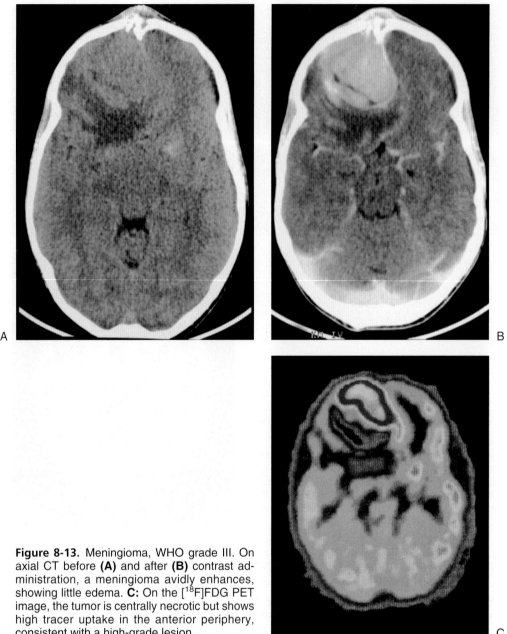

Figure 8-13. Meningioma, WHO grade III. On axial CT before **(A)** and after **(B)** contrast administration, a meningioma avidly enhances, showing little edema. **C:** On the [^{18}F]FDG PET image, the tumor is centrally necrotic but shows high tracer uptake in the anterior periphery, consistent with a high-grade lesion.

could discriminate WHO grade I meningiomas from atypical or anaplastic meningiomas using SUVs and thresholds of 1.05 for primary meningiomas and 0.88 for tumor recurrences. As all histologic subtypes of meningiomas tend to have a very high uptake, diagnosis of tumor recurrence with PET is usually straightforward. Embolization and surgery for symptomatic meningiomas result in a localized defect in [^{18}F]FDG uptake. Recurrent tumor, however, presents with a focus of increased [^{18}F]FDG uptake compared to surrounding gray matter, consistent with tumor recurrence (41) (Fig. 8-14).

[^{18}F]FDG PET probably does not offer significant advantages over CT or MR imaging in diagnosing recurrent meningioma, because RT is seldom applied for this tumor and therefore there are no postirradiation changes to complicate the differential diagnosis. Moreover, the problem of [^{18}F]FDG accumulation in inflammatory cells has also been addressed in imaging of recurrent meningiomas, because false-positive [^{18}F]FDG PET results have been reported (42). In their case report, Fischman et al. (42) described a patient who showed high [^{18}F]FDG uptake in a lesion presumed to be a recurrent atypical meningioma

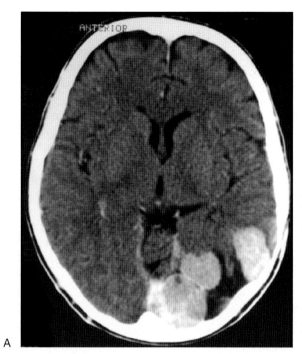
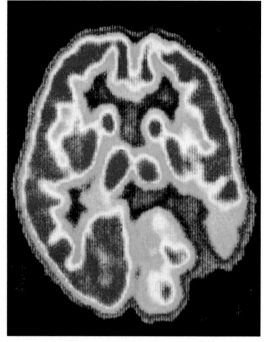

A

B

Figure 8-14. Recurrent right occipital meningioma. **A:** Contrast-enhanced axial CT image demonstrates a multifocal recurrent tumor that avidly enhances. **B:** On axial [^{18}F]FDG PET section, the lesion shows high tracer uptake, consistent with a tumor recurrence.

16 months after primary therapy. However, this lesion proved to be due to radiation necrosis with inflammatory changes on the final histopathologic report.

Other PET Radionuclides. There are no studies dedicated to the imaging of CNS meningiomas with more specific radionuclides. In a small series of meningiomas, studies performed with methionine tagged with carbon 11 ([^{11}C]methionine) showed increased tracer uptake in meningiomas compared to gray matter (43). However, there does not seem to be a clear advantage over using [^{18}F]FDG.

Furthermore, PET in conjunction with 16α[^{18}F]fluoro-17β-estradiol was used to demonstrate a high correlation between tracer uptake and immunohistochemical analysis in meningiomas, thus confirming the presence of estrogen receptors and showing the validity of imaging meningiomas with radioactive estrogen derivatives (44). But as with [^{11}C]methionine, there does not seem to be a substantial advantage in using radionuclides other than [^{18}F]FDG in the primary workup of patients with a presumed meningioma.

LYMPHOMAS

Malignant lymphomas of the CNS are common tumors and can be divided into primary and secondary lymphomas. Primary lymphomas arise in the CNS, showing no evidence of systemic involvement, while secondary lymphomas are primarily systemic. Because primary lymphomas occur mostly in immunocompromised patients, with the acquired immunodeficiency syndrome (AIDS) being the leading cause, the incidence has been increasing over the past decade (45). It is reported that primary intracerebral lymphoma develops in as many as 6% to 12% of AIDS patients (24,28). Other common causes for the development of primary lymphoma are hereditary immune deficiency syndromes and immune suppression associated with organ transplantation, with up to 22% of patients being involved (28). In 55% of this patient population, lymphoma is confined to the CNS.

Of primary intracerebral lymphomas, 98% are B-cell lymphomas, while T-cell lymphomas constitute only 2% and occur mostly in immunocompetent subjects. Secondary involvement of systemic lymphomas occurs in 8% to 22% of patients with non-Hodgkin lymphoma and up to 50% with childhood non-Hodgkin lymphoma (28).

The peak incidence of primary CNS lymphoma in immunocompetent patients is in the sixth to seventh decades, with the men being affected more often. In immunocompromised patients, the peak incidence is much lower: The youngest age of incidence (about 10 years) occurs in inherited immune deficiency syndromes, followed by transplant patients (37 years) and patients with AIDS (39 years). Clinical symptoms of patients with a primary intracerebral lymphoma are nonspecific and may include focal neurologic and neuropsychologic deficits, seizures, or signs of increased intracranial pressure. The most prominent symptom in secondary lymphoma is increased intracranial pressure.

Most primary lymphomas are located supratentorially, predominantly in the deep gray matter (30%) or the periventricular white matter, although they may involve frontal, temporal, parietal, and occipital lobes, as well (46). In up to 50% of patients, lymphomas are multiple, especially in AIDS and organ-transplantation patients. Coating of the ventricles is seen, as well as spread over the corpus callosum. Secondary lymphoma tends to involve the leptomeninges and the cerebrospinal fluid, although parenchymal lesions may be seen.

Neuroimaging

In general, lymphomas in AIDS patients differ in histology and neuroimaging appearance (Table 8-4). On unenhanced CT, primary lymphomas are usually iso- to hyperdense, while in AIDS patients they may also appear hypodense (24). Contrast enhancement is variable but mostly moderate, and may be homogeneous (solitary or multiple) or show a ring-like appearance. This feature is seen predominantly in AIDS patients. A mass effect is seen, but peritumoral edema is usually less severe than in gliomas or metastatic disease. However, in AIDS patients, edema and mass effect may be very extensive.

On MR imaging, signal intensity may be iso- or hypointense on T1-weighted images and is usually high on T2-weighted images; enhancement after contrast administration is marked. Necrotic areas may occur, but only in AIDS patients (47). The ring-like and multiple appearance of primary lymphoma in AIDS patients makes it sometimes impossible to distinguish it from other intracerebral lesions, namely, those of toxoplasmosis (48). Although some typical features have been described for lymphomas (48–50) that are usually not seen in toxoplasmosis, the diagnosis is generally made by stereotactic biopsy or exclusion. However, to avoid stereotactic biopsy, a patient may be given antibiotics against toxoplasmosis, because toxoplasmosis is seen more often than primary intracerebral lymphoma in AIDS patients (51). If no improvement occurs clinically or on CT or MR imaging, the diagnosis of toxoplasmosis should be revised.

PET Imaging

Intracerebral primary lymphoma is a tumor with dense cellularity, a high proliferation rate, and therefore a very high glucose utilization (Fig. 8-15; see Table 8-3). On [18F]FDG PET studies, lymphomas do not differ in appearance from GBM, meningioma, or

TABLE 8-4. *Radiologic differences between non-AIDS and AIDS-induced primary CNS lymphomas*

Features	Non-AIDS	AIDS
Lesions	Single	Multiple
Edema	Moderate	Can be extensive
Mass effect	Moderate	Extensive
Necrosis	No	Yes
Unenhanced CT	Hyperdense	Variable, may be hypodense
T1-/T2-weighted MR	Iso- to hypointense	Hyperintense (T2-weighted, necrosis)
Enhancement (CT/MR)	Homogeneous, solid	Ring-like

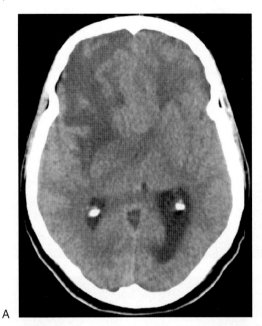
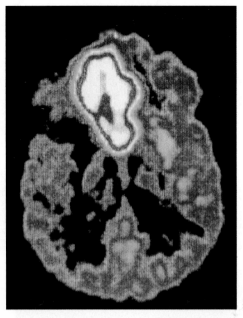

A   B

Figure 8-15. Primary cerebral B-cell lymphoma. **A:** Contrast-enhanced axial CT scan demonstrates a frontal isodense mass lesion showing marked edema. **B:** [^{18}F]FDG PET shows a lesion with very high uptake, suppressing the surrounding cortical gray matter.

metastatic disease. Therefore, the differential diagnosis among these four entities can be made only in conjunction with MR or CT imaging, according to a lesion's appearance and location (Fig. 8-16).

The main role of PET imaging is the differential diagnosis between primary lymphoma in AIDS and other nonneoplastic disorders, particularly toxoplasmosis. Other possible indications are the monitoring of intracerebral lymphomas under chemotherapy or RT (Table 8-5) and the staging of patients with systemic lymphoma who will undergo a PET brain scan in addition to a whole-body scan.

[^{18}F]FDG. Many studies have proved the accuracy of [^{18}F]FDG PET in differentiating primary lymphoma from toxoplasmosis or other nontumorous lesions in AIDS patients (52–54). The amount of [^{18}F]FDG taken up by primary lymphomas in AIDS patients does not differ from that of primary CNS lymphomas in immunocompetent patients. Although the tumor may have a ring-like form, [^{18}F]FDG uptake in the rim is very broad and intense, often suppressing the residual cortical gray matter (Fig. 8-17). This feature can hardly be confounded with other ring-like, nontumorous lesions, such as intracerebral abscess or other infectious diseases, and only a GBM with a large necrotic center should be included in the differential diagnosis. In toxoplasmosis, however, there is either no uptake in the lesion or a very faint rim-like uptake, with activity lying between that of [^{18}F]FDG uptake in white and gray matter (Fig. 8-18). As the diagnostic accuracy of [^{18}F]FDG PET is very straightforward, this imaging modality should be included in the workup of AIDS patients with intracerebral mass lesions to avoid stereotactic biopsy and to spare patients ineffective antitoxoplasmosis drug therapy in case of lymphoma.

In primary, non-AIDS related and secondary lymphomas, brain imaging can be important, as CNS lymphomas are very sensitive to RT. Of nonimmunocompromised patients with primary lymphoma, 85% respond to RT, with an overall survival of 40% to 70%. Therefore, if brain acquisition is performed in addition to a whole-body scan, CNS lymphomas can be detected with a high accuracy due to their very high [^{18}F]FDG uptake compared to adjacent gray matter structures (see Figs. 8-15 and 8-17).

For patients receiving chemotherapy for systemic lymphoma, whole-body [^{18}F]FDG PET can be used to monitor therapy response. The same is true for CNS lymphomas, where early decrease of [^{18}F]FDG uptake in the lesion is consistent with response to therapy (see Table 8-3).

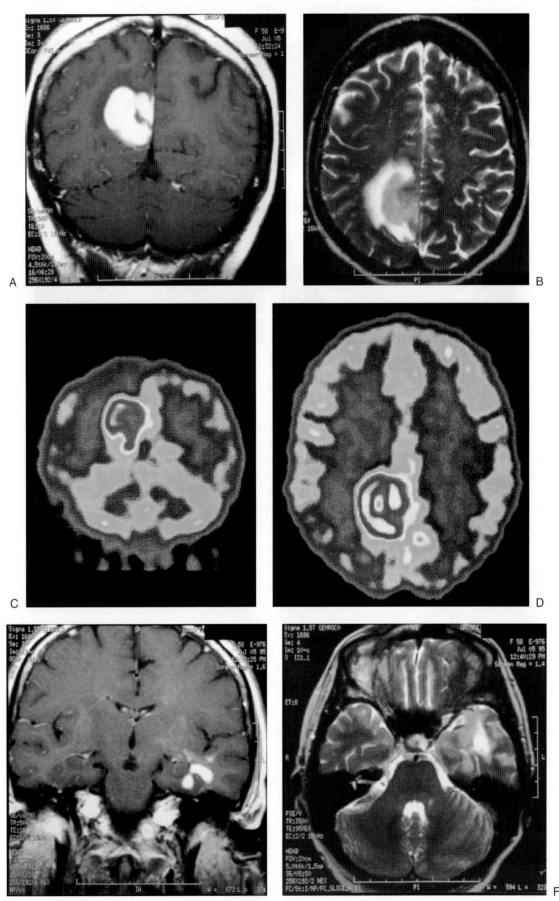

Figure 8-16. Multifocal GBM. T1-weighted, postcontrast coronal **(A)** and T2-weighted axial **(B)** MR images show an avidly enhancing right paracentral mass lesion with edema.

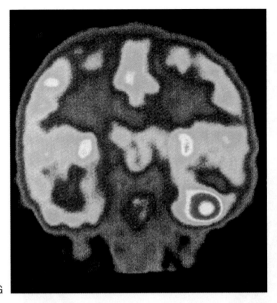
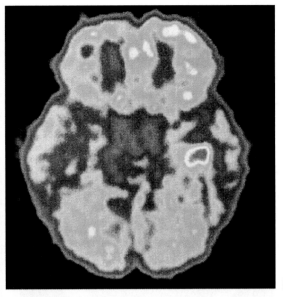

G

H

Figure 8-16. *(Continued)* Coronal **(C)** and axial **(D)** [^{18}F]FDG PET images display a centrally necrotic lesion with very high tracer uptake. The second lesion in the left temporal lobe also avidly enhances on the T1-weighted, postcontrast coronal image **(E)** and shows little edema on the T2-weighted axial image **(F)**; it also shows high [^{18}F]FDG uptake on the coronal **(G)** and axial **(H)** PET sections. This uptake is consistent with a high-grade tumor indistinguishable from CNS lymphoma.

TABLE 8-5. *Appraisal/reimbursement status of PET in tumors and inflammation*

Disease	German consensus classification	USZ classification	Replacement potential	US reimbursement status: Medicare/BC-BS	Swiss reimbursement status
High grade glioma					
Grading	1b	3	2	no/no	yes
Tumor recurrence	1a	4	4	no/no	yes
Tumor residual	1b	4	4	no/no	yes
Determination of best biopsy site	1a	4	4	no/no	yes
Grade change	—	4	4	no/no	no
Low grade glioma					
Grading	1b	4	4	no/no	yes
Tumor recurrence	—	1	3	no/no	yes
Prognostic criteria	—	3	3	no/no	no
Grade change	—	4	3	no/no	no
Other tumors					
Grading	3	3	2	no/no	yes
Tumor recurrence	—	3	2	no/no	yes
Prognostic criteria	—	—	—	no/no	no
Grade change	—	—	—	no/no	no
Brain inflammation	—	2	2	no/no	no

See page 8 for abbreviations and appraisal scheme explanations.

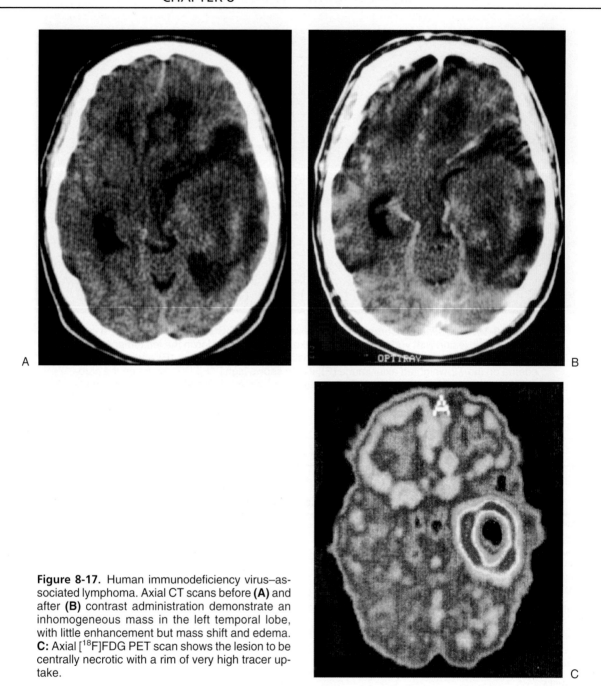

Figure 8-17. Human immunodeficiency virus–associated lymphoma. Axial CT scans before **(A)** and after **(B)** contrast administration demonstrate an inhomogeneous mass in the left temporal lobe, with little enhancement but mass shift and edema. **C:** Axial [^{18}F]FDG PET scan shows the lesion to be centrally necrotic with a rim of very high tracer uptake.

Other PET Radionuclides. [^{11}C]methionine PET has been used successfully for diagnosing lymphomas (before RT) and tumor recurrences, as well as for therapy control (55). However, only a limited number of patients has been studied so far, and further studies need to be performed before a clear statement can be made.

OTHER PRIMARY TUMORS

[^{18}F]FDG is an nonspecific radionuclide, incapable of differentiating tumors histologically. Most [^{18}F]FDG PET scans performed on patients with brain lesions provide only information regarding the aggressivity of the tumor and its extent. There is no extensive experience with [^{18}F]FDG PET for primary brain tumors other than gliomas. This is mainly due to the very low incidence of the vast majority of primary brain tumors. The other rea-

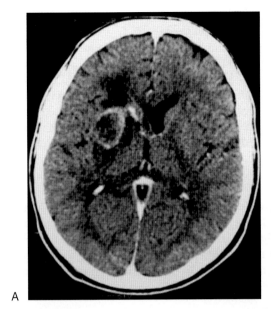
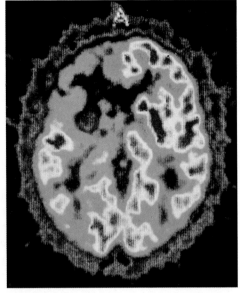

Figure 8-18. Intracerebral lesion in an AIDS patient. **A:** Axial CT scan after contrast administration shows a right paraventricular enhancing lesion that is ametabolic on [^{18}F]FDG PET **(B)**. This finding is consistent with toxoplasmosis.

son might be that in most cases conventional radiology can yield a specific diagnosis because of the very typical features and localization of different types of tumors. [^{18}F]FDG PET's ability to distinguish high-grade from low-grade tumors (tumor grade) is the only aspect of the differential diagnosis for which it might be helpful in therapy management of a patient with an intracerebral brain tumor.

Some case studies have described different types of primary brain tumors, but no definite indication for [^{18}F]FDG PET can be deduced from these. Therefore, nuclear medicine physicians performing [^{18}F]FDG PET on newly diagnosed intracerebral lesions should obtain the postoperative histologic diagnosis to improve the diagnostic accuracy of [^{18}F]FDG PET.

Pituitary Adenomas

Pituitary adenomas can be classified by their histopathology and their size. In autopsy series, asymptomatic microadenomas (<10 mm) occur in 14% to 27% of individuals (24). Macroadenomas are more often seen in men and generally present late in life, while microadenomas with early presentation are more common in women. In nonsecreting pituitary adenomas, patients present with headache, visual-field deficits, and cranial nerve palsy due to suprasellar expansion of the tumor. In hormonally active adenomas, which account for 75% of all adenomas, the clinical symptoms depend on the hormone secreted.

Pituitary adenomas are treated by surgery, with the trans-sphenoidal approach being the most popular technique. However, if the tumor reaches a size not convenient for trans-sphenoidal resection, craniotomy must be performed. In some cases, therapy with bromocriptine can help shrink tumors prior to surgery.

Neuroimaging. On CT, adenomas are of low density, compared to the normal gland, and may show intense enhancement after contrast administration. Pituitary macroadenomas may present with bony changes of the sella, such as focal erosions, enlargement, or thinning. Very small tumors might go undetected by CT scanning.

On MR imaging, microadenomas are usually hypointense on T1-weighted sequences but variable on T2-weighted images. Macroadenomas have generally the same appearance but often demonstrate additional infarction or hemorrhage.

In the differential diagnosis of a pituitary adenoma, one should include metastatic disease, astrocytoma, intrasellar meningioma, and craniopharyngioma. Very rarely, germinomas and melanomas are located in the sellar region; the same holds for nontumorous lesions, such as infections and granulomatous disease.

[¹⁸F]FDG PET. [¹⁸F]FDG PET imaging has been performed in a small number of patients with pituitary adenomas (56,57). Francavilla et al. (56) reported that nonsecreting macroadenomas showed a very high [¹⁸F]FDG uptake compared to surrounding cortical gray matter, whereas hormonally active adenomas demonstrated a reduced [¹⁸F]FDG uptake. This feature might be because nonsecreting adenomas use glucose for growth, while secreting adenomas use glucose for producing hormones. However, no correlation could be found in the amount or type of hormone secreted and the amount of [¹⁸F]FDG uptake. Moreover, in our limited experience with pituitary adenomas, no correlation has been observed between hormonal activity and [¹⁸F]FDG uptake (Figs. 8-19 and 8-20).

A clear-cut indication for [¹⁸F]FDG PET imaging in pituitary adenomas does not exist at present. In differentiating pituitary adenomas from other sellar lesions, [¹⁸F]FDG PET does not offer significant advantages over other neuroimaging modalities. However, one possible indication might be the differential diagnosis between postoperative changes and tumor recurrence of nonsecreting adenomas. CT or MR imaging may not be able to provide the information necessary to make this decision, while with recurrence the tumoral mass would display a high [¹⁸F]FDG uptake on PET.

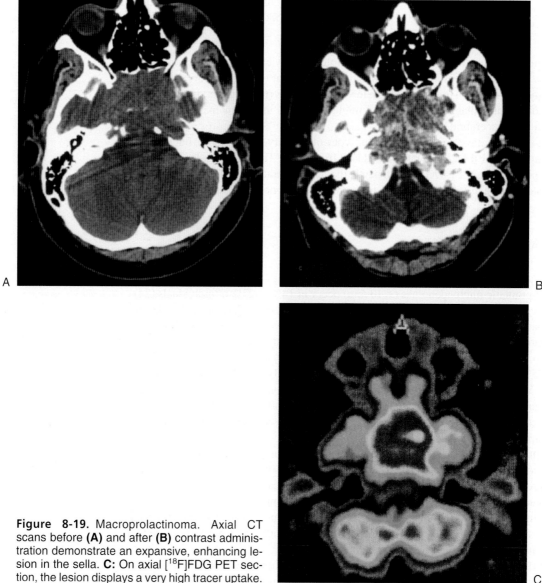

Figure 8-19. Macroprolactinoma. Axial CT scans before **(A)** and after **(B)** contrast administration demonstrate an expansive, enhancing lesion in the sella. **C:** On axial [¹⁸F]FDG PET section, the lesion displays a very high tracer uptake.

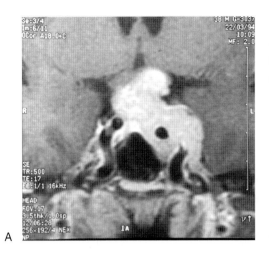
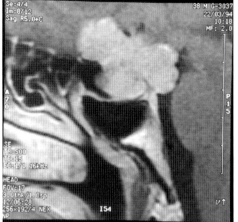

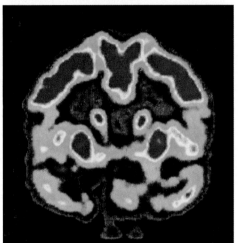

Figure 8-20. Prolactinoma. Contrast-enhanced, T1-weighted coronal **(A)** and sagittal **(B)** MR images demonstrate the tumor. **C:** The same tumor as shown in Fig. 8-19 may display a less pronounced tracer uptake on [^{18}F]FDG PET imaging.

Another possible indication for PET imaging of pituitary adenomas might be the use of [^{11}C]methionine or dopamine D$_2$-receptor ligands, such as [^{11}C]raclopride and [^{18}F]fluoro-ethyl-spiperone (57,58). Here, receptor imaging might help differentiate pituitary adenomas from other sellar/parasellar masses and monitor medical therapy when a dopamine agonist such as bromocriptine is used before surgical intervention. Moreover, pituitary adenomas have been investigated with the monoamine oxidase B inhibitor [^{11}C]-l-deprenyl and proved useful in the differential diagnosis between meningioma and pituitary adenoma (59).

Other Tumors

At our institution, we do not have much experience with other primary intracerebral tumors than those described above. Some single tumors have been imaged (see Fig. 8-11), but not in sufficient number to draw some conclusions for diagnostic purposes. From a review of the literature, however, the same seems to be true for other institutions, from which only case reports have been published (60–62).

METASTASES

In adults, metastases are the most common intracerebral masses, representing up to 40% of intracerebral neoplasms (24). Brain metastases from primary breast, lung, melanoma, kidney, and gastrointestinal tumors are the most common brain metastases and occur as

TABLE 8-6. *Incidence of CNS involvement at time of diagnosis and during tumor growth*

Tumor	At diagnosis (%)	During tumor growth (%)
Lung tumor	10–15	22–10
Breast tumor	1	6–20
Melanoma	6	50
Renal cell tumor	4	11–13
Colorectal tumor	1	—
Sarcoma	1	36

From ref. 63, with permission.

solitary lesions in 30% to 50% of patients (24) (Table 8-6). Multiple metastases from unknown primary sites occur in about 11% of patients (28). If the primary site of a single lesion is not evident from a patient's presentation, the differential diagnosis includes glioma.

Intracranial metastases are found mostly at the gray matter–white matter boundary, the cerebellum, the dura, and less frequently in the basal ganglia. Other sites include the pituitary and pineal glands, the choroid plexus, or preexisting lesions, such as a tumor, infarct, or vascular malformation (28) (Fig. 8-21).

CNS metastases cause nonspecific symptoms that evolve over weeks and include focal neurologic or neuropsychiatric deficits. Spinal metastases may develop over hours and are most often associated with back pain, weakness of extremities, sensory symptoms, or incontinence.

Neuroimaging

On unenhanced CT, metastatic lesions appear rounded and are typically iso- or hypodense. They enhance strongly after contrast administration in a homogeneous or ring-like fashion and are surrounded by edema. Vasogenic edema may be very prominent, except in cortical metastases, where it is usually only minimal or even missing.

On MR imaging, metastases are iso- to hypointense on T1-weighted images and of variable intensity on T2-weighted images, depending on the presence and amount of hemorrhage and necrosis. They show marked enhancement, which may be homogeneous or inhomogeneous, after the injection of low-molecular-weight gadolinium compounds.

[^{18}F]FDG PET

Cerebral metastases are malignant and display a very high mitotic index, usually higher than the primary tumor. Therefore, they most often present as lesions with very high [^{18}F]FDG uptake (see Table 8-3). However, this activity is nonspecific and does not relate to a particular tumor. Again, [^{18}F]FDG PET cannot help in the differential diagnosis between metastases and other high-grade lesions such as lymphoma, meningioma, or GBM. The most important prognostic factor is the number of metastatic lesions and the Karnofsky performance index. The overall median survival of patients with multiple intracerebral metastases is 3 to 6 months (28). Metastatic lesions are usually treated by RT; single metastases can be approached surgically.

The most useful clinical indication for [^{18}F]FDG PET is a whole-body staging scan in patients with malignancies known to metastasize preferably to the brain. In this instance, a separate, three-dimensional brain acquisition should be performed, in addition to the two-dimensional whole-body scan, because otherwise small cortical lesions can easily be missed. Another indication is the monitoring of intracerebral metastases under RT or chemotherapy. The differential diagnosis between postsurgical or postirradiational changes and tumor recurrence is another possible indication for [^{18}F]FDG PET. Here, conventional neuroimaging is known to be less effective than PET because early postsurgical changes, as well as radiation necrosis, cannot be distinguished from tumor recurrence.

Intracerebral metastatic lesions have not been studied very extensively with [^{18}F]FDG

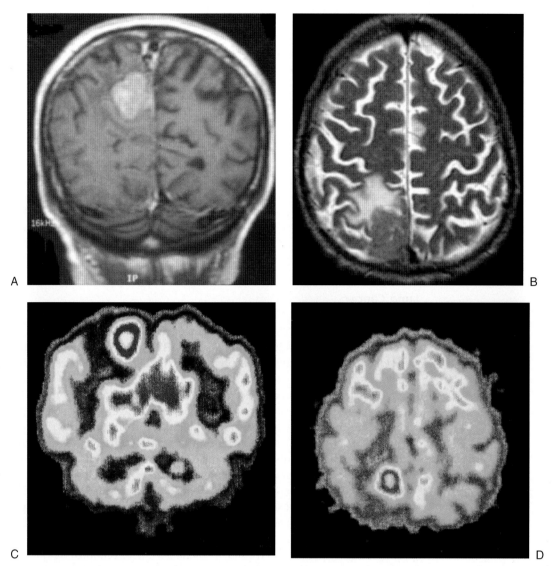

Figure 8-21. Metastatic lesion in a right occipital meningioma, WHO grade I. T1-weighted, Gd-DTPA-enhanced coronal **(A)** and T2-weighted axial **(B)** MR images show a right occipital, contrast-enhancing lesion with little edema. Coronal **(C)** and axial **(D)** [^{18}F]FDG PET images show high tracer uptake.

PET. However, increased, as well as decreased, tracer uptake has been described, depending on tumor location (cortical or white matter), lesion size, histology, and image acquisition. [^{18}F]FDG PET staging for intracerebral metastatic disease can be performed for tumors known for very high [^{18}F]FDG uptake. This is the case in bronchogenic, ovarian, and colon carcinomas and malignant melanoma.

Malignant Melanoma

Malignant melanoma of the skin is the leading cause of death from all lesions arising in the skin, and its incidence continues to increase. Because malignant melanoma responds poorly to RT or chemotherapy, a surgical approach is preferred.

Cutanous melanomas are very easy to diagnose with a thorough clinical examination. However, disease staging is very important because patients with distant metastases have a very poor prognosis, with an overall 5-year survival of less than 10%. Staging is generally performed very extensively and includes clinical examination, CT, MR imaging, and ultrasound. In recent years, [^{18}F]FDG PET imaging has proven to be a very valuable tool in staging patients with metastatic disease and detecting cutaneous lesions as small as 4 mm, as well as organ manifestations of malignant melanoma (64–66) (see Chapter 19: Melanoma; and Fig. 19-1).

Malignant melanoma most frequently spreads along the lymphatic channels, producing satellite, transit, and regional nodal metastases (67). Recurrences, however, tend to spread hematogenously, resulting in cutaneous or visceral metastases. Preferential sites for visceral metastases include liver, lung, bone, and brain. Brain metastases develop in 50% of patients with malignant melanoma, and approximately one-half of deaths occurring in patients with malignant melanoma are related to CNS metastases.

[^{18}F]FDG PET is generally performed as a whole-body procedure in patients with malignant melanoma. However, in high-risk patients (Breslow >1.5 mm), a separate brain scan is usually added to exclude small metastatic lesions, which can reliably be detected down to 1 cm (see Chapter 19). If brain metastases of malignant melanoma are diagnosed, [^{18}F]FDG PET can be used to monitor and follow up the new therapeutic schemes involving immunochemotherapy.

Lung Cancer

Primary lung cancer is a major health problem in the Western hemisphere, with a generally poor prognosis. Only 20% of all patients will have disease confined to the primary lesion at initial diagnosis, 25% will show spread to regional lymph nodes, and 55% will have distant metastatic spread (68).

As the therapeutic approach, as well as the prognosis, depends on tumor histology and disease extent, staging is very important for patient management. Patients with lung carcinoma are subgrouped into those with small cell lung carcinoma (SCLC) and non–small cell lung carcinoma (NSCLC), as the therapeutic approach is different for each group. Patients with NSCLC and local disease are primarily treated surgically, whereas patients with SCLC are subject to RT or chemotherapy.

As the primary diagnosis of lung carcinoma is generally made by a conventional chest radiograph, the extent of disease is determined by CT scan. However, CT imaging is known to have limited sensitivity because lymph nodes of 1 cm or smaller in diameter are not considered pathologic and are therefore missed if microinvasion is present. As a functional imaging method, [^{18}F]FDG PET in conjunction with conventional morphologic imaging has shown to be very accurate in detecting local spread, as well as distant organ manifestations in patients with proven NSCLC (69–71) (see Chapter 15: Tumors of the Chest). Image coregistration helps localize small nodular metastases if surgery is still being considered as the primary therapeutic approach. In general, the area covered in patients imaged with [^{18}F]FDG PET extends from the brain to the urinary bladder and is performed with and without absorption correction. However, if brain metastases, as occur in about 25% of patients, are expected, a separate brain scan that is not routinely performed must be added to improve image resolution (72). If brain metastases are diagnosed, RT is usually given, and [^{18}F]FDG PET can be used to monitor therapy response and differentiate between tumor progression and radiation-induced necrosis (Fig. 8-22).

Breast Cancer

Staging of patients with breast cancer is still a major problem, as the prognosis depends on the multicentricity of the lesion and the extent of axillary lymph node involvement. To date, only surgery provides definitive information regarding lymph node involvement, and no morphologic imaging method has been shown to be nearly as accurate as histology.

Great hope was put in functional imaging methods such as technetium Tc MIBI scintigraphy and [^{18}F]FDG PET for diagnosing and staging breast cancer. Several studies have dealt with staging of patients with breast cancer, showing a very high sensitiv-

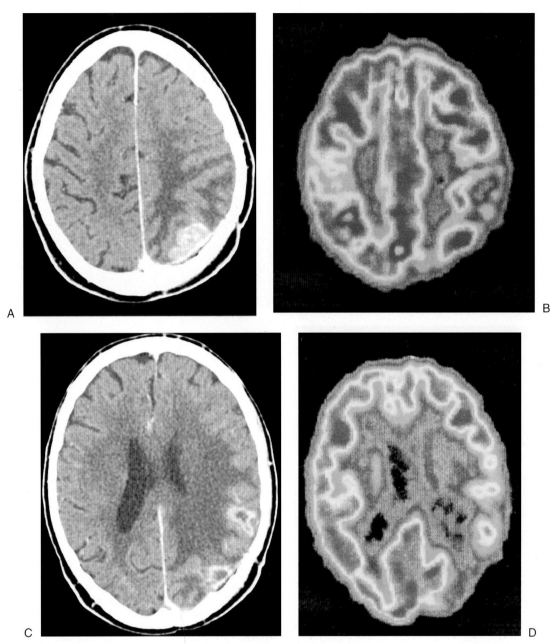

Figure 8-22. Bronchogenic carcinoma after surgical resection and postoperative RT of brain metastases. **A,C:** Contrast-enhanced T1-weighted axial MR images show three contrast-enhancing lesions in the left parietooccipital area. The cranial lesion **(A)** is more compact, whereas the two lesions at the level of the basal ganglia **(C)** are more ring-like in appearance. **B,D:** On [^{18}F]FDG PET images, the more cranial lesion **(B)** is consistent with recurrent disease due to high tracer uptake, and the two lesions at the level of the basal ganglia **(D)** are consistent with radiation necrosis because of low tracer uptake. This presumed diagnosis was histologically proven.

ity and specificity for [^{18}F]FDG PET, even in screening for axillary lymph node metastases (73–75).

Brain imaging is not performed as a regular imaging protocol for patients with breast cancer because brain metastases occur in only 6% to 20% of these patients (67). In general, the diagnosis of a brain metastasis is usually made by conventional CT imaging when neurologic symptoms suggesting cerebral involvement occur. Therefore, no primary role for

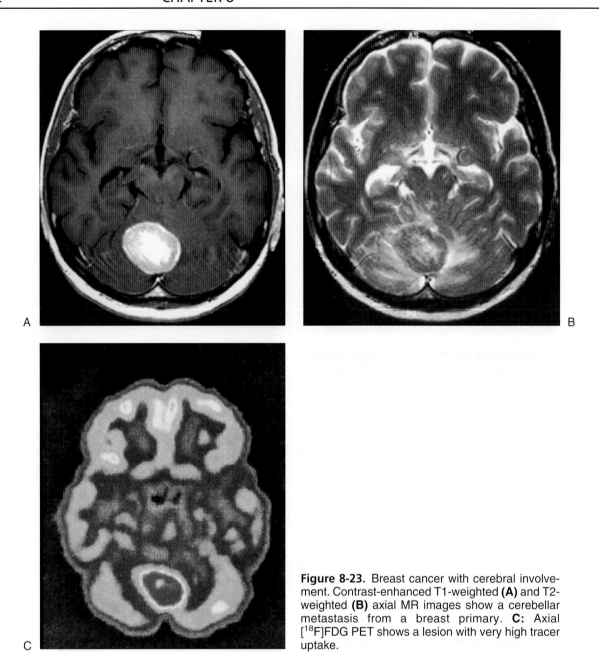

Figure 8-23. Breast cancer with cerebral involvement. Contrast-enhanced T1-weighted **(A)** and T2-weighted **(B)** axial MR images show a cerebellar metastasis from a breast primary. **C:** Axial [^{18}F]FDG PET shows a lesion with very high tracer uptake.

[^{18}F]FDG PET imaging in patients with suggested brain metastases is yet defined. As is true for primary breast cancer, which usually shows high [^{18}F]FDG uptake, metastatic disease also shows high tracer uptake (Fig. 8-23).

Therefore, [^{18}F]FDG PET is mainly used to differentiate RT- or chemotherapy-induced necrosis from recurrent disease. However, as in other primary lesions or other metastases from different tumors, problems are encountered when the lesions are less than 1 cm in size or are located at the boundary between gray and white matter. Here, usually only image coregistration between [^{18}F]FDG PET and CT or MR imaging can provide an accurate diagnosis.

Other Metastatic Tumors

CNS manifestations of other tumors have not been extensively studied with PET. There are some single cases showing the possible utility of this imaging method (Fig. 8-24; see Chapter 14: Extracranial Head and Neck Cancer and Thyroid Cancer; and Fig. 14-2), but

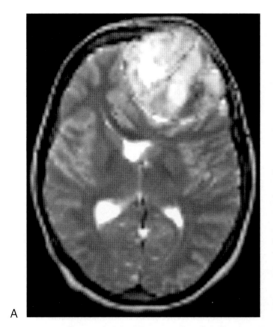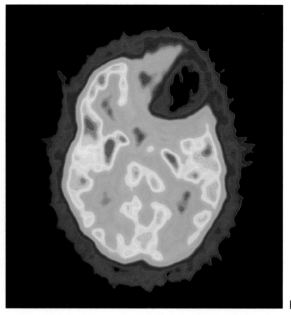

A   B

Figure 8-24. Metastasis of follicular thyroid carcinoma. **A:** T2-weighted axial MR image demonstrates a left frontal mass lesion. **B:** [^{18}F]FDG PET shows the lesion to be partly ametabolic, with the medial rim of the tumor displaying intermediate tracer uptake. The lesion was histologically proven to be metastatic.

more experience must be amassed to prove the accuracy of [18F]FDG PET brain imaging in diagnosing and monitoring brain metastases.

EFFECTS OF RADIATION THERAPY

Many primary intracerebral tumors, as well as intracerebral metastases, are treated either with RT alone or with adjuvant RT after primary surgical resection. RT may cause toxic effects with clinical deterioration and extensive changes on neuroimaging studies. Acute clinical symptoms may develop 1 to 2 weeks after initiation of RT and are usually caused by cerebral edema. Subacute changes usually occur between 3 and 18 months after RT and are attributable to RT effects such as disruption of tumor vascularization, induced cell death, development of necrotic changes, and finally demyelination. Acute and subacute RT effects are usually accompanied by changes in the tumor tissue, as well as the surrounding cortex. These changes are seen on neuroimaging studies as contrast-enhancing lesions, sometimes with edema and mass effect; they are low in attenuation on CT and high in signal intensity on T2-weighted MR images. These acute and subacute changes are usually not distinguishable from ineffective RT treatment or early tumor recurrence (24). In long-term survivors, late changes of RT may develop between 18 and 60 months and include extensive white matter changes, cortical atrophy, hydrocephalus, or hypothalamic dysfunction, depending on the radiation field, radiation dose, and fractionation.

CT and MR imaging have been used in the follow-up of patients after RT. However, tumor recurrence lacks typical features on both imaging modalities; early tumor recurrence is differentiated from RT-induced changes mainly based on clinical experience, serial neuroimaging studies, and responsiveness to steroid therapy.

[^{18}F]FDG PET has proven to be very effective not only for monitoring tumor metabolism under RT but also for assessing RT-induced changes in the tumor bed and surrounding cortical tissue. Several studies have dealt with monitoring of tumor response under RT and have tried to establish prognostic criteria (9,32). On monitoring [^{18}F]FDG PET images, early tumor response to RT will show a decrease in tracer uptake, indicating a cellular response (Fig. 8-25); unchanged or even increased [^{18}F]FDG uptake is consistent with treat-

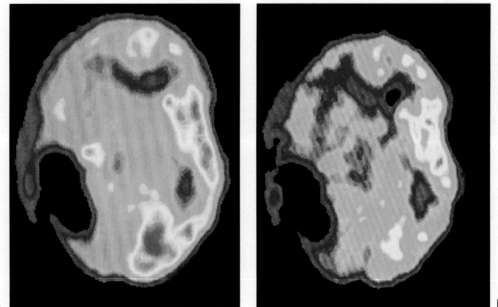

Figure 8-25. Patient with history of right parietal partial surgery and ongoing RT. **A,B:** Both [^{18}F]FDG PET images—one obtained shortly before the start of RT **(A)** and the other 2 weeks into RT (at 30 Gy) **(B)**—are normalized to the ipsilateral cerebellum. There is a marked decrease in tracer uptake in the residual tumor mass at the medial border of the surgical cavity. This finding was interpreted as response to RT.

ment failure (Fig. 8-26). However, some authors have described an inverse effect of a rapid decrease of tumor [^{18}F]FDG uptake on patient survival (76); therefore, further studies are necessary to establish a clear-cut clinical approach in questions regarding tumor response to therapy and the establishment of prognostic criteria.

Several clinical trials have studied the accuracy of [^{18}F]FDG PET in the differential diagnosis between tumor recurrence and RT-induced changes, mainly in glial cell tumors

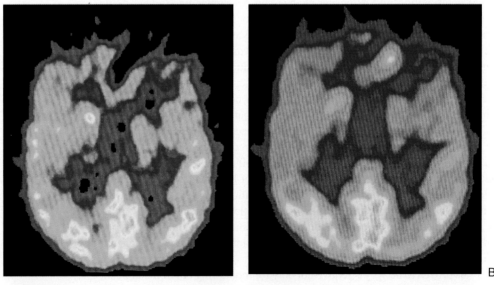

Figure 8-26. Patient with a history of a left frontal GBM, partial surgery, and ongoing RT. **A,B:** Both [^{18}F]FDG PET images—one obtained shortly before the start of RT **(A)** and the other 2 weeks into RT (at 30 Gy) **(B)**—are normalized to the ipsilateral cerebellum. The frontal residual tumor mass has started to fill the surgical cavity and displays higher tracer uptake than before the start of RT. This finding was consistent with tumor progression under RT.

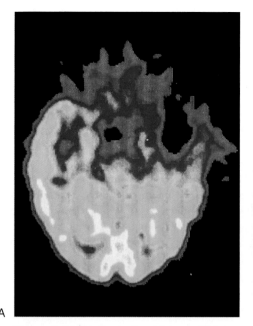
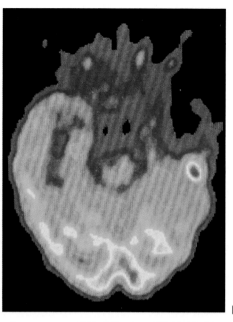

A   B

Figure 8-27. Patient with a history of left temporal surgery and RT. **A,B:** Both [^{18}F]FDG PET images—one obtained shortly after the end of RT **(A)** and the other 12 months after RT **(B)**—are normalized to the ipsilateral cerebellum. A new focus of high tracer uptake is shown at the posterior border of the surgical cavity. This lesion was histologically proven to be recurrent tumor.

(3,4,10,13,36; see "Astrocytomas, Oligodendrogliomas, and Glioblastomas" above). For other, nonglial primary brain tumors, as well as metastatic lesions, with initially high [^{18}F]FDG accumulation, the same pattern must be expected. As the finding of increased [^{18}F]FDG uptake in the tumor bed is virtually diagnostic of tumor recurrence (Fig. 8-27), a defect or substantially reduced uptake is indicative of radiation necrosis (Fig. 8-28; see

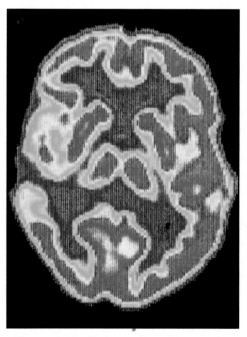
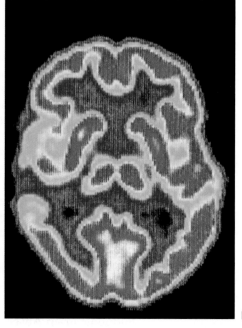

A   B

Figure 8-28. Patient with a history of a right temporal GBM, surgery, RT. **A,B:** Both [^{18}F]FDG PET images—one obtained after completion of RT **(A)** and the other 12 months after RT **(B)**—are normalized to the ipsilateral cerebellum. There is a small region of absent tracer uptake that remains unchanged in size. This region is consistent with the surgical cavity; there are no signs of tumor recurrence.

Table 8-3 and Fig. 8-22C and D). However, some difficulties have been described in differentiating ongoing radiation necrosis from tumor recurrence, not only in glial cell tumors but also in meningiomas (42). Ongoing radiation necrosis contains granulation tissue, and reactive granulocytes are known to accumulate [^{18}F]FDG, therefore producing false-positive results in whole-body (77,78) and brain (42) PET scans. Quantification has been discussed to avoid such pitfalls (78).

Another possibility for avoiding false-positive reports would be the introduction of a more specific radionuclide that accumulates only in tumor cells and not in reactive white cells. This is the case with radiolabeled amino acids, which are used in several centers instead of or in addition to [^{18}F]FDG. Various amino acids have been shown to accumulate in tumors (24). Of them, [^{11}C]methionine has been studied most extensively. There is even some indication that the amount of [^{11}C]methionine uptake correlates with tumor grade (14,43,55,79). Another well studied amino acid is [^{11}C]tyrosine. However, both of these radionuclides have the disadvantage of being bound to ^{11}C, which has a substantially shorter half-life than ^{18}F, thus making it necessary to have a cyclotron close to the imaging center and rapid resynthesis.

INFLAMMATION

Cross-sectional neuroimaging techniques are very sensitive to any intracerebral alterations. Based on the clinical history, physical examination, laboratory results, and CT or MR imaging findings, the differential diagnosis can usually be narrowed quite a bit. Because epidural and subdural infections usually do not produce problems in their differentiation from other, noninfectious diseases, only intraparenchymal lesions are discussed in this section.

The major point of interest is the differential diagnosis between a primary intracerebral neoplasm and an inflammatory or infectious lesion, mainly an abscess. Because of the imaging properties of [^{18}F]FDG PET, neoplastic lesions should easily be separable from nonneoplastic lesions. There are clear-cut features on [^{18}F]FDG images, as well as some pitfalls. As discussed above, high-grade tumors (WHO grades III to IV) usually are distinguished from other intracerebral lesions by their high [^{18}F]FDG uptake compared to cortical gray matter. This is especially true for anaplastic astrocytoma grade III, GBM, meningiomas, lymphomas, some metastases, and juvenile primary brain tumors. However, difficulties have been described in differentiating even high-grade lesions from granulomatous tissue, especially in ongoing radiation-induced necrosis (see Chapter 20: Clinical PET Imaging of Inflammatory Diseases). It is known from experimental studies that inflammatory cells do accumulate [^{18}F]FDG to a higher degree (80,81); therefore quantification is usually recommended to help in the differential diagnosis. Another problem with [^{18}F]FDG PET is the differential diagnosis between low-grade tumors and inflammatory or infectious lesions. Here, [^{18}F]FDG uptake ranges between that of white and gray matter, thus making it impossible to differentiate a nontumorous from an inflammatory or infectious lesion, both usually showing the same accumulation pattern.

As most of the specific infectious diseases can be diagnosed with very high accuracy with conventional imaging methods, [^{18}F]FDG PET does not play an important role, mainly because no histologic differentiation can be obtained by the amount or pattern of [^{18}F]FDG uptake. However, there may be a certain information increase in using [^{18}F]FDG PET if a ring-like enhancing lesion, single or multiple, is observed on CT or MR imaging, because several different pathologic entities must be included in the differential diagnosis in this setting.

Pyogenic Brain Abscess

A pyogenic brain abscess is formed through hematogenous dissemination from a primary site. It most often occurs in septic patients, those with pulmonary, cardiac, or paranasal sinus infections, and individuals who abuse intravenous drugs. Brain abscesses favor the frontal and parietal lobes along the territory supplied by the middle cerebral artery. Single or multiple in number, they usually lie at the junction of the gray and the white matter.

Neuroimaging. Experimental CT imaging has defined four stages of brain abscess formation (82):

1. Early cerebritis: 1 to 3 days;
2. Late cerebritis: 4 to 9 days;
3. Early capsule formation: 10 to 13 days;
4. Late capsule formation: 14 days and onward.

In the cerebritis phase, a low-density lesion with patchy enhancement may be seen. In the late-cerebritis phase, a necrotic center forms within the infectious lesion, surrounded by granulation tissue. Therefore, ring-like enhancement is often present. A mature abscess has low density with considerable edema surrounding it.

On MR imaging, a brain abscess shows low signal intensity on T1-weighted images and high intensity on T2-weighted images in the early-cerebritis phase. After 2 to 3 weeks, the mature abscess appears as a well demarcated, low-intensity mass on T1-weighted sequences with edema beyond it. On T2-weighted images, high signal intensity is seen in the cavity.

As ring-like enhancement is seen in mature abscesses on both CT and MR imaging, several differential diagnoses must be considered; these include infarction, fungal or parasitic infection, primary and metastatic brain tumor, tuberculosis, granuloma, multiple sclerosis, and subacute hematoma. In this clinical setting, [^{18}F]FDG PET in conjunction with conventional neuroimaging might help narrow the differential diagnosis. However, as mentioned above, no clear-cut [^{18}F]FDG PET features for the different pathologic entities have yet been proposed that offer substantial advantages over CT or MR imaging. This is mainly due to the very limited experience with [^{18}F]FDG studies in nontumorous intracerebral lesions, as well as the nonspecific character of this radiopharmaceutical.

[^{18}F]FDG PET. As pyogenic abscesses are surrounded by granulomatous tissue in the late phase of cerebritis, ring-like [^{18}F]FDG uptake might be observed. However, [^{18}F]FDG uptake in granulomatous tissue is inconsistent and may be absent altogether (Fig. 8-29). This feature is probably dependent on the time of scanning and the amount and characteristics of the inflammatory cells. However, intracerebral abscesses usually do not pose difficulties in differentiation from primary or secondary tumors, such as GBM, lymphoma, or metastases, because the ring-like [^{18}F]FDG uptake is never as intense or wide as it is in a tumorous lesion.

Differential Diagnosis of Infectious from Other Lesions Using [^{18}F]FDG PET

Only in AIDS patients can [^{18}F]FDG PET by itself establish the differential diagnosis between an opportunistic infection, such as toxoplasmosis, and primary intracerebral lymphoma (see "Lymphomas" above). For the other pathologic entities mentioned, only limited experience is available, and most of the imaging characteristics are nondifferentiating or not yet scientifically established.

Fungal and Parasitic Infections. For fungal and parasitic infections, the same pattern as in pyogenic brain abscess can be expected. However, there is no experience with [^{18}F]FDG PET in these entities, neither at our institution nor in the literature.

Tuberculosis and Granulomatous Disease. In tuberculosis and granulomatous disease, some experience is available, but mostly in whole-body [^{18}F]FDG PET. However, as both tuberculosis and granulomatous disease have shown high [^{18}F]FDG uptake, the same can be expected in the brain (Fig. 8-30). Here, especially for granulomatous disease, such as sarcoidosis, the differential diagnosis from a high-grade tumor may become a problem because active sarcoidosis usually shows very high [^{18}F]FDG uptake (Fig. 8-31).

Infarction, Multiple Sclerosis, and Subacute Hematoma. The diagnosis of these pathologic entities is usually made by CT or MR imaging. PET is not expected to offer a

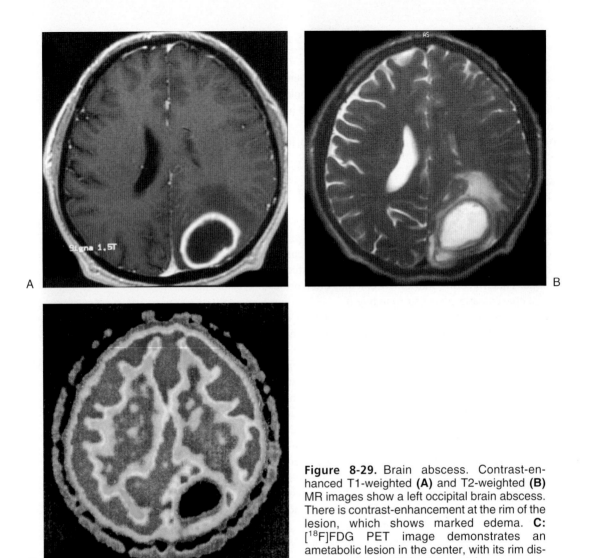

Figure 8-29. Brain abscess. Contrast-enhanced T1-weighted **(A)** and T2-weighted **(B)** MR images show a left occipital brain abscess. There is contrast-enhancement at the rim of the lesion, which shows marked edema. **C:** [^{18}F]FDG PET image demonstrates an ametabolic lesion in the center, with its rim displaying relatively high tracer uptake.

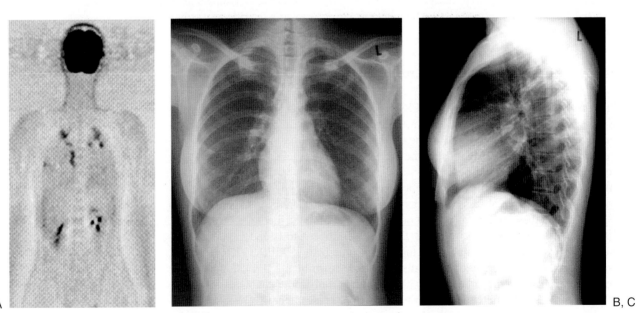

Figure 8-30. Thoracic tuberculosis. **A:** Coronal section of a whole-body [^{18}F]FDG PET scan shows multiple lesions in both lungs displaying high tracer uptake. **B,C:** Plain thoracic x-ray films obtained at the same time as the [^{18}F]FDG PET study.

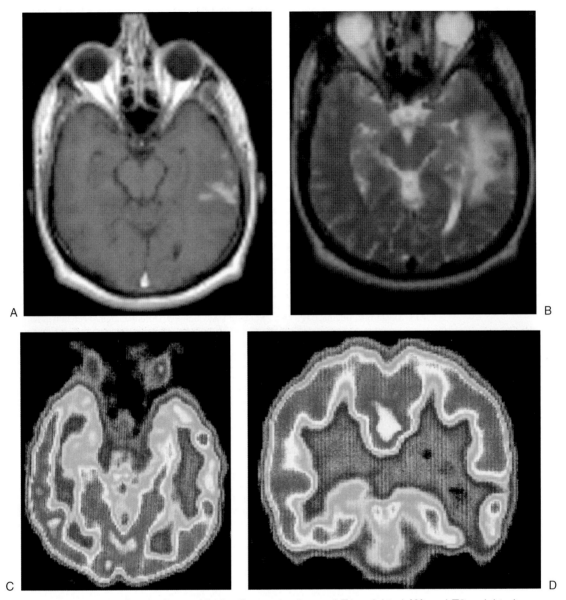

Figure 8-31. Cerebral sarcoidosis. Contrast-enhanced T1-weighted **(A)** and T2-weighted **(B)** axial MR images show an enhancing lesion in the left temporal lobe with marked edema. This lesion was initially believed to be a glioma. On axial **(C)** and coronal **(D)** [^{18}F]FDG PET images, the lesion displays high tracer uptake, which therefore was interpreted as a high-grade tumor.

substantial information increase because no [^{18}F]FDG uptake can be expected in these lesions.

CONCLUSION AND OUTLOOK

[^{18}F]FDG PET in primary and secondary brain tumors is a very promising diagnostic tool, adding substantial information to conventional neuroimaging. However, extensive studies have only been performed on patients with glial cell tumors. With these tumors, [^{18}F]FDG PET staging of primary tumors and differentiation between radiation-induced necrosis and recurrent tumor have proven to be very effective. In the other brain tumors, besides lymphomas and meningiomas, the cases described are very limited. Therefore, information regarding the usefulness of [^{18}F]FDG PET is not yet conclusive and must be improved by larger patient numbers.

REFERENCES

1. Warburg O. On the origin of cancer cells. *Science* 1956;123:309–314.
2. Reivich M, Kuhi D, Wolf A, et al. The (^{18}F)fluorodeoxyglucose method for the measurement of cerebral glucose utilization in man. *Circ Res* 1979;44:127–137.
3. Patronas NJ, Di CG, Brooks RA, et al. Work in progress: [18F] fluorodeoxyglucose and positron emission tomography in the evaluation of radiation necrosis of the brain. *Radiology* 1982;144:885–889.
4. Kim EE, Chung SK, Haynie TP, et al. Differentiation of residual or recurrent tumors from post-treatment changes with F-18 FDG PET. *Radiographics* 1992;12:269–279.
5. Di Chiro G, Oldfield E, Wright DC, et al. Cerebral necrosis after radiotherapy and/or intraarterial chemotherapy for brain tumors: PET and neuropathologic studies. *Am J Roentgenol* 1988;150:189–197.
6. Patronas NJ, Di CG, Kufta C, et al. Prediction of survival in glioma patients by means of positron emission tomography. *J Neurosurg* 1985;62:816–822.
7. Schifter T, Hoffman JM, Hanson MW, et al. Serial FDG-PET studies in the prediction of survival in patients with primary brain tumors. *J Comput Assist Tomogr* 1993;17:509–516.
8. Kim CK, Alavi JB, Alavi A, Reivich M. New grading system of cerebral gliomas using positron emission tomography with F-18 fluorodeoxyglucose. *J Neurooncol* 1991;10:85–91.
9. Blasberg RG. Prediction of brain tumor therapy response by PET. *J Neurooncol* 1994;22:281–286.
10. Glantz MJ, Hoffman JM, Coleman RE, et al. Identification of early recurrence of primary central nervous system tumors by [^{18}F]fluorodeoxyglucose positron emission tomography. *Ann Neurol* 1991;29:347–355.
11. Coleman RE. Single photon emission computed tomography and positron emission tomography in cancer imaging. *Cancer* 1991;67:1261–1270.
12. Alavi JB, Alavi A, Chawluk J, et al. Positron emission tomography in patients with glioma: a predictor of prognosis. *Cancer* 1988;62:1074–1078.
13. Doyle WK, Budinger TF, Valk PE, Levin VA, Gutin PH. Differentiation of cerebral radiation necrosis from tumor recurrence by [^{18}F]FDG and ^{82}Rb positron emission tomography. *J Comput Assist Tomogr* 1987;11:563–570.
14. Kaschten B, Stevenaert A, Sadzot B, et al. Preoperative evaluation of 54 gliomas by PET with fluorine-18-fluorodeoxyglucose and/or carbon-11-methionine. *J Nucl Med* 1998;39:778–785.
15. Delbeke D, Meyerowitz C, Lapidus RL, et al. Optimal cutoff levels of F-18 fluorodeoxyglucose uptake in the differentiation of low-grade from high-grade brain tumors with PET. *Radiology* 1995;195:47–52.
16. Keyes JW Jr. SUV: standard uptake or silly useless value? *J Nucl Med* 1995;36:1836–1839.
17. Kleihues P, Burger PB, Scheithauer BW. Histological typing of tumours of the central nervous system. In: *World Health Organization international histologic classification of tumours*, 2nd ed. Berlin/Heidelberg: Springer-Verlag, 1993, pp. 112.
18. Daumas Duport C, Scheithauer B, O'Fallon J, Kelly P. Grading of astrocytomas: a simple and reproducible method. *Cancer* 1988;62:2152–2165.
19. Wood JR, Green SB, Shapiro WR. The prognostic importance of tumor size in malignant gliomas: a computed tomographic scan study by the Brain Tumor Cooperative Group. *J Clin Oncol* 1988;6:338–343.
20. Wurschmidt F, Bunemann H, Heilmann HP. Prognostic factors in high-grade malignant glioma: a multivariate analysis of 76 cases with postoperative radiotherapy. *Strahlenther Onkol* 1995;171:315–321.
21. McLendon RE, Robinson JS Jr, Chambers DB, Grufferman S, Burger PC. The glioblastoma multiforme in Georgia, 1977-1981. *Cancer* 1985;56:894–897.
22. Leibel SA, Scott CB, Loeffler JS. Contemporary approaches to the treatment of malignant gliomas with radiation therapy. *Semin Oncol* 1994;21:198–219.
23. Prognostic factors for high-grade malignant glioma: development of a prognostic index. A report of the Medical Research Council brain tumour working party. *J Neurooncol* 1990;9:47–55.
24. Grossman RI, Yousem DM. Neoplasms of the brain. In: Thrall, JH ed. *Neuroradiology, the requisites.* St. Louis, MO: Mosby, 1994:67–103.
25. Leeds NE, Elkin CM, Zimmerman RD. Gliomas of the brain. *Semin Roentgenol* 1984;19:27–43.
26. Chamberlain MC, Murovic JA, Levin VA. Absence of contrast enhancement on CT brain scans of patients with supratentorial malignant gliomas. *Neurology* 1988;38:1371–1374. [Erratum: *Neurology* 1988;38:1816.]
27. Ginsberg LE, Fuller GN, Hashmi M, Leeds NE, Schomer DF. The significance of lack of MR contrast enhancement of supratentorial brain tumors in adults: histopathological evaluation of a series. *Surg Neurol* 1998;49:436–440.
28. Kleihues P, Canevee W. *Pathology and genetics of tumours in the nervous system.* Lyons: International Agency for Research on Cancer, 1997.
29. Bicik I, Raman R, Knightly JJ, Di Chiro G, Fulham MJ. PET-FDG of pleomorphic xanthoastrocytoma. *J Nucl Med* 1995;36:97–99.
30. Fulham MJ, Melisi JW, Nishimiya J, Dwyer AJ, Di Chiro G. Neuroimaging of juvenile pilocytic astrocytomas: an enigma. *Radiology* 1993;189:221–225.
31. Mineura K, Sasajima T, Kowada M, et al. Perfusion and metabolim in predicting the survival of patients with cerebral gliomas. *Cancer* 1994;73:2386–2394.
32. Holzer T, Herholz K, Jeske J, Heiss WD. FDG-PET as a prognostic indicator in radiochemotherapy of glioblastoma. *J Comput Assist Tomogr* 1993;17:681–687.
33. Trautmann TG, Shaw EG. Supratentorial low-grade glioma: is there a role for radiation therapy? *Ann Acad Med Singapore* 1996;25:392–396.
34. Francavilla TL, Miletich RS, Di Chiro G, Patronas NJ, Rizzoli HV, Wright DC. Positron emission tomography in the detection of malignant degeneration of low-grade gliomas. *Neurosurgery* 1989;24:1–5.
35. Dooms GC, Hecht S, Brant Zawadzki M, Berthiaume Y, Norman D, Newton TH. Brain radiation lesions: MR imaging. *Radiology* 1986;158:149–155.
36. Garner CM. Positron emission tomography: new hope for early detection of recurrent brain tumors. *Cancer Nurs* 1997;20:277–284.

37. Ishikawa M, Kikuchi H, Miyatake S, Oda Y, Yonekura Y, Nishizawa S. Glucose consumption in recurrent gliomas. *Neurosurgery* 1993;33:28–33,

38. Rigo P, Paulus P, Kaschten BJ, et al. Oncological applications of positron emission tomography with fluorine-18 fluorodeoxyglucose. *Eur J Nucl Med* 1996;23:1641–1674.

39. Di Chiro G, Hatazawa J, Katz DA, Rizzoli HV, De Michele DJ. Glucose utilization by intracranial meningiomas as an index of tumor aggressivity and probability of recurrence: a PET study. *Radiology* 1987;164:521–526.

40. Cremerius U, Bares R, Weis J, et al. Fasting improves discrimination of grade I and atypical or malignant meningioma in FDG-PET. *J Nucl Med* 1997;38:26–30.

41. Shioya H, Mineura K, Sasajima T, et al. [Longitudinal analysis of glucose metabolism in recurrent meningioma]. *No To Shinkei* 1994;46:1088–1093.

42. Fischman AJ, Thornton AF, Frosch MP, Swearinger B, Gonzalez RG, Alpert NM. FDG hypermetabolism associated with inflammatory necrotic changes following radiation of meningioma. *J Nucl Med* 1997;38:1027–1029.

43. Ogawa T, Inugami A, Hatazawa J, et al. Clinical positron emission tomography for brain tumors: comparison of fludeoxyglucose F 18 and l-methyl-^{11}C-methionine, *Am J Neuroradiol* 1996;17:345–353.

44. Moresco RM, Scheithauer BW, Lucignani G, et al. Oestrogen receptors in meningiomas: a correlative PET and immunohistochemical study. *Nucl Med Commun* 1997;18:606–615.

45. Koeller KK, Smirniotopoulos JG, Jones RV. Primary central nervous system lymphoma: radiologic-pathologic correlation. *Radiographics* 1997;17:1497–1526.

46. Jack CR Jr, Reese DF, Scheithauer BW. Radiographic findings in 32 cases of primary CNS lymphoma. *Am J Roentgenol* 1986;146:271–276.

47. Johnson BA, Fram EK, Johnson PC, Jacobowitz R. The variable MR appearance of primary lymphoma of the central nervous system: comparison with histopathologic features. *Am J Neuroradiol* 1997;18:563–572.

48. Balakrishnan J, Becker PS, Kumar AJ, Zinreich SJ, McArthur JC, Bryan RN. Acquired immunodeficiency syndrome: correlation of radiologic and pathologic findings in the brain. *Radiographics* 1990;10:201–215.

49. Laissy JP, Soyer P, Tebboune J, et al. Contrast-enhanced fast MRI in differentiating brain toxoplasmosis and lymphoma in AIDS patients. *J Comput Assist Tomogr* 1994;18:714–718.

50. Laissy JP, Lebtahi R, Cordoliani YS, Henry Feugeas MC, Schouman Claeys E. [The diagnosis of primary cerebral lymphoma in AIDS: the contribution of imaging]. *J Neuroradiol* 1995;22:207–217.

51. Iacoangeli M, Roselli R, Antinori A, et al. Experience with brain biopsy in acquired immune deficiency syndrome-related focal lesions of the central nervous system. *Br J Surg* 1994;81:1508–1511.

52. Heald AE, Hoffman JM, Bartlett JA, Waskin HA. Differentiation of central nervous system lesions in AIDS patients using positron emission tomography (PET). *Int J STD AIDS* 1996;7:337–346.

53. Hoffman JM, Waskin HA, Schifter T, et al. FDG-PET in differentiating lymphoma from nonmalignant central nervous system lesions in patients with AIDS. *J Nucl Med* 1993;34:567–575.

54. Villringer K, Jager H, Dichgans M, et al. Differential diagnosis of CNS lesions in AIDS patients by FDG-PET. *J Comput Assist Tomogr* 1995;19:532–536.

55. Ogawa T, Kanno I, Hatazawa J, et al. Methionine PET for follow-up of radiation therapy of primary lymphoma of the brain. *Radiographics* 1994;14:101–110.

56. Francavilla TL, Miletich RS, DeMichele D, et al. Positron emission tomography of pituitary macroadenomas: hormone production and effects of therapies. *Neurosurgery* 1991;28:826–833.

57. Bergstrom M, Muhr C, Lundberg P0, Langstrom B. PET as a tool in the clinical evaluation of pituitary adenomas. *J Nucl Med* 1991;32:610–615.

58. Lucignani G, Losa M, Moresco RM, et al. Differentiation of clinically non-functioning pituitary adenomas from meningiomas and craniopharyngiomas by positron emission tomography with [18F]fluoro-ethyl-spiperone. *EurJ Nucl Med* 1997;24:1149–1155.

59. Bergstrom M, Muhr C, Jossan S, Lilja A, Nyberg G, Langstrom B. Differentiation of pituitary adenoma and meningioma: visualization with positron emission tomography and [11C]-l-deprenyl. *Neurosurgery* 1992;30:855–861.

60. Shioya H, Mineura K, Kowada M, et al. [Hemocirculation and metabolism in intraventricular tumors: kinetic analysis of glucose metabolism]. *No Shinkei Geka* 1996;24:211–219.

61. Kado H, Ogawa T, Hatazawa J, et al. Radiation-induced meningioma evaluated with positron emission tomography with fludeoxyglucose F 18. *Am J Neuroradiol* 1996;17:937–938.

62. Metsahonkala L, Aarimaa T, Sonninen P, Mikola H, Ruotsalainen U, Bergman J. CT, MRI, and PET in a case of intractable epilepsy. *Childs Nerv Syst* 1996;12:421–424.

63. Chiappa KH, Martin JB, Young RR. Disorders of the central nervous system. In: Braunwald E, Isselbacher KJ, Petersdorf RG, Wilson JD, Martin JB, Fauci AC, eds. *Disorders of the central and peripheral nervous system,* section 1. New York: McGraw Hill.

64. Holder WD Jr, White RL Jr, Zuger JH, Easton EJ Jr, Greene FL. Effectiveness of positron emission tomography for the detection of melanoma metastases. *Ann Surg* 1998;227:764–769.

65. Steinert HC, Huch-Boni RA, Buck A, et al. Malignant melanoma: staging with whole-body positron emission tomography and 2-[F-18]-fluoro-2-deoxy-d-glucose. *Radiology* 1995;195:705–709.

66. Boni R, Boni RA, Steinert H, et al. Staging of metastatic melanoma by whole-body positron emission tomography using 2-fluorine-18-fluoro-2-deoxy-d-glucose. *Br J Dermatol* 1995;132:556–562.

67. Fitzpatrick TB, Sober AJ, Mihm MC Jr. Malignant melanoma of the skin. In: Braunwald E. Isselbacher KJ, Petersdorf RG, Wilson JD, Martin JB, Fauci AC, eds. *Hematology and oncology,* part 9. New York: McGraw Hill.

68. Minna JD. Neoplasms of the lung. In: Braunwald E, Isselbacher KJ, Petersdorf RG, Wilson JD, Martin JB, Fauci AC, eds. *Disorders of the respiratory system.* New York: McGraw-Hill.

69. Bury T, Dowlati A, Paulus P, et al. Whole-body 18FDG positron emission tomography in the staging of non-small cell lung cancer. *Eur Respir J* 1997;10:2529–2534.

70. Steinert HC, Hauser M, Allemann F, et al. Non-small cell lung cancer: nodal staging with FDG-PET versus CT with correlative lymph node mapping and sampling. *Radiology* 1997;202:441–644.

71. Wahl RL, Quint LE, Greenough RL, Meyer CR, White RI, Orringer MB. Staging of mediastinal non-small cell lung cancer with FDG-PET, CT, and fusion images: preliminary prospective evaluation. *Radiology* 1994;191:371–377.

72. Larcos G, Maisey MN. FDG-PET screening for cerebral metastases in patients with suspected malignancy. *Nucl Med Commun* 1996;17:197–198.

73. Noh DY, Yun IJ, Kim JS, et al. Diagnostic value of positron emission tomography for detecting breast cancer. *World J Surg* 1998;22:223–227.

74. Crippa F, Agresti R, Seregni E, et al. Prospective evaluation of fluorine-18-FDG PET in presurgical staging of the axilla in breast cancer. *J Nucl Med* 1998;39:4–8.

75. Adler LP, Faulhaber PF, Schnur KC, Al Kasi NL, Shenk RR. Axillary lymph node metastases: screening with [F-18]2-deoxy-2-fluoro-d-glucose (FDG) PET. *Radiology* 1997;203:323–327.

76. Rozental JM, Cohen JD, Mehta MP, Levine RL, Hanson JM, Nickles RJ. Acute changes in glucose uptake after treatment: the effects of carmustine (BCNU) on human glioblastoma multiforme. *J Neurooncol* 1993;15:57–66.

77. Hautzel H, Muller Gartner HW. Early changes in fluorine-18-FDG uptake during radiotherapy. *J Nucl Med* 1997;38:1384–1386.

78. Dewan NA, Gupta NC, Redepenning LS, Phalen JJ, Frick MP. Diagnostic efficacy of PET-FDG imaging in solitary pulmonary nodules: potential role in evaluation and management. *Chest* 1993;104:997–1002.

79. Ogawa T, Kanno I, Shishido F, et al. Clinical value of PET with 18F-fluorodeoxyglucose and l-methyl-^{11}C-methionine for diagnosis of recurrent brain tumor and radiation injury. *Acta Radiol* 1991;32:197–202.

80. Jones HA, Clark RJ, Rhodes CG, Schofield JB, Krausz T, Haslett C. *In vivo* measurement of neutrophil activity in experimental lung inflammation. *Am J Respir Crit Care Med* 1994;149:1635–1639.

81. Palmer WE, Rosenthal DI, Schoenberg OI, et al. Quantification of inflammation in the wrist with gadolinium-enhanced MR imaging and PET with 2-[F-18]fluoro-2-deoxy-d-glucose. *Radiology* 1995;196:647–655.

82. Grossman RI, Yousem DM. Infectious and noninfectious inflammatory diseases of the brain. In: Grossman RI, Yousem DM, eds. *Neuroradiology, the requisites.* St. Louis, MO: Mosby, 1994:171–199.

83. Pietrzyk U, Herholz K, Fink G, et al. An interactive technique for three-dimensional image registration: validation for PET, SPECT, MRI and CT brain studies. *J Nucl Med* 1994;35:2011–2018.

9

PET Imaging in Epilepsy

Alfred Buck and Heinz-Gregor Wieser

INDICATION

In epilepsy, positron emission tomography (PET) is mainly used to evaluate patients for surgery.

TRACERS AND PARAMETERS OF INTEREST

Most clinical studies in epilepsy patients are conducted with fluorodeoxyglucose tagged with fluorine 18 ($[^{18}F]$FDG). One reason is the relatively wide availability of this tracer. The distribution of benzodiazepine receptors is studied with flumazenil labeled with radioactive carbon (^{11}C-FMZ). This tracer must be synthesized on site before each injection, and its use is therefore restricted to specialized centers. In research, there is a palette of other tracers used to elucidate the pathophysiology of epilepsy.

EPILEPSY

Epilepsy represents a considerable health problem. In the United States, the prevalence is 500 to 800 cases per 100,000. The classifications of epilepsies, seizures, and epileptic syndromes consider the categories *primary generalized* and *partial*. The partial epilepsies are of special interest to functional neuroimaging. Partial seizures originate from distinct foci. The epileptic discharge may remain localized, or it may spread over the whole brain. In the latter case, one talks of *secondary generalization*. If partial seizures involve consciousness, they are referred to as *complex* partial seizures. In general, these originate in the medial temporal lobe (MTL). While most epileptic patients are sufficiently treated with medication, a considerable percentage have a medically intractable disorder. A major subgroup of these patients suffers from temporal lobe epilepsy (TLE), which is commonly as-

A. Buck and H-G. Wieser: Nuclear Medicine, University Hospital, CH-8091 Zurich, Switzerland.

sociated with hippocampal sclerosis. Surgical treatment in these patients has proved to be effective in eliminating seizures. Various surgical strategies exist. The standard procedure consisted initially of removing the anterior two-thirds of the affected temporal lobe, so-called Falconer's *en bloc* anterior temporal lobe resection. At the University Hospital in Zurich, the standard operation since 1975 has been the selective amygdalohippocampectomy (AHE), a procedure pioneered by Wieser and Yasargil (1). Surgical therapy is less often performed for extratemporal refractory epilepsy, although this is changing with improved methods for presurgical evaluation. In general, [^{18}F]FDG PET has proved to be useful in candidates for epilepsy surgery.

TEMPORAL LOBE EPILEPSY

Preoperative Evaluation

The aims of the preoperative evaluation are to maximize the chance of achieving postsurgical freedom from seizures or at least a substantial reduction in seizure frequency, and to minimize postsurgical deficits. A prerequisite for surgery is that the seizures always originate from a stable focus. Patients displaying bilateral disease must be excluded from operative treatment because the neuropsychologic deficits following a bilateral operation would be prohibitive. The preoperative workup of patients with TLE differs somewhat among centers. At our institution, it includes noninvasive as well as invasive electroencephalographic (EEG) recording of interictal and ictal events, long-term video monitoring, magnetic resonance (MR) imaging, and [^{18}F]FDG PET. All these modalities yield complementary information.

[^{18}F]FDG PET

The typical interictal finding in TLE is reduced tracer uptake in the affected temporal lobe. The area of hypometabolism usually extends beyond the MTL and often includes the lateral temporal cortex, as illustrated in Figs. 9-1 to 9-4. A likely reason for this phe-

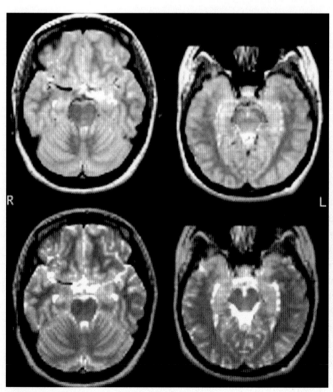

A

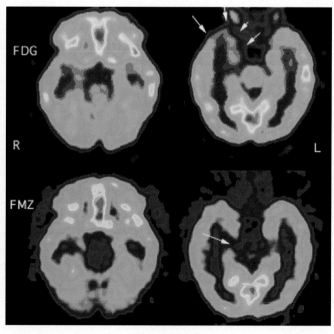

B

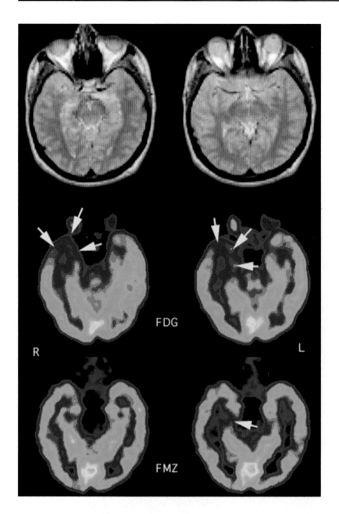

Figure 9-2. Transaxial slices of T1-weighted MR (TR 500 ms/TE 40 ms), [^{18}F]FDG PET, and ^{11}C-FMZ imaging in a patient with right-sided TLE; all images are coregistered. The MR image demonstrates no marked pathology. [^{18}F]FDG uptake is reduced in the MTL and LTL, whereas the reduction in ^{11}C-FMZ uptake is limited to a circumscribed area in the MTL *(arrows)*. No other abnormalities are noticed on either the [^{18}F]FDG or the ^{11}C-FMZ images. Electrophysiology also demonstrated seizures originating from the right MTL. This patient was an ideal candidate for surgery. Following selective AHE, he became seizure-free.

nomenon is deafferentation of the cortex functionally connected with the epileptogenic focus. Besides the abnormality in the MTL, hypometabolic regions reported in TLE include the thalamus, basal ganglia, and parts of the frontal lobe (2). These examples illustrate that [^{18}F]FDG PET is not suitable for localizing the seizure-onset zone *per se*. The important PET information is the lateralization and the exclusion of pathology on the contralateral side. The incidence of an ipsilateral temporal lobe hypometabolism in patients with TLE is in the range of 60% to 90% (3–10).

^{11}C-FMZ PET

^{11}C-FMZ is a benzodiazepine receptor antagonist that is an excellent PET marker for cerebral benzodiazepine receptor density. Because the receptors are located on neurons, reduction in receptor density may indicate neuronal loss, as is typical in a sclerotic region. Examples of ^{11}C-FMZ PET imaging in patients with TLE are shown in Figs. 9-1 to 9-4. Whereas glucose metabolism is depressed well beyond the sclerotic MTL, ^{11}C-FMZ

Figure 9-1. A: T1-weighted **(top)** and T2-weighted **(bottom)** MR images in a patient with right-sided TLE; **left:** the original transaxial images; **right:** the images reoriented parallel to the long axis of the temporal lobes. There is no evident abnormality on visual inspection. Volumetry of the hippocampal area might have revealed hippocampal atrophy. **B:** [^{18}F]FDG and ^{11}C-FMZ PET images; **left:** transaxial sections; **right:** images oriented along the long axis of the temporal lobes. Hippocampal sclerosis, typical of TLE, is evident. Hypometabolism extends beyond the medial region into the LTL. In contrast, the reduction in ^{11}C-FMZ uptake is restricted to a small area in the MTL corresponding to the sclerotic tissue *(white arrows)*.

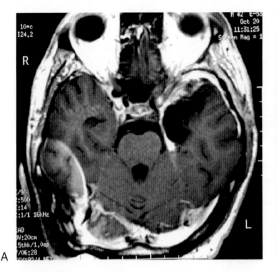

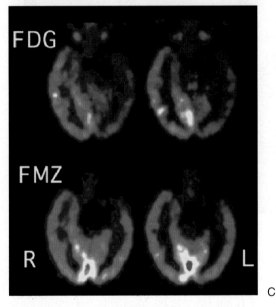

Figure 9-3. Patient with TLE who was not seizure-free following selective AHE. **A:** T1-weighted, gadolinium (Gd-)enhanced MR image (TR 500 ms/TE 14 ms) demonstrates the mediotemporal defect 1 year following left-sided surgery. Gd-enhancement of the dura along the area of resection corresponds to normal postoperative changes. No pathology is evident in the lateral temporal cortex. The artefact on the right corresponds to a susceptibility effect caused by the reservoir of a shunt. **B:** Proton-weighted MR image (TR 3500 ms/TE 15 ms) above the area of resection shows no pathology within the white matter and cortex of the LTL. **C:** Coregistered transaxial [18F]FDG PET and 11C-FMZ PET slices aligned along the long axis of the temporal lobe. The question was whether PET could identify the pathology responsible for the persistent postoperative seizures. [18F]FDG uptake is massively depressed in the greater part of the LTL and absent in the operated MTL. The finding in the LTL raises the question whether it is merely due to functional deafferentation or whether there might be some neuronal damage potentially responsible for the persisting seizures. Normal 11C-FMZ uptake in the LTL makes the latter most unlikely.

demonstrates a circumscribed defect limited to the affected MTL. An interesting case is demonstrated in Fig. 9-3. This patient was not seizure-free following selective AHE. In addition to absent tracer uptake in the operated area, [18F]FDG PET demonstrated widespread depression in almost the whole lateral temporal lobe (LTL). Although extended reduction in [18F]FDG uptake is typical in TLE, the degree and area of reduction exceeded the usual pattern. The question therefore arose whether there might be neuronal damage in the LTL. Structural damage in this area was excluded on MR imaging (see Fig. 9-3B). Normal 11C-FMZ uptake in the LTL clearly demonstrated neuronal integrity. That reduced 11C-FMZ uptake is restricted to abnormal tissue was demonstrated in several studies (11,12) and confirmed using the more objective method of statistical parametric mapping (13).

MR Imaging

The main rationale for MR imaging in epilepsy patients is to identify or exclude underlying pathologies such as tumors, vascular lesions, and migrational disorders. In TLE, the

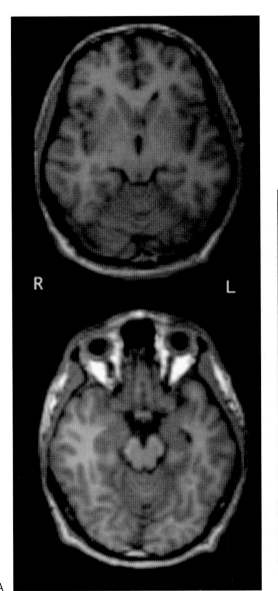

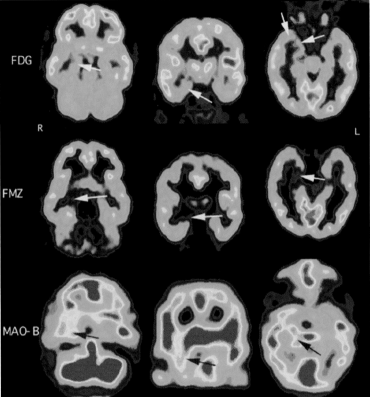

Figure 9-4. A: T1-weighted MR image (TR 500 ms/TE 20 ms) in a patient with right-sided TLE; **top:** image oriented along the canthomeatal line; **bottom:** image aligned along the long axis of the temporal lobes. No pathology is evident on the images. **B (top two rows):** [18F]FDG and 11C-FMZ images; **third row:** SPECT images of the distribution of the tracer [123I]Ro 43-0463, a marker for the enzyme MAO-B. [18F]FDG uptake is reduced in the MTL and part of the right LTL. 11C-FMZ demonstrates a circumscribed reduction in the MTL. In contrast to the reduced uptake of [18F]FDG and 11C-FMZ, [123I]Ro 43-0463 uptake is increased in the MTL, which is best appreciated by the asymmetry in MTL uptake. This most likely reflects hippocampal sclerosis because MAO-B is predominantly located in glial cells. Neither tracer shows abnormalities on the contralateral side, which was in keeping with the electrophysiologic data. Following selective AHE, the seizures subsided.

most common pathology is hippocampal sclerosis, which resisted reliable evaluation with MR imaging until 1990. This has changed with advances in MR imaging technology. Qualitative and quantitative approaches for assessing hippocampal sclerosis exist, and the latter are more accurate and measure hippocampal volume. In a study with 41 patients, it was shown that hippocampal volume ratios yielded the correct lateralization of the seizure focus in 76% of patients (14). Although useful, the technique of hippocampal volumetry is rather laborious and therefore not always possible in a clinical setting.

EXTRATEMPORAL EPILEPSIES

[^{18}F]FDG PET

In frontal lobe epilepsy (FLE), the area of hypometabolism may also exceed structural abnormalities. However, it is not uncommon that the hypometabolic zone is restricted to an underlying structural pathology (15,16). Hypometabolic areas are found in approximately 60% of patients with FLE, most of whom also demonstrate a structural abnormality on MR imaging. In general, it seems that the epileptogenic focus is contained within the hypometabolic area, if one exists. Given the high incidence of positive MR imaging scans, the value of [^{18}F]FDG PET in FLE seems mainly in the exclusion of other pathologic areas.

Most malformations of cortical development are identified with MR imaging, and the additional value of [^{18}F]FDG PET seems limited to special cases. For instance, metabolic abnormalities in the contralateral hemisphere of patients with hemimegalencephaly have been associated with a poorer prognosis following surgery (17).

^{11}C-FMZ PET

There are indications that ^{11}C-FMZ might be of high clinical value also in the evaluation of extratemporal epilepsies. In a preliminary series of six patients with FLE, ^{11}C-FMZ PET demonstrated circumscribed lesions consistent with clinical and EEG data (18). In two of four patients who were also scanned with [^{18}F]FDG, the area of reduced tracer uptake was more extensive than the one delineated with ^{11}C-FMZ. MR imaging was read as normal in five patients, underlining the usefulness of ^{11}C-FMZ PET.

MR Imaging

As in TLE, MR imaging is the method of choice to delineate structural abnormalities. An interesting entity often leading to seizures involves malformations of cortical development (MCD). These include schizencephaly, agyria, diffuse and focal macrogyria, focal polymicrogyria, minor gyral abnormalities, subependymal gray matter heterotopias, bilateral subcortical laminar heterotopias, tuberous sclerosis, focal cortical dysplasias, and dysembryoblastic neuroepithelial tumors. Such malformations were found in more than 4% of 303 patients with epileptic seizures referred for MR imaging (19). MCD can also be found in the temporal lobe. In a series of 222 patients with seizures originating from the temporal lobe, MCD were diagnosed in 7% (20). These included focal cortical dysplasia, nodular heterotopia, abnormal gyration, limited schizencephaly, and hippocampal malformations.

OTHER TRACERS USED IN THE INVESTIGATION OF EPILEPSY

All tracers mentioned in this section shed new light on the pathophysiology of epilepsies; however, their clinical use has yet to be demonstrated. Studies using ^{11}C-carfentanil have shown that opioid receptors are increased in the ipsilateral temporal lobe of patients with TLE (21). It has been speculated that an upregulation of the opioid receptors serves to limit the spread of seizures. Other opioid receptor subtypes have been studied with ^{11}C-diprenorphine and [^{18}F]cyclofoxy. These studies demonstrated that the various subtypes of opioid receptors are differentially affected in TLE.

A few studies investigated the distribution of the enzyme monoamine oxidase B (MAO-B). This enzyme is mainly located on glial cells. Since these are increased in sclerotic tissue, the demonstration of elevated MAO-B concentration may positively identify epileptogenic foci in patients with TLE. Studies using [^{11}C]deuterium-deprenyl indeed demonstrated increased binding in the MTL of patients with TLE (22). This finding was confirmed in a single photon emission computed tomography (SPECT) study with the ligand [^{123}I]Ro 43-0463 that binds reversibly to MAO-B. This study further revealed increased MAO-B in the ipsilateral putamen (23).

ICTAL STUDIES

Whereas interictal studies commonly show decreased metabolism, blood flow, or receptor densities in epileptogenic tissue, ictal studies demonstrate increased blood flow early after the onset of a seizure. This can be demonstrated using SPECT and tracers such as technetium Tc 99m hexamethylpropyleneamine oxime (^{99m}Tc-HMPAO) or ^{99m}Tc-ethylenedicysteine diethylester (^{99m}Tc-ECD). SPECT is superior to PET in this regard, because the tracers can be injected in the neurology ward while the patient is monitored. Imaging can then be performed hours later after the patient has been stabilized. This is possible because ^{99m}Tc-HMPAO and ^{99m}Tc-ECD get trapped in the brain within 2 minutes following injection, and the activity distribution hours later still reflects the distribution at the time of injection. Ictal SPECT has established itself as a highly accurate method of identifying seizure foci, especially when combined with interictal studies. In TLE, identification of the seizure focus was possible in up to 90% of patients (24–29). Ictal SPECT has also proved its value in the evaluation of extratemporal epilepsies, where 92% of foci were correctly identified (30).

Ictal studies are more difficult to perform with PET. The half-life of ^{15}O$_2$ is so short that imaging would have to be performed immediately after injection. This is clinically impractical because the patient would have to remain positioned in the PET scanner until a seizure occurs. However, it is possible to perform ictal PET scans in selected cases, as demonstrated in Fig. 9-5C. This patient suffered from Rasmussen's encephalitis. The pathophysiology of this rare disease is not clear. One hypothesis assumes the involvement of autoantibodies against a subpopulation of the glutamate receptors, in particular GluR3. Normally, such antibodies cannot penetrate the blood–brain barrier (BBB). However, if the BBB is disturbed, such antibodies may enter brain tissue and lead to inflammation, causing further damage to the BBB and thus continually worsening the disease. Sometimes, the only effective therapy is hemispherectomy. Patients with Rasmussen's encephalitis suffer from intractable epileptic seizures. In this patient, the seizures occurred almost continuously (epilepsia partialis continua). It was therefore easy to perform ictal scanning. PET scanning with [^{18}F]FDG and ammonia tagged with nitrogen 13 ([^{13}N]ammonia) demonstrated increased metabolism and blood flow in the affected areas, namely, the right frontal lobe. Of interest is the additional activation of the contralateral cerebellum. This is most probably due to crossed cerebrocerebellar pathways. If these pathways are interrupted, as they would be with a brain tumor, one often observes a deactivation of the contralateral cerebellum. The clinical value of PET in this patient was the confirmation of unilateral neocortical disease, which is a prerequisite for surgical therapy.

IMAGING PROTOCOLS

[^{18}F]FDG PET

Patient preparation: A catheter is placed in a cubital vein for tracer injection; injection should occur in a quiet room, with the patient keeping eyes closed for 20 minutes afterward;

Injected activity: depends on the scanner;

—Three-dimensional (3D) acquisition: 200 MBq;

—Two-dimensional (2D) acquisition: 400 MBq;

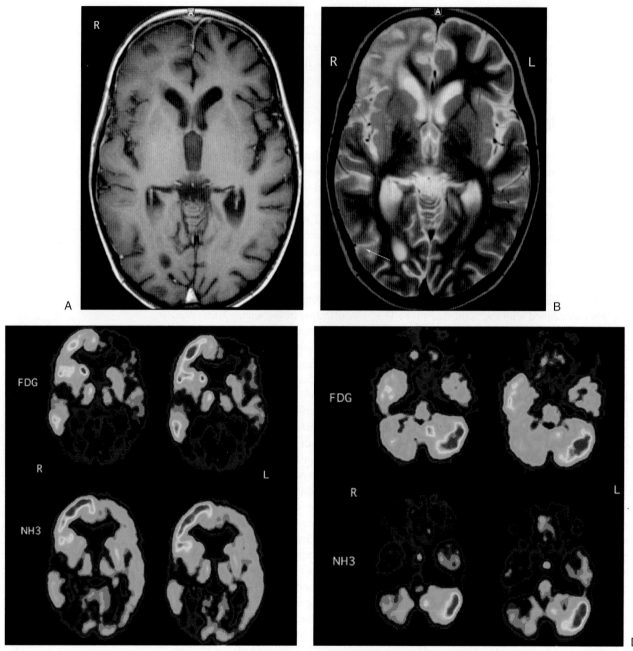

Figure 9-5. A: T1-weighted transaxial MR image (TR 600 ms/TE 20 ms) in a patient with epileptic seizures due to Rasmussen's encephalitis. Cortex and subcortical white matter are indistinguishable due to hypointensity of the right frontal subcortical white matter. **B:** The corresponding T2-weighted transaxial MR image (TR 3800 ms/TE 80 ms) more clearly delineates the pathology caused by Rasmussen's encephalitis. There is cortical and subcortical increase in signal intensity in the right frontal and insular region, putamen, caudate, external capsule, and anterior limb of the internal capsule. The cortical–subcortical border is partly erased along the superior temporal gyrus *(arrow)*, showing an additional region of involvement. The sylvian fissure is slightly widened, indicating atrophy adjacent to pathologic signal. **C:** Coregistered transaxial [^{18}F]FDG and [^{13}N]ammonia PET scans. Increased [^{18}F]FDG uptake in the right frontal lobe, caudate, and parts of the LTL corresponds to practically continuous epileptic discharges. [^{13}N]ammonia may be used to trace cerebral perfusion. The uptake pattern shows increased perfusion in the active epileptogenic zones. The important information in this case is the absence of epileptogenic activity in the contralateral hemisphere. The patient was scheduled for left hemispherectomy. Evidence of contralateral epileptogenic activity would have been a clear contraindication for the surgical procedure. **D:** Increased perfusion and metabolism in the contralateral cerebellum most probably correspond to activations via crossed cerebrocerebellar pathways.

TABLE 9-1. *Appraisal/reimbursement status of PET in focal epilepsy*

Disease	German consensus classification	USZ classification	Replacement potential	US reimbursement status: Medicare/BC-BS	Swiss reimbursement status
Temporal lobe FDG	1a	3	3	no/yes	yes
Extratemporal lobes FDG	1b	3	3	no/yes	yes
Focal epilepsy Flumazenil	1b	—	—	no/no	

See page 8 for abbreviations and appraisal scheme explanations.

Imaging: single scan, 40 to 60 minutes following injection;
Image fusion: Coregistration with MR imaging is desirable in selected cases.

¹¹C-FMZ PET

Patient preparation: A catheter is placed in a cubital vein for tracer injection;
Injected activity: depends on the scanner;
—3D acquisition: 400 MBq;
—2D acquisition: 800 MBq;
Imaging: single scan, 40 to 60 minutes following injection;
Image fusion: Coregistration with MR imaging is desirable in selected cases.

The above protocols are suggestions for the clinical use of these tracers. If quantitation is required, the protocols would have to be modified, and arterial blood sampling might be necessary.

CLINICAL USEFULNESS

A consensus meeting of the German Society for Nuclear Medicine in 1997 rated the procedures as indicated in Table 9-1.

REFERENCES

1. Wieser HG, Yasargil MG. Selective amygdalohippocampectomy as surgical treatment of mesiobasal limbic epilepsy. *Surg Neurol* 1982;17:445–457.
2. Henry TR, Mazziotta JC, Engel J Jr. Interictal metabolic anatomy of mesial temporal lobe epilepsy. *Arch Neurol* 1993;50:582–589.
3. Kuhl DE, Engel J Jr, Phelps ME, Selin C. Epileptic patterns of local cerebral metabolism and perfusion in humans determined by emission computed tomography of 18FDG and ¹³NH₃. *Ann Neurol* 1980;8:348–360.
4. Engel J Jr, Kuhl DE, Phelps ME, Crandall PH. Comparative localization of epileptic foci in partial epilepsy by PCT and EEG. *Ann Neurol* 1982;12:529–537.
5. Engel J Jr, Brown WJ, Kuhl DE, et al. Pathological findings underlying focal temporal lobe hypometabolism in partial epilepsy. *Ann Neurol* 1982;12:518–528.
6. Engel J Jr, Kuhl DE, Phelps ME, Mazziotta JC. Interictal cerebral glucose metabolism in partial epilepsy and its relation to EEG changes. *Ann Neurol* 1982;12:510–517.
7. Theodore WH, Newmark ME, Sato S, et al. [¹⁸F]fluorodeoxyglucose positron emission tomography in refractory complex partial seizures. *Ann Neurol* 1983;14:429–437.
8. Franck G, Sadzot B, Salmon E, et al. Regional cerebral blood flow and metabolic rates in human focal epilepsy and status epilepticus. *Adv Neurol* 1986;44:935–948.
9. Abou Khalil BW, Siegel GJ, Sackellares JC, et al. Positron emission tomography studies of cerebral glucose metabolism in chronic partial epilepsy. *Ann Neurol* 1987;22:480–486.
10. Gaillard WD, White S, Malow B, et al. FDG-PET in children and adolescents with partial seizures: role in epilepsy surgery evaluation. *Epilepsy Res* 1995;20:77–84.
11. Henry TR, Frey KA, Sackellares JC, et al. *In vivo* cerebral metabolism and central benzodiazepine-receptor binding in temporal lobe epilepsy. *Neurology* 1993;43:1998–2006.
12. Savic I, Ingvar M, Stone Elander S. Comparison of [¹¹C]flumazenil and [¹⁸F]FDG as PET markers of epileptic foci. *J Neurol Neurosurg Psychiatry* 1993;56:615–621.
13. Koepp MJ, Richardson MP, Brooks DJ, et al. Cerebral benzodiazepine receptors in hippocampal sclerosis: an objective *in vivo* analysis. *Brain* 1996;119:1677–1687.
14. Jack CR Jr, Sharbrough FW, Twomey CK, et al. Temporal lobe seizures: lateralization with MR volume measurements of the hippocampal formation. *Radiology* 1990;175:423–429.

15. Engel J Jr, Henry TR, Swartz BE. Positron emission tomography in frontal lobe epilepsy. *Adv Neurol* 1995;66:223–238.
16. Henry TR, Sutherling WW, Engel J Jr, et al. Interictal cerebral metabolism in partial epilepsies of neocortical origin. *Epilepsy Res* 1991;10:174–182.
17. Rintahaka PJ, Chugani HT, Messa C, Phelps ME. Hemimegalencephaly: evaluation with positron emission tomography. *Pediatr Neurol* 1993;9:21–28.
18. Savic I, Thorell JO, Roland P. [^{11}C]flumazenil positron emission tomography visualizes frontal epileptogenic regions. *Epilepsia* 1995;36:1225–1232.
19. Brodtkorb E, Nilsen G, Smevik O, Rinck PA. Epilepsy and anomalies of neuronal migration: MRI and clinical aspects. *Acta Neurol Scand* 1992;86:24–32.
20. Lehericy S, Dormont D, Semah F, et al. Developmental abnormalities of the medial temporal lobe in patients with temporal lobe epilepsy. *Am J Neuroradiol* 1995;16:617–626.
21. Frost JJ, Mayberg HS, Fisher RS, et al. Mu-opiate receptors measured by positron emission tomography are increased in temporal lobe epilepsy. *Ann Neurol* 1988;23:231–237.
22. Kumlien E, Bergstrom M, Lilja A, et al. Positron emission tomography with [^{11}C]deuterium-deprenyl in temporal lobe epilepsy. *Epilepsia* 1995;36:712–721.
23. Buck A, Frey LD, Bläuenstein P, et al. Monoamine oxidase B single photon emission tomography with [^{123}I]Ro 43-0463: imaging in volunteers and patients with temporal lobe epilepsy. *Eur J Nucl Med* 1998;25:464–470.
24. Rowe CC, Berkovic SF, Sia ST, et al. Localization of epileptic foci with postictal single photon emission computed tomography. *Ann Neurol* 1989;26:660–668.
25. Newton MR, Berkovic SF, Austin MC, et al. Ictal, postictal, and interictal single-photon emission tomography in the lateralization of temporal lobe epilepsy. *Eur J Nucl Med* 1994;21:1067–1071.
26. Rowe CC, Berkovic SF, Austin MC, McKay WJ, Bladin PF. Patterns of postictal cerebral blood flow in temporal lobe epilepsy: qualitative and quantitative analysis. *Neurology* 1991;41:1096–1103.
27. Duncan R, Patterson J, Roberts R, Hadley DM, Bone I. Ictal/postictal SPECT in the pre-surgical localisation of complex partial seizures. *J Neurol Neurosurg Psychiatry* 1993;56:141–148.
28. Harvey AS, Bowe JM, Hopkins IJ, et al. Ictal 99mTc-HMPAO single photon emission computed tomography in children with temporal lobe epilepsy. *Epilepsia* 1993;34:869–877.
29. Cross JH, Gordon I, Jackson GD, et al. Children with intractable focal epilepsy: ictal and interictal ^{99m}Tc HMPAO single photon emission computed tomography. *Dev Med Child Neurol* 1995;37:673–681.
30. Newton MR, Berkovic SF, Austin MC, et al. SPECT in the localisation of extratemporal and temporal seizure foci. *J Neurol Neurosurg Psychiatry* 1995;59:26–30.

10

PET Imaging in Cerebrovascular Disease

Alfred Buck and Yasuhiro Yonehawa

INDICATIONS

A major indication for positron emission tomography (PET) is the hemodynamic evaluation of cerebral perfusion before surgical treatment. Imaging in acute stroke may be useful but should be limited to specialized stroke centers.

AVAILABLE TRACERS AND PARAMETERS OF INTEREST

The most common tracer used to evaluate cerebral perfusion is oxygen 15–labeled water ([^{15}O]water), which most often is intravenously injected as a bolus. Some groups use [^{15}O]carbon dioxide, which is inhaled through a special delivery system. In the body, [^{15}O]carbon dioxide is almost immediately converted to [^{15}O]water. Another PET perfusion tracer is [^{15}O]butanol. Cerebral blood volume (CBV) is typically altered in chronic cerebrovascular disease (CVD). It can be measured with [^{15}O]carbon monoxide. Recent studies demonstrated that the density of benzodiazepine receptors is a good predictor of potentially salvageable tissue following stroke. It can be assessed with flumazenil labeled with radioactive carbon (^{11}C-FMZ). Another crucial measure for the survival of tissue is oxygen metabolism, which is evaluated using ^{15}O$_2$.

METHODOLOGY

Perfusion

The kinetic behavior of diffusible perfusion tracers such as [^{15}O]water is crucially different from tracers that are trapped, such as technetium Tc 99m hexamethylpropyle-

A. Buck: Nuclear Medicine, University Hospital, CH-8091 Zurich, Switzerland.
Y. Yonehawa: Neurosurgery Department, University Hospital, CH-8091 Zurich, Switzerland.

neamine oxime (^{99m}Tc-HMPAO) used in single photon emission computed tomography (SPECT). This difference warrants a completely different acquisition protocol. Since ^{99m}Tc-HMPAO uptake does not change following injection, imaging can be performed as a single scan from minutes to hours following injection. In contrast, [^{15}O]water is washed in and out of tissue within minutes. Together with the short physical half-life of [^{15}O], this mandates that imaging be performed within minutes following injection. A detailed description of the methods used for [^{15}O]water PET imaging is given at the end of this chapter (see "Appendix: Detailed Methodology for Quantitative Perfusion Imaging").

Cerebral Blood Volume

Following inhalation as a bolus, [^{15}O]carbon monoxide is irreversibly bound to hemoglobin. Its distribution is therefore restricted to intravascular space. Thus, the ratio of the [^{15}O]carbon monoxide concentration in the brain and in blood directly yields CBV.

PET IMAGING IN CHRONIC CEREBROVASCULAR DISEASE

Stenoses of the larger arteries feeding the brain are common. An important clinical aspect in this regard concerns the hemodynamic significance. There are two mechanisms by which atherosclerotic plaques may lead to symptoms such as transient ischemic attacks or stroke. Emboli may break loose from plaques and cause symptoms. Another possibility is that a stenosis is severe enough to lead to compromised cerebral perfusion in areas fed by the affected artery. The cerebral vascular response to reduced perfusion is complex. As a first response, the brain increases the oxygen extraction fraction. Another response is vessel dilatation in an attempt to reduce vascular resistance and counteract reductions in perfusion. When the potential of these mechanisms is fully exploited and perfusion still decreases, the patient becomes symptomatic. For instance, if perfusion is just sufficient with maximum oxygen extraction and fully dilated vessels, any further stress will lead to decompensation. Such patients may benefit from a revascularization procedure, such as endarterectomy or extracranial-to-intracranial (EC-IC) bypass surgery. Improvement in cerebral perfusion following revascularization has been demonstrated in several studies (1–6).

Several methods and parameters exist for evaluating patients with chronic CVD. Based on the physiologic regulation of cerebral blood flow (CBF), the assessment of CBV and perfusion are useful. This is illustrated in Fig. 10-1. The images on the left sketch the vascular autoregulation occurring in CVD. The most common site for stenoses is the carotid bifurcation. The regulatory steps include increased oxygen extraction and vessel dilatation to reduce vascular resistance. The latter step is synonymous with an increase in CBV. One method for evaluating the hemodynamic situation is indeed based on the measurement of CBV. The ratio of CBV to CBF is an especially useful measure. The critical situation is reached when the vessels are fully dilated and CBF continues to decrease. This situation is reflected in an increasing CBI/CBF ratio. Alternatively, one can measure the hemodynamic behavior during induced vasodilatation. A strong stimulus for vasodilatation is an increase in arterial carbon dioxide (P_aCO_2). Hypercapnia can be induced by inhalation of a carbon dioxide–enriched air mixture or by administering acetazolamide (Diamox). In healthy subjects, reduced vascular resistance due to induced vasodilatation leads to an increase in CBF. The CBI/CBF ratio during hypercapnia and at baseline is often referred to as the cerebral perfusion reserve capacity. The situation with a stenosis is illustrated at the bottom of Fig. 10-1. The situation may be such that regional CBF (rCBF) is normal at baseline due to chronic vasodilatation on the compromised side. Blood-flow images will reveal symmetric perfusion in both hemispheres. Inducing hypercapnia will dilate vessels on the healthy side but not, or only to a lesser degree, on the affected side. Blood flow will therefore predominantly increase on the healthy side, leading to a marked asymmetry in rCBF. Blood-flow

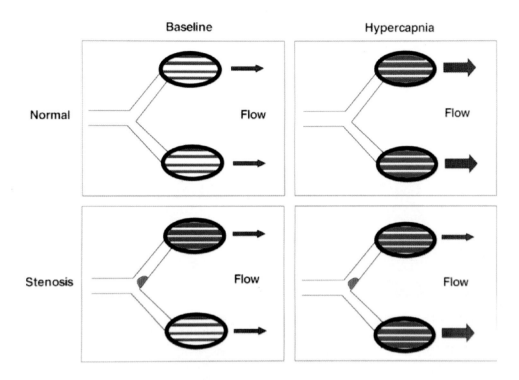

Figure 10-1. Vascular response to hypoxia and hypercapnia. **Top row:** In the normal brain, hypercapnia induces vasodilatation and subsequent symmetric increase in blood flow. **Bottom left:** In chronic CVD, a severe stenosis may lead to vasodilatation in an attempt to reduce vascular resistance and maintain adequate blood flow. The flow may still be symmetric. If the vessels are maximally dilated on the compromised side, hypercapnia will only dilate vessels on the healthy side, leading to asymmetric increase of blood flow **(bottom right)**.

imaging with SPECT primarily allows the qualitative assessment of CBF. The assessment of the hemodynamic situation with that modality most often relies on the evaluation of the CBV/CBF ratio or the asymmetry index during baseline and induced hypercapnia. A common problem arises if there is bilateral or even more extended disease. In that case, hypercapnia-induced blood flow increase may be uniformly impaired, not leading to marked asymmetries. In these situations, the CBV/CBF ratio may be a more reliable measure for the hemodynamic situation. The most accurate evaluation is probably quantitative assessment of the hemodynamics, as is possible with PET. Examples are demonstrated in Figs. 10-2 to 10-5.

The benefit of surgical treatment of occlusive CVD is still inconclusive. One large international trial failed to demonstrate the effectiveness of EC-IC bypass surgery for preventing cerebral ischemia in patients with arteriosclerotic CVD (7). However, one criticism of that study is that the patients' preoperative hemodynamic status was not fully assessed. It may be possible that a quantitative evaluation of the hemodynamic situation may better select patients who can potentially benefit from bypass surgery. A more recent study in 12 patients demonstrated hemodynamic improvement following bypass surgery using quantitative oxygen 15 water ([$H_2^{15}O$]water) PET (8). A Japanese trial involving patients with low rCBF demonstrated no benefit of EC-IC bypass surgery in terms of stroke prevention, although a significant improvement of rCBF was found in the surgical group (9). It is obvious that larger studies are needed to resolve this issue.

(text continues on page 129)

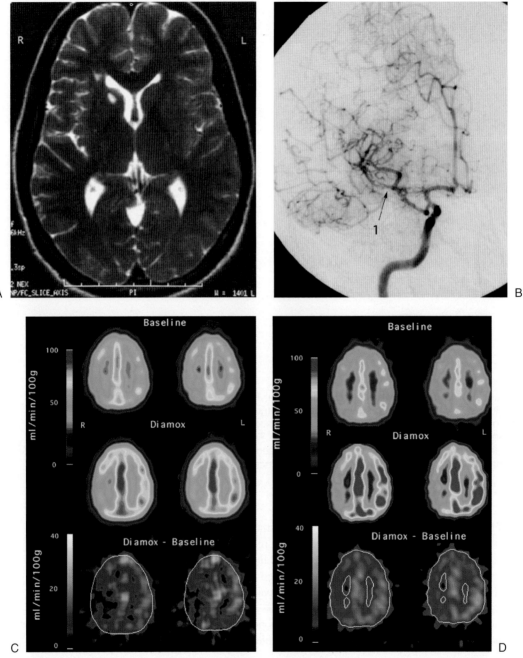

Figure 10-2. A: T2-weighted axial MR image demonstrates enhanced signal in the left caudate, indicating infarction. **B:** Preoperative angiogram shows stenosis of the right MCA *(arrow 1)*. **C:** Preoperative quantitative evaluation of CBF with [$H_2^{15}O$]water PET. **Bottom row:**
The difference between blood flow during hypercapnia (acetazolamide) and baseline. Note
the reduced baseline flow and the absent increase during hypercapnia in most of the right
MCA territory. **D:** Quantitative evaluation of CBF with [$H_2^{15}O$]water PET following EC-IC bypass from the superficial temporal artery to the MCA. There is marked improvement in
hemodynamic situation. This is best appreciated on the difference images. Although there
is still impaired perfusion reserve in the posterior part of the MCA territory, the situation has
clearly improved in the anterior part.

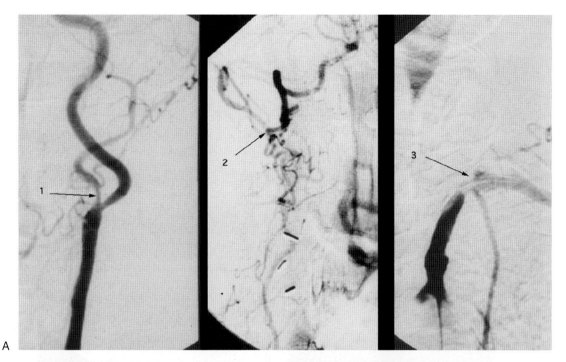

A

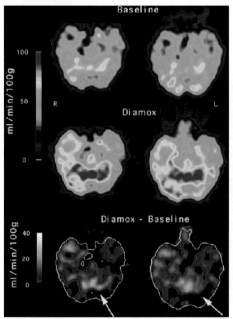

B

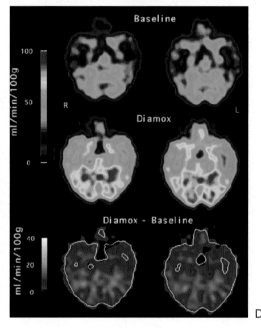

D

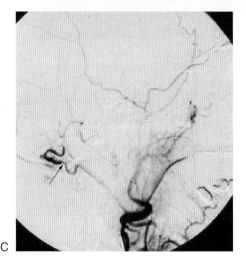

C

Figure 10-3. A: Preoperative angiograms demonstrate a stenosis of the left ICA *(1)* and the right vertebral artery *(2)* and a complete occlusion of the left vertebral artery *(3)*. **B:** Preoperative quantitative evaluation of CBF with [H₂¹⁵O]water PET. **Bottom row:** The difference between blood flow during hypercapnia (acetazolamide) and baseline. Note the absent increase in blood flow during hypercapnia in parts of the left cerebellum *(arrows)*. **C:** Angiogram following EC-IC bypass from the occipital artery to the posteroinferior cerebellar artery. The *arrow* points to the anastomosis at the occipital artery. **D:** Quantitative evaluation of CBF with [H₂¹⁵O]water PET following bypass surgery. The hemodynamic situation has completely normalized.

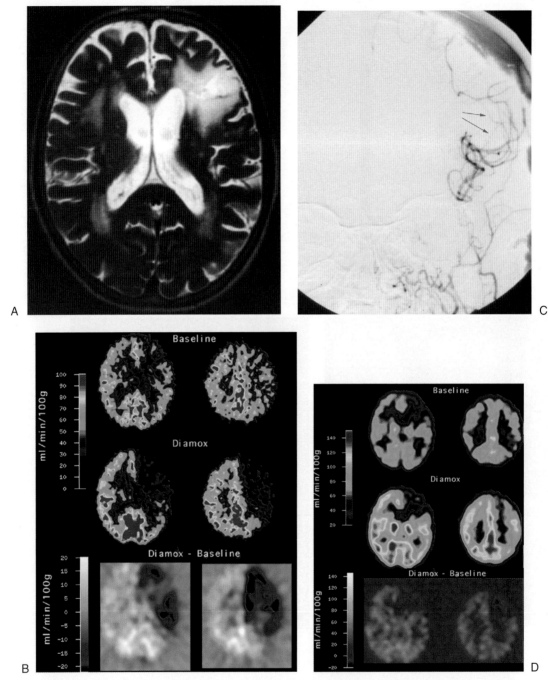

Figure 10-4. A: T2-weighted MR image demonstrates infarction in the left frontal lobe. **B:** Preoperative quantitative evaluation of CBF with [$H_2^{15}O$]water PET. **Bottom row:** The difference between blood flow during hypercapnia (acetazolamide) and baseline. Note the actual decrease in blood flow during hypercapnia in the anterior left frontal cortex (steal phenomenon), indicating a severely compromised hemodynamic situation. **C:** Postoperative angiogram shows adequate blood supply to the left MCA territory *(arrows)* from the bypass (superficial temporal artery to MCA). **D:** Quantitative evaluation of CBF with [$H_2^{15}O$]water PET following bypass surgery demonstrates a complete normalization of the hemodynamics in the posterior part of the right MCA territory and residual impairment in the anterior part.

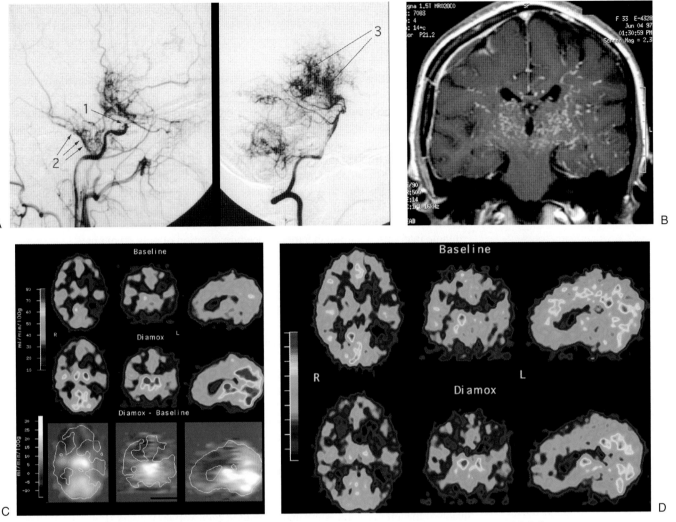

Figure 10-5. A: Lateral projections of common carotid **(left)** and vertebral **(right)** angiograms. The late arterial phase reveals an occlusion of the ICA *(1)* distal to the origin of the ophthalmic artery. A collateral network is present, supplied by meningocortical branches *(2)* and thalamoperforating arteries *(3)*. In conjunction with dilated lenticulostriate branches, the collateral network gives rise to the typical puff-of-smoke appearance of moyamoya disease. **B:** Gd-enhanced T1-weighted MR image (TR 500 ms/TE 14 ms) shows flow visualized within numerous dilated thalamoperforating and lenticulostriate branches. **C:** Quantitative hemodynamic evaluation with [H$_2$^{15}O]water PET. The baseline scan shows absent perfusion in the temporolateral, frontal, and parietal areas of the left hemisphere, corresponding to infarction. Following administration of acetazolamide, perfusion does not appropriately increase in most of the brain, except in the cerebellum, thalamus, and striatum. There is even decreased perfusion in a right frontal area, best appreciated on the difference images. **D:** Qualitative hemodynamic evaluation. In contrast to part **C**, the qualitative count images (accumulated over 60 seconds following arrival of the bolus in the brain) are shown.

Other Imaging Modalities

Computed tomography (CT) and magnetic resonance (MR) imaging are used to assess possible chronic manifestations of CVD. Angiography is used to assess the morphology of vessels and identify the location and degree of stenoses. It may be possible that MR angiography may gain a major role in this area. Perfusion measurements can be performed with xenon-enhanced CT. However, this method is less validated than [H$_2$^{15}O]water PET and often does not allow assessment of the whole brain simultaneously.

SPECT allows qualitative assessment of hemodynamics using tracers such as ^{99m}Tc-HMPAO or ^{99m}Tc-ECD. The major advantage of SPECT is its wide availability.

Differences in uptake patterns at baseline and during hypercapnia allow conclusions regarding the perfusion reserve capacity. CBV can be assessed using ^{99m}Tc-labeled erythrocytes. The disadvantages of SPECT compared to $[H_2{}^{15}O]$water PET can be summarized as follows:

SPECT is qualitative in character, although attempts in the area of quantitation have been published.

Under physiologic conditions, SPECT perfusion tracers are only 60% to 70% extracted, and intracellular trapping requires an intact metabolism. In pathologic situations, extraction and intracellular trapping may be altered. Thus, altered uptake may not only reflect changed blood flow. In this regard, $[H_2{}^{15}O]$water PET is ideal, as it does not require an intact metabolism and its extraction fraction is high.

Assessment of the perfusion reserve capacity relies on two scans, one at baseline and one during hypercapnia. With SPECT, these scans have to be acquired on separate days due to the relatively long half-life of ^{99m}Tc. With $[H_2{}^{15}O]$water, injections can follow at 15-minute intervals, resulting in a total procedure duration of only 30 minutes.

Examples

Case A. The case of a 23-year-old woman is illustrated in Fig. 10-2. T2-weighted MR imaging of the brain demonstrated an infarct in the right caudate (Fig. 10-2A). Angiography revealed a stenosis of the right middle carotid artery (MCA) (Fig. 10-2B). The results of the hemodynamic $[H_2{}^{15}O]$water PET evaluation are shown in Fig. 10-2C. The baseline examination revealed a reduced CBF in the greater part of the right MCA territory. Following administration of acetazolamide, there was no CBF increase in that area, indicating a severely compromised hemodynamic situation. Following EC-IC bypass surgery from the superficial temporal artery to the MCA, the hemodynamic situation improved, as illustrated by the postoperative PET evaluation (Fig. 10-2D). The improvement is best appreciated on the difference images. Although perfusion reserve capacity in the posterior part of the MCA territory is still impaired, the situation has clearly improved in the anterior part.

Case B. Figure 10-3 illustrates the case of a 78-year-old woman who had complete occlusion of the left vertebral artery and a stenosed right vertebral artery (Fig. 10-3A). There was another stenosis in the internal carotid artery (ICA). The preoperative $[H_2{}^{15}O]$water PET evaluation demonstrated a normal perfusion pattern at baseline but a severely decreased perfusion reserve capacity in parts of the cerebellum (Fig. 10-3B). The hemodynamic situation normalized completely following EC-IC bypass surgery from the occipital artery to the posteroinferior cerebellar artery (Fig. 10-3C). The postoperative PET assessment showed a normal perfusion pattern and perfusion reserve capacity (Fig. 10-3D).

Case C. This case demonstrates the usefulness of a fully quantitative assessment of CBF. The patient was a 67-year-old woman who suffered from syncope and episodes of motor aphasia. Angiography revealed an occlusion of the left ICA and a 50% stenosis of the right ICA. MR imaging demonstrated an infarction in the left frontal lobe (Fig. 10-4A). The preoperative $[H_2{}^{15}O]$water PET examination showed an almost normal perfusion at baseline and severely pathologic behavior during hypercapnia in the territory of the left MCA (Fig. 10-4B). The red areas in the subtraction images indicate that CBF even decreased during hypercapnia (steal phenomenon), demonstrating a severely compromised hemodynamic situation. Demonstration of an actual decrease requires some sort of quantitation. A qualitative assessment would only have demonstrated an asymmetry during hypercapnia. The patient's symptoms disappeared following EC-IC bypass surgery from the superficial temporal artery to the left middle cerebral artery. Postoperative angiography revealed good blood supply from the bypass to the left MCA territory (Fig. 10-4C). The postoperative PET assessment demonstrated normalized hemodynamics in the posterior left MCA territory (Fig. 10-4D). As expected, no changes occurred in the left frontal infarction area.

IMAGING OF MOYAMOYA DISEASE

Named by Suzuki and Takaku (10), moyamoya disease is characterized by abnormal vascular networks at the base of the brain. *Moyamoya* means "something hazy, just like a puff of cigarette smoke drifting in the air." The abnormal vessels are thought to function as collaterals in the presence of stenotic or occlusive lesions at the terminal parts of the ICAs. The clinical hallmarks of this disease depend on age. Younger patients most often suffer from the consequences of hemodynamic insufficiency, such as transient ischemic attacks. These are characteristically triggered by hyperventilation leading to hypocapnia, a vaso-constrictive stimulus. Older patients often present with intracranial bleeding.

CT

Forty percent of cases presenting with cerebral ischemia have been reported to demonstrate abnormal findings on CT. These findings include the following:

Low-density areas in the cortex and/or white matter, usually not in the basal ganglia;
Dilatation of the convolutions and sulci;
Mild ventricular dilatation;
High-density areas corresponding to hemorrhage (in order of frequency) in the basal ganglia, thalamus, ventricle, subcortical areas, and cortex.

MR Imaging and MR Angiography

MR imaging may detect infarcts not seen on CT. MR imaging and MR angiography are increasingly used instead of conventional angiography, especially in children. The clear advantage is noninvasiveness.

Cerebral Angiography

Angiography is still the most common method of diagnosing moyamoya disease. In addition to the cardinal finding of stenosis or occlusion at the terminal parts of the ICAs and abnormal vascular networks, the following may also be observed in typical and advanced cases, indicating the presence of a transdural collateral circulation:

Ethmoidal moyamoya: abnormal vessels at the base of the brain anteriorly;
Vault moyamoya: transdural anastomoses at the cranial vault originating from the following arteries: anterior falcal, middle meningeal, ethmoidal, occipital, tentorial, and superficial temporal.

In addition, cerebral aneurysms are detected in 4% to 14% of patients with moyamoya disease.

[^{15}O]water PET

A typical example of moyamoya disease is illustrated by the case of a 25-year-old woman shown in Fig. 10-5. An abnormal vascular network was clearly seen on angiography (Fig. 10-5A). Gadolinium (Gd)-enhanced T1-weighted MR imaging (TR 500 ms/TE 14 ms) showed flow visualized within many dilated thalamoperforating and lenticulostriate branches (Fig. 10-5B). On hemodynamic [^{15}O]water PET evaluation, the baseline scan demonstrated absent perfusion in the temporolateral, frontal, and parietal areas of the left hemisphere, corresponding to infarction (Fig. 10-5C). Following administration of acetazolamide, perfusion did not appropriately increase in most of the brain, except the cerebellum, thalamus, and striatum. There was even a decrease in perfusion in a right frontal area, best appreciated on the difference images. This hemodynamic information is important in the planning of surgical procedures. A comparison of parts C and D in Fig. 10-5 demonstrates the superiority of quantitative perfusion imaging. The images in part D represent the counts accumulated over 60 seconds following the arrival of the bolus in the brain. The images are scaled to the maximum of each image. Although they demonstrate relatively decreased tracer uptake in large frontal, temporal, and parietal areas, the absolute decrease in the right frontal cortex and the normal increase in the cerebellum, thalamus, and striatum are not appreciated.

ACUTE ISCHEMIC STROKE

PET Imaging

Acute stroke is a common complication of CVD that often leads to death or severe handicap. In contrast to myocardial infarction, the therapeutic window for treatment is much shorter because of the higher vulnerability of neurons to hypoxia. However, double-blind trials with thrombolytic agents have lately shown promise (11). These positive findings are explained by experimental results, including [^{15}O]water PET studies that demonstrated that larger areas with vital tissue could potentially be salvaged by some kind of reperfusion therapy. In this regard, other imaging modalities seem of limited value, since the tissue at risk cannot be adequately defined with CT or MR imaging. Here, PET is the modality of choice. However, due to its limited availability, its use will be restricted to a few centers. Another limiting factor is the short time window available for potential thrombolytic therapy. Nevertheless, PET imaging has contributed valuable insights into the pathophysiology of stroke.

In acute ischemic stroke, the evaluation of perfusion and oxygen metabolism is of special interest. The affected tissue in stroke consists of various zones. If no reperfusion occurs within a short time, the most hypoperfused tissue will become necrotic. This zone is often surrounded by a region of tissue at risk called the penumbra. This tissue may survive, depending on the postinfarction course of reperfusion. PET measurements have shown that perfusion values less than 12 mL/min/100 g lead to irreversible damage. Values between 12 and 25 mL/min/100 g are typical for the penumbra and can be tolerated for hours (12). One of the most important parameters regarding tissue vitality is the rate of oxygen metabolism. Values less than 65 μmol/min/100 g lead to irreversible damage. Serial studies in stroke patients demonstrated that the oxygen metabolic rate may deteriorate during the 2 weeks following stroke onset, especially in the penumbra (13,14). Another promising approach to detecting viable tissue in stroke relies on the evaluation of benzodiazepine receptors with ^{11}C-FMZ. It was shown that the pattern of tracer uptake could separate vital from irreversibly damaged tissue (15). These results underline the importance of the penumbra. It is this zone that draws most attention in newer thrombolytic approaches.

Other Imaging Modalities

In the diagnostic workup of acute stroke, CT is used to exclude hemorrhage. This is important because bleeding may alter patient management. Ischemic stroke may evade detection at very early stages. Angiography is necessary if intraarterial thrombolysis is being considered.

Standard MR imaging fails to detect early ischemic lesions. At later stages, MR imaging is the method of choice for investigating the number and extent of infarct areas. Structural MR imaging is more sensitive than CT, especially in the cerebellum, brain stem, and deep white matter (16–18). Where available, MR imaging combined with MR angiography is ideal for delineating infarction beyond 12 hours after infarction onset. Recent progress in functional MR methods now also allow investigation of early infarction. Diffusion-weighted imaging (DWI) is sensitive to the self-diffusion of water and can detect an ischemic lesion at the earliest periods studied (19–21). These methods are especially useful in stroke centers where new methods of treatment are developed.

Perfusion SPECT also allows exact delineation of the stroke area at very early stages. However, if the choice exists between MR imaging including DWI, and SPECT, the former is superior; it delivers morphologic and angiographic information in the same session.

EXAMPLE PROTOCOLS

Quantitative Evaluation of Perfusion

The following is a protocol used at the University Hospital in Zurich to assess cerebral perfusion reserve capacity. It is based on the autoradiographic method.

Patient Preparation

Catheters are placed in the radial artery for blood sampling and in a cubital vein for injection.
Blood sampling is most easily performed with a continuous sampling device. Manual drawing of blood samples and counting in a well counter are impractical for [^{15}O]water.

Data Acquisition

Injection of 700 MBq [^{15}O]water. Although the injection can be performed manually, it is advantageous to use an automatic injection device.
Acquisition of one 60-second scan following the arrival of the bolus in the brain.
Performance of continuous blood sampling with a special sampling device.
Acquisition of a 10-minute transmission scan for photon attenuation correction.
At the beginning of the transmission scan, acetazolamide, 1 g, is injected as a slow bolus over 2 minutes.
Thirteen minutes following the start of acetazolamide injection, the second scan is initiated as described in 1-3 above.

The whole procedure lasts approximately 30 minutes.
Data Analysis. Following reconstruction, the data are exported and processed in a flexible analysis tool (22). In a preprocessing step, delay and dispersion of the arterial input curve are corrected using the method described by Meyer (23). The parametric flow maps are then smoothed with a gaussian filter, and subtraction images calculated ($\text{flow}_{\text{Diamox}} - \text{flow}_{\text{baseline}}$).

Measurement of Blood Volume

Patient Preparation. A catheter is placed in a cubital vein for continuous blood sampling.

Data Acquisition

Acquisition of a 10-minute transmission scan for photon attenuation correction.
Inhalation of 1,000 MBq [^{15}O]carbon monoxide as a bolus.
Acquisition of five 60-second scans immediately following inhalation.
Drawing of continuous venous blood samples 3 to 5 minutes following inhalation with a continuous sampling device.

The whole procedure lasts approximately 20 minutes.
Data Analysis. Following reconstruction, the time course of the activity in the brain is assessed by defining a region of interest that can encompass a whole transaxial slice. The purpose is to find the time point after which full equilibrium is achieved and the activity remains constant. This point is usually reached after 2 to 3 minutes. Then, all scans acquired after this time point can be summed. The division of this summation image and the mean radioactivity in the blood during the equilibrium period directly yield the blood vol-

TABLE 10-1. *Appraisal/reimbursement status of PET in cerebrovascular disease*

Disease	German consensus classfication	USZ classification	Replacement potential	US reimbursement status: Medicare/BC-BS	Swiss reimbursement status
Acute stroke	2a	—	—	no/no	no
Chronic CVD (before surgery)	2b	3	3	no/no	yes

See page 8 for abbreviations and appraisal scheme explanations.

ume. Depending on the required accuracy, it must be considered that the hematocrit in arterial and venous blood is slightly different. The easiest way to correct for the difference is to use a fixed correction factor. Alternatively, arterial or arterialized blood could be sampled.

CLINICAL USEFULNESS

A consensus meeting of the German Society for Nuclear Medicine in 1997 rated the procedures as indicated in Table 10-1.

APPENDIX: DETAILED METHODOLOGY FOR QUANTITATIVE PERFUSION IMAGING

Diffusible tracers display typical time–activity curves (TACs) following injection. An example for [^{15}O]water is shown in the bottom part of Fig. 10-6. Displayed are the TACs in arterial plasma and tissue in a simulated situation. The arterial time activity curves (TACs) shows a relatively sharp peak. The tissue TACs follow the arterial curve with dispersion. At the higher flow rate, the initial increase is steeper, the peak is higher, and the subsequent decline (washout) is faster than at the lower blood flow. Based on these kinetics, there exist several possibilities for assessing perfusion. It can easily be shown that the area below the TAC during the initial increase is closely related to perfusion. Due to washout, this area will underestimate true perfusion, and this effect is more pronounced the longer the integration time is. Nevertheless, the integration of activity during the first 60 seconds following the arrival of the bolus in the brain is a reasonable measure of perfusion. Full quantitation requires the application of a mathematical model.

An example for [H$_2$^{15}O]water is demonstrated in the top half of Fig. 10-6. The model consists of an arterial input, a tissue compartment, and the venous outflow. It is assumed that tracer distribution in the accessible part of the tissue compartment is homogeneous and that the concentration is equal to the venous outflow. The partition coefficient p is the fraction of tissue space that is actually permeated by the tracer. For water, it is in the range 80% to 90%. The kinetics is then described by a single differential equation that contains only one unknown, flow F. The solution of the differential equation can be written as a convolution with the arterial input curve. If one measures the tissue TAC and the arterial input curve, flow F can be calculated by some standard method of parameter estimation. Probably, the simplest way is the autoradiographic method, which requires only one static scan besides arterial blood sampling. The value of F is then adjusted by a fitting routine so that the model value fits the measured value. Somewhat more complex are the methods that use a series of scans. The advantage of such methods is that they allow estimation of the partition coefficient along with flow. This may be advantageous in situations where the partition coefficient is altered. For all methods that make use of an arterial input curve, one must consider that the arterial input curve is measured at a place distant from the brain, often the radial artery. Therefore, the delay and shape of the measured input curve may differ from those of the true input curve in the brain. Further distortions happen if an automatic sampling device is used.

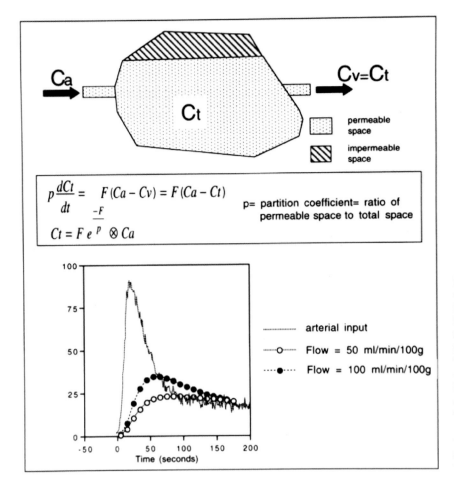

Figure 10-6. Upper: Model used for the quantitation of the $H_2^{15}O$ kinetics. The tissue compartment is fed by an arterial inflow with concentration C_a. It is assumed that the concentration in the venous outflow (C_v) equals the concentration in the permeable part of tissue space (C_t). The differential equations describing the kinetics and the solution are indicated below the model, operation of convolution; p, partition coefficient for water. **Lower:** Arterial input and tissue TACs for two different flow values. Note the steeper rise and decline at the higher flow rate.

REFERENCES

1. Vorstrup S, Brun B, Lassen NA. Evaluation of the cerebral vasodilatory capacity by the acetazolamide test before EC-IC bypass surgery in patients with occlusion of the internal carotid artery. *Stroke* 1986;17: 1291–1298.
2. Tsuda Y, Yamada K, Hayakawa T, et al. Cortical blood flow and cognition after extracranial-intracranial bypass in a patient with severe carotid occlusive lesions: a three-year follow-up study. *Acta Neurochir (Wien)* 1994;129:198–204.
3. Cikrit DF, Burt RW, Dalsing MC, et al. Acetazolamide-enhanced single photon emission computed tomography (SPECT) evaluation of cerebral perfusion before and after carotid endarterectomy. *J Vasc Surg* 1992;15:747–753.
4. Cikrit DF, Harris VJ, Hemmer CG, et al. Comparison of spiral CT scan and arteriography for evaluation of renal and visceral arteries. *Ann Vasc Surg* 1996;10:109–116.
5. Tatemichi TK, Desmond DW, Prohovnik I, Eidelberg D. Dementia associated with bilateral carotid occlusions: neuropsychological and haemodynamic course after extracranial to intracranial bypass surgery. *J Neurol Neurosurg Psychiatry* 1995;58:633–636.
6. Muraishi K, Kameyama M, Sato K, et al. Cerebral circulatory and metabolic changes following EC/IC bypass surgery in cerebral occlusive diseases. *Neurol Res* 1993;15:97–103.
7. The EC/IC Bypass Study Group. Failure of extracranial-intracranial arterial bypass to reduce the risk of ischemic stroke: results of an international randomized trial. *N Engl J Med* 1985;313:1191–1200.
8. Kuwabara Y, Ichiya Y, Sasaki M, et al. PET evaluation of cerebral hemodynamics in occlusive cerebrovascular disease pre- and postsurgery. *J Nucl Med* 1998;39:760–765.
9. The Japanese Extracranial-Intracranial Arterial Bypass Study Group. [Extracranial-intracranial arterial bypass in Japan: results of a prospective multicenter trial.] *Jpn J Stroke* 1997;19:217–224. [English abstract.]
10. Suzuki J, Takaku A. Cerebrovascular "moyamoya" disease: disease showing abnormal net-like vessels in base of brain. *Arch Neurol* 1969;20:288–299.
11. Marler JR, Brott T, Broderick J, et al. Tissue plasminogen activator for acute ischemic stroke. *N Engl J Med* 1995;333:1581–1587.
12. Heiss WD. Experimental evidence of ischemic thresholds and functional recovery. *Stroke* 1992;23:1668–1672.

13. Hakim AM, Evans AC, Berger L, et al. The effect of nimodipine on the evolution of human cerebral infarction studied by PET. *J Cereb Blood Flow Metab* 1989;9:523–534.

14. Heiss WD, Huber M, Fink GR, et al. Progressive derangement of periinfarct viable tissue in ischemic stroke. *J Cereb Blood Flow Metab* 1992;12:193–203.

15. Heiss WD, Grond M, Thiel A, et al. Permanent cortical damage detected by flumazenil positron emission tomography in acute stroke. *Stroke* 1998;29:454–461.

16. Ramadan NM, Deveshwar R, Levine SR. Magnetic resonance and clinical cerebrovascular disease: an update. *Stroke* 1989;20:1279–1283.

17. Amarenco P, Kase CS, Rosengart A, et al. Very small (border zone) cerebellar infarcts: distribution, causes, mechanisms and clinical features. *Brain* 1993;116:161–186.

18. Yuh WT, Crain MR, Loes DJ, et al. MR imaging of cerebral ischemia: findings in the first 24 hours. *Am J Neuroradiol* 1991;12:621–629.

19. Moseley ME, Kucharczyk J, Mintorovitch J, et al. Diffusion-weighted MR imaging of acute stroke: correlation with T2-weighted and magnetic susceptibility-enhanced MR imaging in cats. *Am J Neuroradiol* 1990;11:423–429.

20. Moseley ME, Mintorovitch J, Cohen Y, et al. Early detection of ischemic injury: comparison of spectroscopy, diffusion-, T2-, and magnetic susceptibility-weighted MRI in cats. *Acta Neurochir Suppl (Wien)* 1990;51:207–209.

21. Moseley ME, Cohen Y, Mintorovitch J, et al. Early detection of regional cerebral ischemia in cats: comparison of diffusion- and T2-weighted MRI and spectroscopy. *Magn Reson Med* 1990;14:330–346.

22. Burger C, Buck A. Requirements and implementation of a flexible kinetic modeling tool. *J Nucl Med* 1997;38:1818–1823.

23. Meyer E. Simultaneous correction for tracer arrival delay and dispersion in CBF measurements by the $H_2{}^{15}O$ autoradiographic method and dynamic PET. *J Nucl Med* 1989;30:1069–1078.

11

PET Imaging in Dementias

Michele Arigoni and Alfred Buck

Dementia is defined as a chronic, acquired, global, and progressive impairment of intellect, memory, and personality without impairment of consciousness. Dementing diseases can be classified into two main categories: (a) diseases in which dementia is the only symptom (Alzheimer's disease, Pick's disease, multiinfarct dementia) and (b) diseases in which dementia is associated with other clinical or laboratory signs (i.e., infection, subdural hematoma, brain tumor, metabolic disorder, electrolyte imbalance, nutritional deficiency, Parkinson's disease, Huntington's disease, normal pressure hydrocephalus). Because of its effects on the ability to function in society, dementia not only affects the patient but also the people in his or her environment. The prevalence of dementias increases with age (3% of the population older than 65 years, 10% older than 75 years) (1), and dementing diseases will thus become a growing sociologic health problem in the aging society of developed countries. Indeed, the number of affected elderly people will likely double between 1981 and 2001 (2).

INDICATION FOR POSITRON EMISSION TOMOGRAPHY

The diagnostic assessment in dementia includes a detailed history, a physical (especially neurologic) examination, blood and cerebrospinal fluid (CSF) screening, and computed tomography (CT) or magnetic resonance (MR) imaging. These tools are very useful in detecting most of the treatable causes of disorientation and loss of memory. For the remaining dementing diseases, such as neurodegenerative disorders and some cerebrovascular diseases, the definitive diagnosis is often based on biopsy or postmortem histopathologic findings. Functional imaging such as positron emission tomography (PET) in combination with morphologic imaging, such as CT or MR, is believed to help identify the cause of dementia and determine the neurophysiologic mechanisms underlying the disorder.

M. Arigoni and A. Buck: Nuclear Medicine, University Hospital, CH-8091 Zurich, Switzerland.

NORMAL AGING

Histopathologic findings show that the brain undergoes a number of age-related changes, including neuron loss, ventricular enlargement, and cortical atrophy.

CT and MR imaging are valuable techniques for identifying brain volume loss and ventricular enlargement. In a MR imaging study involving 76 normal subjects, it was shown that the volumes of the cerebral hemispheres, the frontal and temporal lobes, and the amygdalo–hippocampal complex decrease with age, while the ventricular volume increases (3). PET studies using fluorodeoxyglucose tagged with fluorine 18 ([18F]FDG) show a reduced metabolic rate in the elderly brain compared to young controls (4). However, when corrected for brain atrophy with CT or MR imaging, this age-related effect disappears (5). Effects due to atrophy should therefore always be taken into account in the interpretation of [18F]FDG PET scans in elderly patients.

ALZHEIMER'S DISEASE

Alzheimer's disease (AD) is the most common cause of dementia. The clinical diagnostic criteria require progressive, chronic, cognitive deficits in patients aged 40 to 90 years without identifiable underlying cause (6). Although these criteria permit accurate identification of AD patients with severe disease, it is very difficult to diagnose patients with early disease and to differentiate this from other forms of neurodegenerative disorders.

Although the diagnosis is made based on microscopic criteria, the brain in AD patients often shows characteristic changes on gross examination, such as cortical atrophy in the frontal, temporal, and parietal cortices, as well as frequent enlargement of the lateral and the third ventricles (7,8). Analyzing the atrophy pattern on CT or MR images helps distinguish AD from normal age-related atrophy. With appropriate scan angles, it is possible to evaluate the temporal lobe and the hippocampus. The sizes of the sylvian fissure, the temporal horn, the temporal sulcus, and the suprasellar cistern characterize temporal lobe atrophy and aid in differentiating an AD-affected brain from a normal brain (9). Further, atrophy of the hippocampus present in AD patients is detected by enlargement of the choroid–hippocampal fissure (10). Atrophy analysis by hand-drawn regions of interest in specific regions, such as the hippocampus and the temporal role, helps identify AD, but this method is observer-dependent (11,12).

Different [18F]FDG PET studies comparing AD patients with age-matched normal controls showed a 20% to 30% decrease in whole-brain tracer uptake, with prominent hypometabolism in the bilateral parietal and temporal lobes (13–15) (Fig. 11-1). The visual and motor cortices appear to be spared by this reduced [18F]FDG uptake. Studies of cerebral blood flow with PET using radioactively labeled water or with single photon emission computed tomography with technetium Tc 99m hexamethylpropyleneamine oxime (99mTc-HMPAO) show a similar picture, with relative hypoperfusion in the parietal and temporal lobes (16,17). The biparietal pattern, although highly predictive of AD, is not pathognomonic. In a study involving 129 patients with dementia, Salmon et al. (18) found that 97% of clinically or pathologically diagnosed AD subjects had an abnormal [18F]FDG distribution, with 66% showing the typical bilateral pattern. The specificity of bilateral temporoparietal involvement appears to be 68%. When followed with repeat scans, patients with atypical patterns tended to evolve to the characteristic [18F]FDG distribution. With disease progression, the hypometabolism and the hypoperfusion extended to the frontal regions (15) (Fig. 11-2A). The magnitude and the extent of the hypometabolism have been shown to correlate with the severity of the dementia symptoms (19).

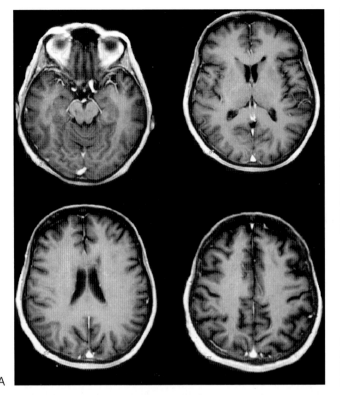

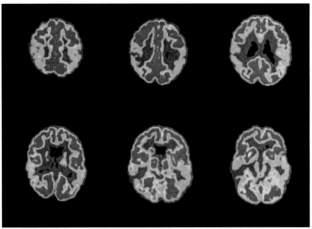

A

B

Figure 11-1. AD: 60-year-old man with progressive cortical dementia. **A:** MR image shows cortical atrophy. **B:** [^{18}F]FDG PET shows the typical bilateral temporoparietal hypometabolism.

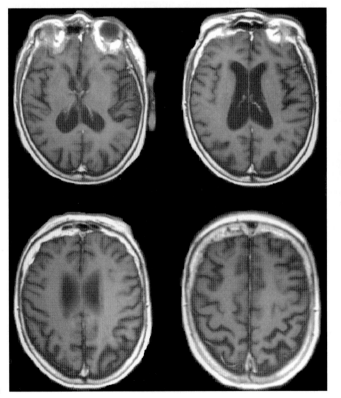

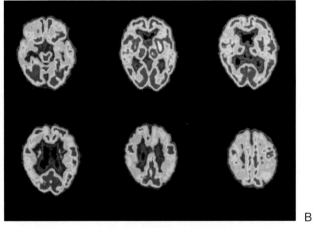

A

B

Figure 11-2. AD: 67-year-old woman with severe dementia, apatia, and increasing disorientation. **A:** MR image shows pronounced cortical atrophy. **B:** [^{18}F]FDG PET yields diffuse cortical hypometabolism with spared motor and visual cortex.

Different investigators have shown that [^{18}F]FDG PET appears to be a valuable tool in predicting AD in patients with mild dementia (20). This clearly shows the utility and advantage of PET in the assessment of demented patients. Since the introduction of new therapies for AD, such as the cholinesterase inhibitors, early diagnosis could be of importance in the success of treatment. PET also appears to be a good modality for assessing the effect of these new treatments. Indeed, when treated with cholinesterase inhibitors, AD patients showed improved cerebral glucose metabolism (21).

Neuroreceptor imaging is a promising tool in the diagnosis of AD. Different studies have identified alterations in the neurotransmission of the cholinergic, serotonergic, and GABAergic systems (22–24). However, these types of PET examinations are not yet part of clinical routine.

MULTIINFARCT DEMENTIA

After AD, multiinfarct dementia (MID) is the second most common cause of dementia, accounting for about 13% to 24% of cases. MID is caused by multiple infarcts that are usually distributed asymmetrically throughout the cortex. Clinically, symptoms tend to progress stepwise, in contrast to the constant disease progression in AD. CT and MR imaging have been shown to be sensitive in detecting MID. Vascular dementia is supported by the demonstration of vascular lesions by CT or T1-weighted MR imaging (25–27). The absence of vascular lesions in these imaging studies is sufficient to exclude a vascular etiology for the dementia. [^{18}F]FDG PET studies of patients with MID show multiple, scattered, focal areas of hypometabolism corresponding to the lesions seen on MR imaging (27,28) (Fig. 11-3). Dementia severity was found to correlate with the total volume of hypometabolic brain tissue. The lesions seen in PET studies appear to be larger than the corresponding MR lesions, and thus can be of help in early diagnosis. Furthermore, MID and AD commonly coexist, making it necessary to combine [^{18}F]FDG PET and MR imaging findings to establish the diagnosis (27).

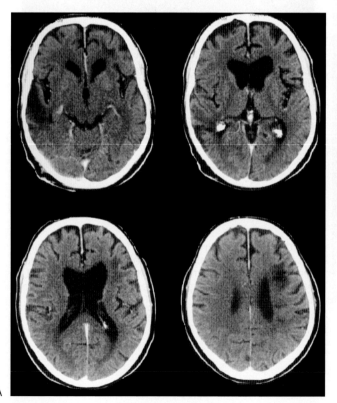

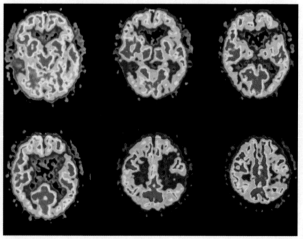

Figure 11-3. MID: 63-year-old man with stepwise progressive apraxia and impaired memory. **A:** CT shows various infarcts in the right temporal lobe, as well as left frontal. **B:** [^{18}F]FDG PET with concordant scattered hypometabolic areas in the bilateral parietal lobes, as well as left frontal and right temporolateral.

A

B

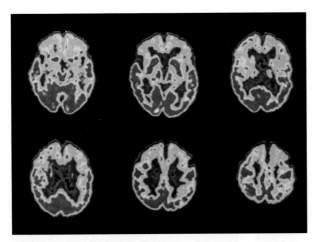

Figure 11-4. Pick's disease: 67-year-old paraspastic woman with dementia. [^{18}F]FDG PET shows bifrontal hypometabolism **(A)**, as well as in the anterior temporal lobes **(B)**, with normal temporoparietal [^{18}F]FDG uptake.

FRONTOTEMPORAL DEMENTIA

Frontotemporal dementia (FTD) defines a group of dementing diseases characterized by atrophy of the frontal and the temporal lobes. Pick's disease, the best known member of this group, is a neurodegenerative disease associated with atrophy, neuronal loss, gliosis, and the presence of Pick bodies on histopathologic examination. These alterations affect predominantly the frontal and the temporal lobes in patients in mid- to late adulthood.

Clinically, the distinction between Pick's disease and AD is difficult. Frontal or temporal atrophy, as well as widening of the interhemispheric fissure frontally, with compensatory enlargement of the frontal horn, can be seen in MR images or CT (29). Differentiation between AD and FTD can be difficult on the basis of these findings. In [^{18}F]FDG PET studies, patients with Pick's disease show symmetric reduction in glucose metabolism in both frontal and anterior temporal lobes (30) (Fig. 11-4). These same regions also appear to have reduced perfusion (31). This pattern allows Pick's disease to be distinguished from AD, which is important because AD patients could benefit from specific treatment, in contrast to persons suffering from Pick's disease. However, other disorders, such as schizophrenia, also manifest with a bilateral frontal hypometabolism, but these should not present a problem in being clinically differentiated from Pick's disease.

PARKINSON'S DISEASE

Parkinson's disease (PD) is a neurodegenerative disorder of dopaminergic neurons in the substantia nigra, characterized by the triad consisting of hypokinesis, tremor, and rigidity. Dementia will develop in approximately 20% to 40% of patients with PD (32). Currently, MR imaging findings show no significant difference between patients with PD and age-matched controls. [^{18}F]FDG PET studies of demented patients with PD show a uniform cerebral hypometabolism, with parietal predilection similar to the pattern seen in AD patients. Indeed, histopathologic findings of demented patients with PD show the typical alterations characteristic not only of PD but often also of AD (33). The two types of dementia are almost indistinguishable by [^{18}F]FDG PET, but because of the motor dysfunction in PD, this poses no problem for the differential diagnosis (34,35). Functional imaging with ^{18}F-dopa to evaluate presynaptic function showed reduced radioligand uptake in the basal ganglia of PD patients (36). Imaging of the dopamine receptor system with the D_2-receptor antagonist [^{11}C]raclopride has yielded variable results and must still be investigated (37).

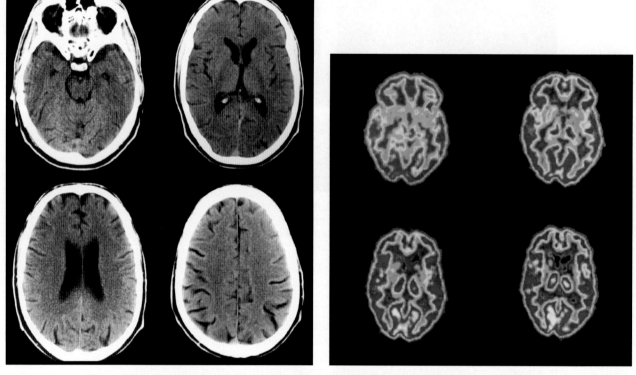

A

B

Figure 11-5. HD: 50-year-old man with clinically suspected HD confirmed by molecular genetic tests. **A:** [^{18}F]FDG PET shows hypometabolism in the striatum bilaterally, but it is more pronounced in the caudate nucleus. **B:** CT shows no particular abnormalities.

HUNTINGTON'S DISEASE

A genetic disorder involving an autosomal dominantly-inherited defect on chromosome 4, Huntington's disease (HD) is characterized by progressive motor dysfunction, including chorea and akinetic rigidity, behavioral disturbances, and progressive cognitive deterioration; onset is in the third or forth decade. Although chorea is the hallmark of this disease, intellectual deterioration can precede the development of this motor abnormality. Histopathologically, there is neuronal loss and gliosis in the striatum of patients with HD. Accordingly, [^{18}F]FDG PET studies show a substantial decrease in perfusion and glucose metabolism in the caudate nucleus and the putamen (38,39) (Fig. 11-5). These findings often precede the striatal atrophy seen in CT and MR imaging (39). The hypometabolism is not confined to the striatum but can also affect various cortical regions, and the degree of dementia was found to correlate with the decreased [^{18}F]FDG uptake in the frontal, parietal, and temporal lobes (38).

PROGRESSIVE SUPRANUCLEAR PALSY

Clinically, progressive supranuclear palsy (PSP) is characterized by ocular movement disorders, parkinsonism, and dementia. The typical onset of symptoms is in the sixth or seventh decade. Histopathologic findings show cell loss in different brain regions, such as the brain stem, pallidus, and substantia nigra, usually with sparing of the cortex. Midbrain atrophy, particularly of the tectum, and enlargement of the aqueduct of Sylvius, quadrigeminal cistern, and posterior third ventricle—observed in MR images—mirror the neuropathologic changes (40). Glucose hypometabolism of the superior frontal cortex, as well as of the basal ganglia, the thalamus, and the pons, has been demonstrated by [^{18}F]FDG

PET (41,42). A similar distribution has been reported for cerebral blood flow. PSP patients can thus be clearly differentiated from those suffering from AD. The pattern of [^{18}F]FDG distribution is similar to but lesser in extent than that observed in patients with Pick's disease; however, clinically the two diseases can easily be differentiated.

NORMAL PRESSURE HYDROCEPHALUS

Normal pressure hydrocephalus (NPH) is an important cause of dementia because it is potentially treatable. Clinically, the triad of dementia, ataxia, and urinary incontinence characterizes NPH. Although the ventricles are dilated, the CSF pressure appears to be normal. Although the clinical and radiologic diagnostic criteria are clear, there are cases in which identification of NPH can be difficult. The diagnosis is nevertheless important, because the patient may benefit from a CSF shunt. The success of shunting is highest for patients with a history of prior meningitis or subarachnoid hemorrhage. MR imaging and CT findings in patients with NPH show variable grades of ventricular enlargement with rounding of the anterior third ventricle and increased size of the temporal horns and the sylvian fissure (43). A good parameter for hydrocephalus is the increased ratio of the maximum frontal ventricular horn width to the transverse inner diameter of the calvaria. A CSF flow void within the aqueduct and the third ventricle can be seen in MR images (44). [^{18}F]FDG PET studies in NPH patients yield a diffuse reduced cortical perfusion and metabolism without any regional predilection (45,46) (Figs. 11-6 and 11-7). The ventricular dilation, when massive, can also be identified with PET. Selection of patients for shunting is based on clinical, CSF, and imaging findings combined with response to spinal tap and CSF removal.

ALCOHOL-RELATED DEMENTIA

Dementia with impaired orientation can develop in patients with a long history of alcoholism. In PET studies involving alcoholic patients, investigators found a decrease in

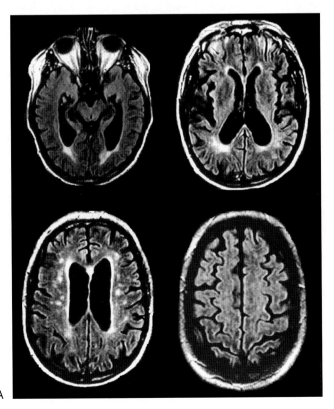

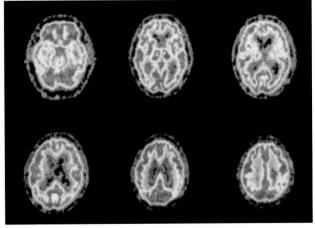

A

B

Figure 11-6. NPH: 68-year-old woman with dementia and extrapyramidal symptoms. Enlarged ventricles and cortical atrophy can be seen on both MR imaging **(A)** and [^{18}F]FDG PET **(B)** without focal hypometabolism.

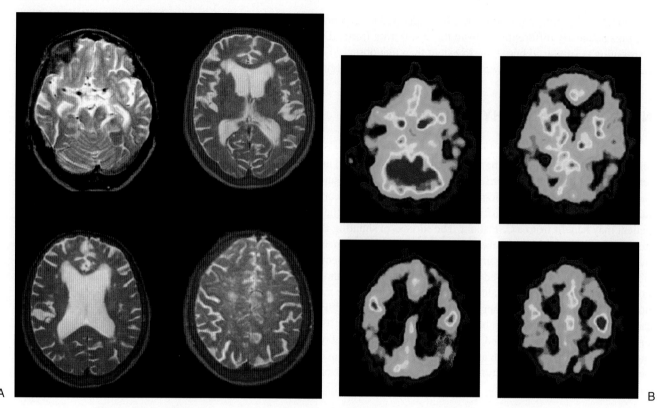

A

B

Figure 11-7. NPH: 75-year-old woman with dementia, incontinence, and extrapyramidal symptoms. **A:** MR image yields enlarged ventricles. **B:** [$H_2^{15}O$]water PET shows enlarged ventricles and reduced cortical perfusion in the cortex.

whole-brain metabolism and especially in cortical and subcortical brain regions (47). Other studies have reported a more pronounced hypometabolism in the left hemisphere. Chronic alcoholic patients with cerebellar degeneration show a hypometabolism in the superior vermis compared to age-related control subjects. A study comparing the effect of alcohol administration to chronic alcoholics and to normal subjects found reduced glucose metabolism in the occipital, prefrontal, and cerebellar cortices, which, interestingly, are the regions with the highest density of GABAergic receptors (48).

CREUTZFELD-JAKOB DISEASE

Creutzfeld-Jakob disease (CJD) is caused by a transmissible prion. The disease is characterized by a subacute spongiform encephalophaty and a rapidly increasing dementia, with patients dying shortly after diagnosis. CJD being relatively new, only a few PET studies with proven autoptic of bioptic diagnosis have been carried out. It seems that CJD patients show decreased [^{18}F]FDG uptake. but the pattern is not yet clear. Perfusion also appears to be reduced (49).

DEMENTIA RELATED TO ACQUIRED IMMUNODEFICIENCY SYNDROME

Different neurologic dysfunctions can arise in patients infected with the human immunodeficiency virus (HIV). These conditions can be caused directly by HIV, by a secondary opportunistic infection such as toxoplasmosis, or by neoplasms associated with the ac-

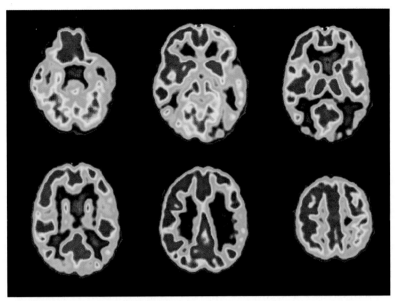

Figure 11-8. AIDS-related dementia: 32-year-old HIV-positive patient with dementia. [^{18}F]FDG PET shows hypometabolism bilaterally in the temporal, occipital, and parietal lobes, as well as the left frontal.

quired immunodeficiency syndrome (AIDS). AIDS-related dementia is thought to be directly caused by HIV and is one of the AIDS-defining criteria. It can occur as the only symptom or in association with other clinical manifestations of AIDS. The prevalence of dementia in AIDS patients is thought to be at least 5%. [^{18}F]FDG PET findings in patients suffering from AIDS-related dementia show decreased glucose metabolism and perfusion in the cerebral cortex (50) (Fig. 11-8).

PATIENT PREPARATION AND IMAGING PROTOCOL

No real specific patient preparation is needed for cerebral [^{18}F]FDG PET in patients with dementing diseases. In contrast to PET studies in oncology and cardiology, fasting prior to examination is not required. Good hydration is useful to help wash out activity from the patient's body and reduce the radiation dose. A delay of 30 to 40 minutes should be observed between injection of the usual [^{18}F]FDG dose of 100 to 200 MBq and the start of the scan to allow the tracer to accumulate in brain tissue. During this uptake phase, the patient rests calmly with minimal sensory input (i.e., eyes closed, minimal ambient noise). The brain is then scanned in three-dimensional mode for 20 minutes. For transmission correction, a transmission scan of 10 minutes' duration is also carried out. In specific cases, a special scan plane can be chosen for the reconstructed images, for example, to show the temporal lobes in their full extent.

For perfusion studies, oxygen 15 water ([H$_2$^{15}O]water) is used at the University Hospital in Zurich; the half-life of the isotope is approximatively 2 minutes. No patient preparation is required, unless quantitative flow maps are to be produced, in which case an arterial catheter is necessary for arterial sampling. Because only relative perfusion is usually needed, qualitative PET scanning is sufficient. A dose of 800 MBq of [H$_2$^{15}O]water is injected into the antecubital vein by an automated device. While the patient lies calmly without unnecessary sensory input, scanning of the brain is carried out for 60 seconds, starting from the time of initial increase of activity in the brain. A 10-minute transmission scan is added to correct for absorption effects.

TABLE 11-1. *Appraisal/reimbursement status of PET in the dementias*

Disease	German consensus classification	USZ classification	Replacement potential	US reimbursement status: Medicare/BC-BS	Swiss reimbursement status
Dementias	1a	3	3	yes/yes	yes (<70y)

See page 8 for abbreviations and appraisal scheme explanations.

CLINICAL CONSEQUENCES

In summary, PET is a useful tool in the diagnosis of dementing diseases, when combined with morphologic neuroimaging techniques such as CT or MR imaging. Comparing MR imaging and PET findings allows the physiologic effects of morphologically identifiable brain lesions to be estimated. For some diseases, such as Pick's disease, PET seems to be superior in differentiating a disorder from other causes of dementia (31). Furthermore, it appears that abnormal findings in PET often precede alterations that can be found in CT or MR imaging, thus leading to an early diagnosis (21,51,52).

Unfortunately, most of the causes of dementia that have been discussed are untreatable. Nevertheless, for some dementing diseases, newer treatments appear to be able to slow the disease course. Indeed, AD patients profit from therapy with drugs that enhance cholinergic activity, such as the cholinesterase inhibitors or muscarinic cholinergic agonists. Early diagnosis in these patients can lead to an early start of treatment. In MID patients, lesions demonstrated by PET appear to be larger and thus more easily identified than they are in MR imaging or CT, and early diagnosis leads to antithrombotic prophylaxis and to a reduction of risk factors, such as hypertonia or diabetes mellitus. This permits slowing or even stopping disease progression. In NPH, PET helps select patients who might benefit from a shunting operation (45).

If the diagnosis is not clear, PET findings often help direct the subsequent investigation. A hypometabolic focus in the striatum for example is suggestive of HD, which can be proved by genetic tests. Diagnosing HD is very important because genetic counseling is necessary not only for the patient but also his relatives.

PET seems to be a useful tool for understanding the pathophysiologic mechanisms of underlying diseases, which could be helpful in developing new treatment strategies. Moreover, PET appears to be a possible method for monitoring drug effects in dementing diseases. An increase in glucose metabolism has been observed after administration of tacrine (Cognex), a cholinesterase inhibitor, and of piracetam in patients with AD (21,51).

Neuroreceptor imaging is a promising modality. For the time being, the data analysis is still time-consuming and clinically feasible only in a few cases. Nevertheless, it is of great interest in assessment of the pathophysiology of many diseases.

REFERENCES

1. Henderson AS. The epidemiology of Alzheimer's disease. *Br Med Bull* 1986;42:3–10.
2. Ineichen B. Measuring the rising tide: how many dementia cases will there be by 2001? *Br J Psychiatry* 1987;150:193–200.
3. Coffey CE, Wilkinson WE, Parashos IA, et al. Quantitative cerebral anatomy of the aging human brain: a cross-sectional study using magnetic resonance imaging. *Neurology* 1992;42:527–536.
4. Hoffman JM, Guze BH, Baxter LR, Mazziotta JC, Phelps ME. [^{18}F]-fluorodeoxyglucose (FDG) and positron emission tomography (PET) in aging and dementia: a decade of studies. *Eur Neurol* 1989;29(suppl 3):16–24.
5. Yoshii F, Barker WW, Chang JY, et al. Sensitivity of cerebral glucose metabolism to age, gender, brain volume, brain atrophy, and cerebrovascular risk factors. *J Cereb Blood Flow Metab* 1988;8:654–661.
6. McKhann G, Drachman D, Folstein M, Katzman R, Price D, Stadlan EM. Clinical diagnosis of Alzheimer's disease: report of the NINCDS-ADRDA work group under the auspices of Department of Health and Human Services task force on Alzheimer's disease. *Neurology* 1984;34:939–944.
7. Mirra SS, Hart MN, Terry RD. Making the diagnosis of Alzheimer's disease: a primer for practicing pathologists. *Arch Pathol Lab Med* 1993;117:132–144.

8. Mirra SS, Heyman A, McKeel D, et al. The consortium to establish a registry for Alzheimer's disease (CERAD). Part II. Standardization of the neuropathologic assessment of Alzheimer's disease. *Neurology* 1991;41:479–486.
9. Kido DK, Caine ED, LeMay M, Ekholm S, Booth H, Panzer R. Temporal lobe atrophy in patients with Alzheimer disease: a CT study. *Am J Neuroradiol* 1989;10:551–555.
10. George AE, de-Leon MJ, Stylopoulos LA, et al. CT diagnostic features of Alzheimer disease: importance of the choroidal/hippocampal fissure complex. *Am J Neuroradiol* 1990;11:101–107.
11. Jack CR Jr, Petersen RC, O'Brien PC, Tangalos EG. MR-based hippocampal volumetry in the diagnosis of Alzheimer's disease. *Neurology* 1992;42:183–188.
12. Kesslak JP, Nalcioglu O, Cotman CW. Quantification of magnetic resonance scans for hippocampal and parahippocampal atrophy in Alzheimer's disease. *Neurology* 1991;41:51–54.
13. Friedland RP, Jagust WJ, Huesman RH, et al. Regional cerebral glucose transport and utilization in Alzheimer's disease. *Neurology* 1989;39:1427–1434.
14. Heiss WD, Kessler J, Szelies B, Grond M, Fink G, Herholz K. Positron emission tomography in the differential diagnosis of organic dementias. *J Neural Transm Suppl* 1991;33:13–19.
15. Kumar A, Schapiro MB, Grady C, et al. High-resolution PET studies in Alzheimer's disease. *Neuropsychopharmacology* 1991;4:35–46.
16. Montaldi D, Brooks DN, McColl JH, et al. Measurements of regional cerebral blood flow and cognitive performance in Alzheimer's disease. *J Neurol Neurosurg Psychiatry* 1990;53:33–38.
17. Holman BL, Johnson KA, Gerada B, Carvalho PA, Satlin A. The scintigraphic appearance of Alzheimer's disease: a prospective study using technetium-99m-HMPAO SPECT. *J Nucl Med* 1992;33:181–185.
18. Salmon E, Sadzot B, Maquet P, et al. Differential diagnosis of Alzheimer's disease with PET. *J Nucl Med* 1994;35:391–398.
19. Duara R, Grady C, Haxby J, et al. Positron emission tomography in Alzheimer's disease. *Neurology* 1986;36:879–887.
20. Rapoport SI, Horwitz B, Grady CL, Haxby JV, DeCarli C, Schapiro MB. Abnormal brain glucose metabolism in Alzheimer's disease, as measured by positron emission tomography. *Adv Exp Med Biol* 1991;291:231–234.
21. Nordberg A. Clinical studies in Alzheimer patients with positron emission tomography. *Behav Brain Res* 1993;57:215–224.
22. Weinberger DR, Gibson R, Coppola R, et al. The distribution of cerebral muscarinic acetylcholine receptors *in vivo* in patients with dementia: a controlled study with [123]IQNB and single photon emission computed tomography. *Arch Neurol* 1991;48:169–176.
23. Blin J, Baron JC, Dubois B, et al. Loss of brain 5-HT2 receptors in Alzheimer's disease: *in vivo* assessment with positron emission tomography and [18F]setoperone. *Brain* 1993;116:497–510.
24. Meyer M, Koeppe RA, Frey KA, Foster NL, Kuhl DE. Positron emission tomography measures of benzodiazepine binding in Alzheimer's disease. *Arch Neurol* 1995;52:314–317.
25. Roman GC, Tatemichi TK, Erkinjuntti T, et al. Vascular dementia: diagnostic criteria for research studies: report of the NINDS-AIREN international workshop. *Neurology* 1993;43:250–260.
26. Chui HC, Victoroff JI, Margolin D, Jagust W, Shankle R, Katzman R. Criteria for the diagnosis of ischemic vascular dementia proposed by the state of California Alzheimer's disease diagnostic and treatment centers. *Neurology* 1992;42:473–480.
27. Duara R, Barker W, Loewenstein D, Pascal S, Bowen B. Sensitivity and specificity of positron emission tomography and magnetic resonance imaging studies in Alzheimer's disease and multi-infarct dementia. *Eur Neurol* 1989;29(suppl 3):9–15.
28. Gibbs JM, Frackowiak RS, Legg NJ. Regional cerebral blood flow and oxygen metabolism in dementia due to vascular disease. *Gerontology* 1986;32(suppl 1):84–88.
29. Knopman DS, Christensen KJ, Schut LJ, et al. The spectrum of imaging and neuropsychological findings in Pick's disease. *Neurology* 1989;39:362–368.
30. Kamo H, McGeer PL, Harrop R, et al. Positron emission tomography and histopathology in Pick's disease. *Neurology* 1987;37:439–445.
31. Miller BL, Cummings JL, Villanueva-Meyer J, et al. Frontal lobe degeneration: clinical, neuropsychological, and SPECT characteristics. *Neurology* 1991;41:1374–1382.
32. Mayeux R, Chen J, Mirabello E, et al. An estimate of the incidence of dementia in idiopathic Parkinson's disease. *Neurology* 1990;40:1513–1517.
33. Perry EK, McKeith I, Thompson P, et al. Topography, extent, and clinical relevance of neurochemical deficits in dementia of Lewy body type, Parkinson's disease, and Alzheimer's disease. *Ann N Y Acad Sci* 1991;640:197–202.
34. Peppard RF, Martin WR, Clark CM, Carr GD, McGeer PL, Calne DB. Cortical glucose metabolism in Parkinson's and Alzheimer's disease. *J Neurosci Res* 1990;27:561–568.
35. Eidelberg D, Moeller JR, Dhawan V, et al. The metabolic topography of parkinsonism. *J Cereb Blood Flow Metab* 1994;14:783–801.
36. Leenders KL, Salmon EP, Tyrrell P, et al. The nigrostriatal dopaminergic system assessed *in vivo* by positron emission tomography in healthy volunteer subjects and patients with Parkinson's disease. *Arch Neurol* 1990;47:1290–1298.
37. Brooks DJ, Ibanez V, Sawle GV, et al. Striatal D_2 receptor status in patients with Parkinson's disease, striatonigral degeneration, and progressive supranuclear palsy, measured with 11C-raclopride and positron emission tomography. *Ann Neurol* 1992;31:184–192.
38. Kuwert T, Lange HW, Langen KJ, Herzog H, Aulich A, Feinendegen LE. Cortical and subcortical glucose consumption measured by PET in patients with Huntington's disease. *Brain* 1990;113:1405–1423.
39. Hayden MR, Martin WR, Stoessl AJ, et al. Positron emission tomography in the early diagnosis of Huntington's disease. *Neurology* 1986;36:888–894.
40. Savoiardo M, Girotti F, Strada L, Ciceri E. Magnetic resonance imaging in progressive supranuclear palsy and other parkinsonian disorders. *J Neural Transm Suppl* 1994;42:93–110.

41. Goffinet AM, DeVolder AG, Gillain C, et al. Positron tomography demonstrates frontal lobe hypometabolism in progressive supranuclear palsy. *Ann Neurol* 1989;25:131–139.

42. Foster NL, Gilman S, Berent S, Morin EM, Brown MB, Koeppe RA. Cerebral hypometabolism in progressive supranuclear palsy studied with positron emission tomography. *Ann Neurol* 1988;24:399–406.

43. Larsson A, Wikkelso C, Bilting M, Stephensen H. Clinical parameters in 74 consecutive patients shunt operated for normal pressure hydrocephalus. *Acta Neurol Scand* 1991;84:475–482.

44. Bradley WG Jr, Whittemore AR, Watanabe AS, Davis SJ, Teresi LM, Homyak M. Association of deep white matter infarction with chronic communicating hydrocephalus: implications regarding the possible origin of normal-pressure hydrocephalus. *Am J Neuroradiol* 1991;12:31–39.

45. Brooks DJ, Beaney RP, Powell M, et al. Studies on cerebral oxygen metabolism, blood flow, and blood volume, in patients with hydrocephalus before and after surgical decompression, using positron emission tomography. *Brain* 1986;109:613–628.

46. Jagust WJ, Friedland RP, Budinger TF. Positron emission tomography with [^{18}F]fluorodeoxyglucose differentiates normal pressure hydrocephalus from Alzheimer-type dementia. *J Neurol Neurosurg Psychiatry* 1985;48:1091–1096.

47. Samson Y, Baron JC, Feline A, Bories J, Crouzel C. Local cerebral glucose utilisation in chronic alcoholics: a positron tomographic study. *J Neurol Neurosurg Psychiatry* 1986;49:1165–1170.

48. Volkow ND, Hitzemann R, Wolf AP, et al. Acute effects of ethanol on regional brain glucose metabolism and transport. *Psychiatry Res* 1990;35:39–48.

49. Friedland RP, Prusiner SB, Jagust WJ, Budinger TF, Davis RL. Bitemporal hypometabolism in Creutzfeldt-Jakob disease measured by positron emission tomography with [18F]-2-fluorodeoxyglucose. *J Comput Assist Tomogr* 1984;8:978–981.

50. Rottenberg DA, Sidtis JJ, Strother SC, et al. Abnormal cerebral glucose metabolism in HIV-1 seropositive subjects with and without dementia. *J Nucl Med* 1996;37:1133–1140.

51. Heiss WD, Szelies B, Kessler J, Herholz K. Abnormalities of energy metabolism in Alzheimer's disease studied with PET. *Ann N Y Acad Sci* 1991;640:65–71.

52. Rapoport SI. Discriminant analysis of brain imaging data identifies subjects with early Alzheimer's disease. *Int Psychogeriatr* 1997;9(suppl 1):229–235.

Clinical PET Imaging of the Heart

PART III

Clinical PET Imaging of the Heart

12

Coronary Artery Disease

Philipp A. Kaufmann

This chapter presents an overview of the impact of positron emission tomography (PET) on the evaluation of patients with coronary artery disease (CAD). After a short description of tracers and technique, the utility and accuracy of PET for diagnosis, risk assessment, and prognosis are considered and compared to other available techniques. With the development of PET technology, accuracy in diagnosis and prognosis has improved. In addition, PET provides an elegant tool for assessing metabolic processes in myocardial cells. This enables the distinction of viable myocardium from nonviable left ventricular (LV) segments after myocardial infarction (MI). Accurate assessment of the extent of dysfunctional but viable myocardium (hibernating myocardium) is important in patients with a large MI and LV dysfunction. With combined information from PET and coronary angiography, the best revascularization strategy can be found. For the detection of viable myocardium, PET offers a positive predictive value of 85% to 90% and negative predictive value of 70% to 75%.

CAD detection and risk assessment continue to be mainstays of modern cardiology. They have gained in importance because of the broad range of therapeutic options now available to patients with CAD. These options range from cardiac surgery and catheter revascularization to modern pharmacologic treatment, and, most likely in the foreseeable future, to gene therapy.

Basically, there are two possible bases on which to describe stenosis severity: anatomic or physiologic determinants. The "gold standard" for the evaluation of CAD remains coronary angiography, which provides exact information on the location and anatomic severity of epicardial coronary artery stenoses. However, the interpretation of coronary angiographic images is affected by considerable interobserver variability (1), which is underlined by the poor agreement of angiographic results *in vivo* with those postmortem (2,3). Furthermore, the physiologic significance of any lesion may be difficult to assess from angiographic images alone, and perfusion abnormalities may occur in the absence of arteriographically assessable stenoses. In fact, angiographic evidence of stenosis severity is reported to show no or poor correlation with clinical or physiologic parameters such as coronary flow reserve and reactive hyperemia (4). Even the introduction of quantitative coronary angiography has not improved the predictive value of angiography: This explains

P. A. Kaufmann: Nuclear Medicine and Cardiology, University Hospital, CH-8091 Zurich, Switzerland.

the increasing importance of cardiac nuclear perfusion imaging in cardiovascular medicine. PET represents the most advanced scintigraphic technique, allowing accurate qualitative and quantitative assessment of regional myocardial tracer distribution. It has gained increasing clinical acceptance in cardiology.

At present, two specific clinical applications of PET have been proposed for the evaluation of patients with CAD by the joint task force of the American College of Cardiology (ACC) and the American Heart Association (AHA) (5):

Noninvasive detection of CAD and estimation of disease severity;
Assessment of myocardial viability in patients with CAD and LV dysfunction.

MYOCARDIAL PERFUSION TRACERS

Currently, various radionuclides are available for PET cardiac perfusion studies (see Table 3-1). Typically, the positron-emitting radionuclides used in PET studies have short physical half-lives. These should be compared with the half-lives of radionuclides routinely used in diagnostic nuclear medicine, such as technetium Tc 99m and thallium Tl 201, which have half-lives of 6.0 and 73.5 hours, respectively. The short half-lives of positron-emitting radionuclides provide a number of practical advantages, particularly reduction of patient radiation exposure and acquisition of repeated myocardial blood flow (MBF) measurements in the same patient in the same scanning session within a reasonable time (1 to 2 hours).

None of the tracers tested thus far has all the characteristics required for optimal quantitation: short physical half-life, minimal radiation dose, uptake directly related to flow and independent of metabolic conditions, and availability without a cyclotron. At present, quantification requires sophisticated mathematical analysis, rapid data acquisition free of detector saturation, and, depending on the technique, concomitant administration of a blood pool tracer.

The three most common tracers are ammonia tagged with nitrogen 13 ($[^{13}N]$ammonia), rubidium Rb 82 (^{82}Rb), and oxygen 15–labeled water ($[^{15}O]$water). They have been selected for their physical and biochemical properties. Their physiologic characteristics show remarkable differences. $[^{15}O]$water is essentially freely diffusible in the heart, with minimal effect of flow on uptake and nearly 100% extraction (6). However, it also remains in the blood pool, contaminating the image with uptake within the ventricular chambers and surrounding structure.

By contrast, $[^{13}N]$ammonia provides high image contrast because it is rapidly cleared from the blood and avidly retained in myocardial tissue. Due to its tissue solubility, it diffuses readily into cells, where most is trapped as glutamate. At physiologic pH, ammonia is primarily found in the form of NH_4^+. Its concentration in the myocardium depends not only on flow but also on the amount of $[^{13}N]$ammonia administered as a function of time (input function), its extraction at the instantaneous flow, and metabolic state.

The potassium analogue ^{82}Rb can be eluted from a strontium Sr 82 generator system, avoiding the need for an on-site cyclotron. The extraction is flow-related at high flow rates, and therefore a correction of ^{82}Rb uptake for extraction is needed. The mean positron energy emitted by ^{82}Rb is higher than that with $[^{13}N]$ammonia. Thus, the distance traversed by ^{82}Rb positrons in tissue is longer, resulting in a lower theoretical limit of resolution. Together with the lower count rate due to the shorter half-life, image quality is reduced compared to that with $[^{13}N]$ammonia.

By displaying data in the format of slices with discrete thickness, tomographic imaging allows better discrimination of myocardial and other nonmyocardial structures and individual coronary artery beds, and is inherently quantitative. A standardized nomenclature for tomographic views (short axis, vertical long axis, and horizontal long axis; see Fig. 6-5) and displays has been developed for different tomographic imaging techniques, including single photon emission computed tomography (SPECT), PET, computed tomography, and magnetic resonance (MR) imaging, by the Committee on Advanced Cardiac Imaging and Technology, the Council on Clinical Cardiology, the AHA in collaboration with the

Cardiovascular Imaging Committee of the ACC, and the Board of Directors of the Cardio-vascular Council of the Society of Nuclear Medicine (7).

EVALUATION OF CORONARY ARTERY DISEASE: ROLE OF PET

In a large number of studies, several primary clinical applications of PET perfusion imaging in CAD have been established:

Accurate, noninvasive diagnosis of CAD in symptomatic or asymptomatic patients, including those with balanced three-vessel disease;

Assessment of physiologic stenosis severity for identification of the culprit lesion as a target for revascularization procedures in patients with documented CAD;

Assessment of response to antiischemic and thrombolytic treatment, as well as percutaneous transluminal angioplasty and surgical interventions designed to augment perfusion and improve function;

Follow-up of progression or regression of CAD during risk-factor modification;

Evaluation of collateral function.

Detection of CAD with PET

In daily clinical routine, diagnostic visual qualitative evaluation of [^{13}N]ammonia or ^{82}Rb PET perfusion images has proven feasible and accurate using a subjective scoring method rather than absolute flow quantification (8). The procedure is performed using a PET perfusion agent at rest and during pharmacologic vasodilation. The short half-lives of these agents permit rapid sequential examinations, such as rest–dipyridamole studies, within a short time frame (1 to 2 hours). After intravenous administration, both [^{13}N]ammonia and ^{82}Rb distribute in proportion to regional blood flow. Images of the heart show deficits in regions where blood flow is relatively reduced and in zones of nonviable myocardium (e.g., previous MI). Pharmacologically induced myocardial hyperemia is commonly used to cause regional inhomogeneities in the perfusion pattern related to coronary stenoses (Figs. 12-1 and 12-2). Physical exercise in PET studies is less feasible and has therefore only rarely been used.

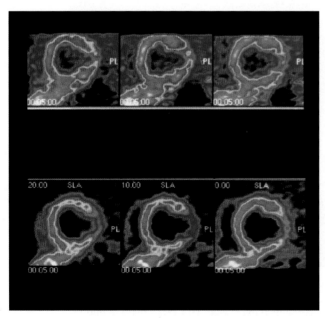
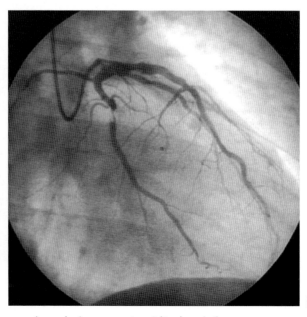

A   B

Figure 12-1. A: Short-axis projection of a [^{13}N]ammonia perfusion scan at rest **(top)** and after dipyridamole stress **(bottom)** in a patient with a lateral MI. A matched lateral defect and additional adjacent stress-induced defects were found. **B:** Coronary angiogram of the left coronary circulation shows a high-grade stenosis of the circumflex coronary artery.

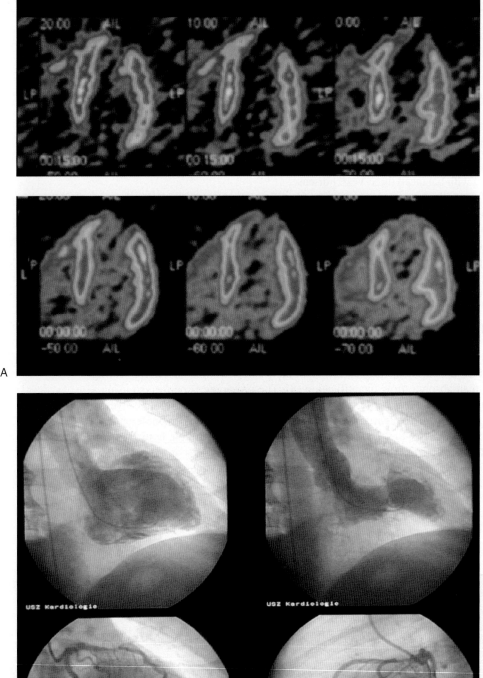

Figure 12-2. Cardiac horizontal long-axis view in a patient with a large anterior MI. **A: top:** [^{13}N]ammonia PET imaging shows a matched large anterior defect with no perfusion; **bottom:** [^{18}F]FDG PET shows no glucose uptake, indicating a scar. **B:** Comparison of end-diastolic **(left)** and end-systolic **(right)** LV angiography (right anterior oblique projection) shows massive dyskinesia of the anterior wall; angiogram also shows a proximal left anterior descending artery stenosis **(bottom)**.

Pharmacologic Stress. The common drugs used as substitutes for exercise stress testing are dipyridamole (Persantine), adenosine (Adenocard), and dobutamine (Dobutrex). Since the introduction of dipyridamole-induced coronary vasodilation as an adjunct to ^{201}Tl myocardial perfusion imaging (9), pharmacologic interventions have become an important tool in the noninvasive diagnosis of CAD.

Intravenous dipyridamole induces coronary vasodilation indirectly by inhibiting cellular uptake of adenosine. This subsequently causes an increase in blood and tissue levels of adenosine, a potent, direct coronary vasodilator that markedly increases coronary blood flow. Pharmacologically induced flow increase is of lesser magnitude through stenotic arteries, thus creating heterogeneous myocardial perfusion that can be visualized with a perfusion tracer. This mechanism may exist independently of myocardial ischemia, but in some patients true myocardial ischemia can occur with either dipyridamole or adenosine because of a coronary steal phenomenon. The accuracy of myocardial perfusion imaging with pharmacologic and physical stress has been found to be equal (10). Left bundle branch block may lead to false-positive septal defects when physical but not when pharmacologic stress is used (11). Before using dipyridamole or adenosine, patients must fast for 4 to 8 hours because of potential side effects of the stressors, such as nausea, vomiting, and hypotension. In addition, they must refrain from caffeine-containing foods and beverages or aminophylline-containing drugs within 24 hours before the imaging study to prevent interference with the hyperemic effect.

High doses of dobutamine (20 to 40 g/kg/min) elicit a secondary increase in MBF by increasing the three main determinants of myocardial oxygen demand, namely, heart rate, systolic blood pressure, and myocardial contractility. Although the achieved flow increase (two- to threefold above baseline) is less than what is elicited by the above mentioned direct vasodilators, it is sufficient to cause heterogeneous perfusion using radionuclide imaging. Overall, accuracy is in the same range as testing with exercise, dipyridamole, or adenosine. Despite frequent side effects, it appears to be relatively safe.

Accuracy. Several studies have demonstrated the high diagnostic accuracy of using ^{82}Rb or [^{13}N]ammonia for the detection of CAD. After animal studies indicated that this technique is sensitive for the detection of regional coronary artery lesions, the first clinical study by Schelbert et al. (12) confirmed these observations, demonstrating the high sensitivity and specificity of this approach in a selected patient population. A similar diagnostic performance was found using ^{82}Rb and [^{13}N]ammonia in a larger patient population (8). These promising results have been reproduced by several groups using either [^{13}N]ammonia or ^{82}Rb (13,14). From these studies, an average sensitivity of 92% and specificity of 88% can be derived.

Although these data indicate the diagnostic superiority of PET over SPECT imaging, one has to interpret these data with caution for several reasons: Most reports on the diagnostic accuracy of myocardial perfusion imaging have used sensitivity and specificity values requiring binary (positive or negative) classification of both perfusion imaging and coronary

TABLE 12-1. *Assessment of hibernating myocardium: prognostic impact of PET*

Study	n	Follow-up (y)	Clinical outcome
Eitzman et al. (26)	82	1	Cardiac events with revascularization 23% vs. 50% without revascularization
Tamaki et al. (27)	84	2	Enhanced [^{18}] FDG uptake best prognostic predictor
Yoshida and Gould (28)	35	3	Viability and infarct size best prognostic predictor
DiCarli et al. (29)	79	1	Survival rate after revascularization 88% vs. 58% without revascularization
Lee et al. (30)	129	2	Nonfatal cardiac events after revascularization 88% vs. 58% without revascularization

angiographic results. This approach, however, has several inherent limitations that need to be mentioned:

1. CAD is not an all-or-none condition but has a continuous spectrum of severity by both SPECT and PET.
2. My colleagues and I (15) and others (16) have shown that percentage diameter narrowing is not an adequate standard for quantifying stenosis severity because of the hemodynamic importance of absolute diameter, integrated length effects, shape, and functional integrity of the endothelium.
3. As with any test in medicine, sensitivity and specificity values are determined by the prevalence and—in perfusion imaging—the severity of the disease in the study population (17).

Furthermore, it is very difficult to perform a true comparative study between clinically established diagnostic tests and new imaging modalities. The results of the established tests are most likely used in the clinical decision-making process (e.g., indication for coronary angiography). This has been referred to as verification or posttest bias affecting the apparent accuracy of a test (18). This bias results when a newly introduced technology is evaluated after physicians have begun to rely on its results and no longer require verification of them. Thus, patients with positive tests are more likely to have their results verified (in this case, by undergoing angiography), while those with negative tests are rarely referred for subsequent studies. This practice will increase apparent sensitivity because false-negative results are unlikely to be discovered. Conversely, specificity will decrease because true-negative results will be less likely to be confirmed and therefore will be underrepresented.

An elegant possibility to overcome some of these problems is to directly compare PET with SPECT imaging in the same patient population. However, only few such studies exist: The first study in 51 selected patients with a prevalence for CAD of greater than 90% reported a sensitivity of 96% for ^{201}Tl SPECT and 98% for [82]Rb PET (19). The lack of difference between the two techniques could be explained by the magnitude of the defects, which were large enough to be detected equally even by the inferior technique (20). A global specificity for this study is not available due to the low number (n=3) of patients without CAD. In a study from the Cleveland Clinic, [82]Rb PET proved to be significantly more sensitive than ^{201}Tl SPECT (95% versus 79%) using coronary angiography as the "gold standard" (13). In a study from the University of Michigan, there was a significant improvement in specificity when ^{201}Tl SPECT (53%) and [82]Rb PET (85%) were compared (14).

Based on available results of PET studies, a joint task force of the ACC and the AHA, together with the Society of Nuclear Medicine, has appreciated a sensitivity of 87% to 97% and a specificity of 78% to 100% for PET compared to a sensitivity of 89% and a specificity of 76% for SPECT (5). Although it is clear that PET provides valuable diagnostic information, larger, more definitive comparative studies with comparable expertise in both PET and SPECT imaging are required to determine the relative diagnostic efficacy of the two techniques. Thus, at present, PET is a competitive tool for the evaluation of CAD. Its replacement potential will mainly depend on its cost effectiveness compared to SPECT.

PET and Preclinical CAD

PET has been shown to allow noninvasive and accurate quantitative measurement of regional MBF if suitable tracers are used and appropriate mathematical models are applied. Baseline and hyperemic MBF measurements allow the assessment of coronary vasodilator reserve ($CVR = MBF_{hyperemia}/MBF_{baseline}$), an integrated parameter of endothelial function and vascular smooth muscle relaxation. PET has been widely used to assess CVR in healthy volunteers and patients with CAD, coronary risk factors, or other cardiac diseases (21). In the past few years, remarkable advances have been achieved in vascular biology. Critical mechanisms in the evolution of CAD have been unraveled, and fundamentals of combating CAD and preventing, or even reversing, its progression have been established.

In this particular area, PET can play a potentially pivotal role in risk stratification, disease management, and monitoring of effects of different interventions. Initial findings have been promising. For example, measurement of CVR with PET has been used to assess the effect of pharmacologic interventions, such as alpha- and beta-blockade, lipid lowering, and cardiovascular conditioning. PET-based measurement of MBF offers a means of probing coronary vasomotion and, even more important, a test of early, evolving but preclinical atherosclerosis.

Hibernating Myocardium

Clinical Context. The assessment of myocardial viability is an issue of emerging clinical relevance in the current era of thrombolytic therapy and coronary revascularization in selected patients. There is a subset of patients in whom LV function improves significantly after coronary revascularization procedures. These clinical observations have led to the concept that myocardium may adapt to chronic ischemia by decreasing its contractility, matching the reduced perfusion with reduced energy demand and thereby preserving viability. This response of myocardial tissue to chronic reduction in coronary blood flow has been described as "hibernating myocardium" (22). If the ischemia is relieved, the myocardium regains normal contractility. From the earliest days of coronary artery bypass grafting, it was reported that impaired ventricular function was improved by operation, supporting the hypothesis of jeopardized but viable myocardium. Myocardium in which normal contractility may be restored often coexists with areas of infarcted, or scar, tissue, leading to the definition of hypoperfused hibernating myocardium as viable myocardium. To identify viable myocardium is of most value in patients with the greatest impairment of LV function and areas of myocardial asynergy, where revascularization improves contractility to the greatest degree and improves survival, although the risk associated with coronary revascularization in these patients is higher.

Diagnostic Role of PET. Much effort has gone into developing strategies to assess myocardial viability with a view to identifying patients who are most likely to benefit from aggressive revascularization. PET has led the way in this regard and has provided insight into the pathophysiology of the adaptation. Using fluorodeoxyglucose tagged with fluorine 18 ([18F]FDG), which measures myocardial glucose utilization, it is possible to identify myocardial tissue that is hypoperfused at rest with preserved or increased glucose uptake. Once it has been phosphorylated by hexokinase, [18F]FDG is not metabolized further and therefore accumulates in tissue, providing a strong positive signal that can be readily identified. Thus, an increased uptake of [18F]FDG in relation to myocardial perfusion, or flow–metabolism mismatch, is indicative of hibernating myocardium (Fig. 12-3), whereas matched defects are indicative of scar (Fig. 12-4). The positive and negative predictive values have been reported to range from 80% to 85% (23,24). Early after MI, the positive predictive value might be low due to reactive inflammation with increased glucose and [18F]FDG uptake (25), suggesting that a viability study should not be carried out within the first couple of weeks after an acute MI.

Prognostic Impact of PET. The prognostic relevance of PET is an important issue not only in the clinical context but also in view of its cost effectiveness. Several studies have documented PET's diagnostic usefulness with respect to hibernating myocardium as a beneficial effect on prognosis (see Table 12-1). Eitzman et al. (26) reported on a follow-up study of 82 patients after MI. Cardiac events (MIs and cardiac deaths) were more numerous in patients with hibernating myocardium. Only 13% of the patients in revascularized group experienced a cardiac event, compared to 50% in the nonrevascularized group. In a study involving 84 patients with CAD by Tamaki et al. (27), a regional increase in [18F]FDG uptake was found to be the best predictor of cardiac events over a period of 2 years after MI. In a follow-up study over 3 years in 35 patients, Yoshida and Gould (28) found that viability and infarct size as assessed by PET were stronger predictive indicators than LV ejection fraction. DiCarli et al. (29) studied the 1-year follow-up in 79 patients with severely depressed LV function. They found that among patients with hibernating

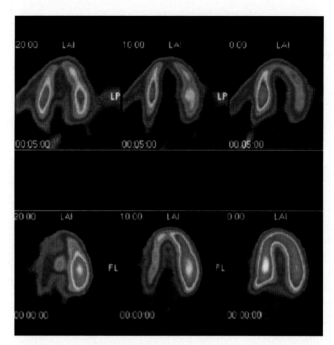

Figure 12-3. Horizontal long-axis view of [^{13}N]ammonia **(top)** and [^{18}F]FDG **(bottom)** scans in a patient after anterior MI. Note the perfusion defect anteriorly with preserved [^{18}F]FDG uptake. This is the classic flow–metabolism mismatch indicative of hibernating myocardium.

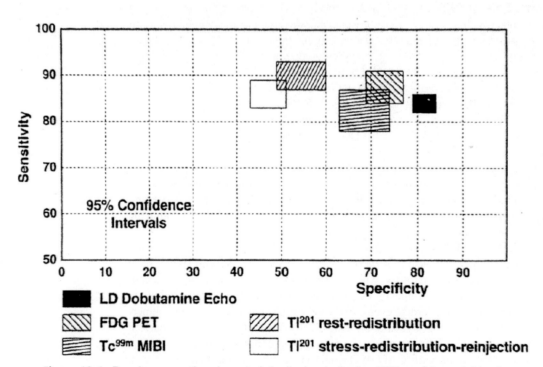

Figure 12-4. Receiver-operating characteristic display, indicating 95% confidence intervals for each technique. The most effective modalities are located closer to the upper right corner of the graph. In this display, the smaller the square, the better the technique. A square (as opposed to a rectangle) indicates a good balance between sensitivity and specificity. A small symbol reflects narrow confidence intervals (LD, low dose). (From ref. 30, with permission.)

TABLE 12-2. *Appraisal/reimbursement status of PET in heart disease*

Disease	German consensus classification	USZ classification	Replacement potential	US reimbursement status Medicare/BC-BS	Swiss reimbursement status
Heart Imaging					
Coronary artery disease (CAD); unclear other investigations	1a	3	3	yes/yes	no
Before heart transplantation	—	4	3	yes/yes	yes
Hibernating myocardium	1a	4	3	yes/yes	yes
Coronary three vessel disease	—	4	3	yes/yes	yes

See page 8-6 abbreviations and appraisal scheme explanations.

myocardium, those who had not had revascularization had a lower survival rate after 1 year (59%), compared to those who had revascularization (88%). Lee et al. (30) compared the effect of medical versus surgical treatment in 129 patients with hibernating myocardium over a period of 2 years after MI. In the medically treated group, 48% had nonfatal cardiac events, but only 8% in the surgically treated group had done so. These studies are summarized in Table 12-1 to underline their importance for clinical decision making, despite their retrospective nature. There have been no prospective studies of the prognostic implication of revascularizing hibernating myocardium. However, the higher mortality in patients with evidence of hibernating myocardium who do not undergo revascularization supports the concept that revascularization improves the prognosis in such patients.

Comparison to Other Techniques. Nuclear imaging techniques for detecting hibernating myocardium rely on the demonstration of membrane integrity or residual metabolic activity within the hibernating areas. Thus, various radionuclides with different physical and physiologic characteristics can be used for this purpose. Both ^{201}Tl-chloride and ^{99m}Tc-sestamibi have proven useful for assessing myocardial viability. In addition, echocardiography performed during the infusion of increasing doses of dobutamine is a widely used and accurate method of detecting hibernating myocardium and predicting regional and global recovery of function after revascularization. However, none of the currently available techniques for the identification of myocardial viability can be considered unequivocally superior to the others (31). All these techniques have equivalent sensitivity, but the specificity is highest with dobutamine echocardiography and lowest with ^{201}Tl studies. The accuracy of these techniques may vary with the severity of LV dysfunction. In the absence of a prospective evaluation of cost effectiveness, the initial approach to the preoperative study of patients with CAD and LV dysfunction can be either stress echocardiography or nuclear imaging with SPECT or PET, depending on availability and expertise. Other promising new approaches currently under evaluation are metabolic imaging with SPECT, myocardial contrast echocardiography, and MR imaging.

REFERENCES

1. Zir LM, Miller SW, Dinsmore RE, Gilbert JP, Harthorne JW. Interobserver variability in coronary angiography. *Circulation* 1976;53:627–632.
2. McPherson DD, Hiratzka LF, Lamberth WC, et al. Delineation of the extent of coronary atherosclerosis by high-frequency epicardial echocardiography. *N Engl J Med* 1987;316:304–309.
3. Mann JM, Davies MJ. Assessment of the severity of coronary artery disease at postmortem examination: are the measurements clinically valid? *Br Heart J* 1995;74:528–530.
4. Gould KL, Kirkeeide RL, Buchi M. Coronary flow reserve as a physiologic measure of stenosis severity. *J Am Coll Cardiol* 1990;15:459–474.
5. Guidelines for the American College of Cardiology/American Heart Association task force on assessment of diagnostic and therapeutic cardiovascular procedures (committee on radionuclide imaging), developed in collaboration with the American Society of Nuclear Cardiology. *J Am Coll Cardiol* 1995;25:521–547.
6. Bergmann SR, Fox KA, Rand AL, et al. Quantification of regional myocardial blood flow *in vivo* with H$_2$^{15}O. *Circulation* 1984;70:724–733.
7. Committee on Advanced Cardiac Imaging and Technology, Council on Clinical Cardiology, American Heart Association; Cardiovascular Imaging Committee, American College of Cardiology; and Board of Directors,

Cardiovascular Council, Society of Nuclear Medicine. Standardization of cardiac tomographic imaging. *Circulation* 1992;86:338–339.

8. Demer LL, Gould KL, Goldstein RA, et al. Assessment of coronary artery disease severity by positron emission tomography: comparison with quantitative arteriography in 193 patients. *Circulation* 1989;79:825–835.

9. Gould KL, Westcott RJ, Albro PC, Hamilton GW. Noninvasive assessment of coronary stenoses by myocardial imaging during pharmacologic coronary vasodilatation. II. Clinical methodology and feasibility. *Am J Cardiol* 1978;41:279–287.

10. Nguyen T, Heo J, Ogilby JD, Iskandrian AS. Single-photon emission computed tomography with thallium-201 during adenosine-induced coronary hyperemia: correlation with coronary arteriography, exercise thallium imaging and two-dimensional echocardiography. *J Am Coll Cardiol* 1990;16:1375–1383.

11. Rockett JF, Wood WC, Moinuddin M, Loveless V, Parrish B. Intravenous dipyridamole thallium-201 SPECT imaging in patients with left bundle branch block. *Clin Nucl Med* 1990;15:401–407.

12. Schelbert HR, Wisenberg G, Phelps ME, et al. Noninvasive assessment of coronary stenoses by myocardial imaging during pharmacologic coronary vasodilation. VI. Detection of coronary artery disease in human beings with intravenous N-13 ammonia and positron computed tomography. *Am J Cardiol* 1982;49:1197–1207.

13. Go RT, Marwick TH, MacIntyre WJ, et al. A prospective comparison of rubidium-82 PET and thallium-201 SPECT myocardial perfusion imaging utilizing a single dipyridamole stress in the diagnosis of coronary artery disease. *J Nucl Med* 1990;31:1899–1905.

14. Stewart RE, Schwaiger M, Molina E, et al. Comparison of rubidium-82 positron emission tomography and thallium-201 SPECT imaging for detection of coronary artery disease. *Am J Cardiol* 1991;67:1303–1310.

15. Kaufmann P, Frielingsdorf J, Mandinov L, Hess OM. Influence of the culprit lesion on clinical symptoms of coronary artery disease, with special emphasis on exercise data. *Coron Artery Dis* 1998;9:185–190.

16. Brown BG, Bolson E, Frimer M, Dodge HT. Quantitative coronary arteriography: estimation of dimensions, hemodynamic resistance, and atheroma mass of coronary artery lesions using the arteriogram and digital computation. *Circulation* 1977;55:329–337.

17. Turner DA, Battle WE, Deshmukh H, et al. The predictive value of myocardial perfusion scintigraphy after stress in patients without previous myocardial infarction. *J Nucl Med* 1978;19:249–255.

18. Rozanski A, Diamond GA, Berman D, Forrester JS, Morris D, Swan HJ. The declining specificity of exercise radionuclide ventriculography. *N Engl J Med* 1983;309:518–522.

19. Tamaki N, Yonekura Y, Senda M, et al. Value and limitation of stress thallium-201 single photon emission computed tomography: comparison with nitrogen-13 ammonia positron tomography. *J Nucl Med* 1988;29:1181–1188.

20. Gould KL. Clinical cardiac positron emission tomography: state of the art. *Circulation* 1991;84(suppl):I.22–I.36.

21. Camici P, Chiriatti G, Lorenzoni R, et al. Coronary vasodilation is impaired in both hypertrophied and non-hypertrophied myocardium of patients with hypertrophic cardiomyopathy: a study with nitrogen-13 ammonia and positron emission tomography. *J Am Coll Cardiol* 1991;17:879–886.

22. Rahimtoola S. The hibernating myocardium. *Am Heart J* 1989;117:211–221.

23. Tillisch J, Brunken R, Marshall R, et al. Reversibility of cardiac wall-motion abnormalities predicted by positron tomography. *N Engl J Med* 1986;314:884–888.

24. Lucignani G, Paolini G, Landoni C, et al. Presurgical identification of hibernating myocardium by combined use of technetium-99m hexakis 2-methoxyisobutylisonitrile single photon emission tomography and fluorine-18 fluoro-2-deoxy-d-glucose positron emission tomography in patients with coronary artery diesase. *Eur J Nucl Med* 1992;19:874–881.

25. Schwaiger M, Brunken R, Grover-McKay M, et al. Regional myocardial metabolism in patients with acute myocardial infarction assessed by positron emission tomography. *J Am Coll Cardiol* 1986;8:800–808.

26. Eitzman D, al-Aouar Z, Kanter HL, et al. Clinical outcome of patients with advanced coronary artery disease after viability studies with positron emission tomography. *J Am Coll Cardiol* 1992;20:559–565.

27. Tamaki N, Kawamoto M, Takashashi N, et al. Prognostic value of an increase in fluorine-18 deoxyglucose uptake in patients with myocardial infarction: comparison with stress thallium imaging. *J Am Coll Cardiol* 1993;22:1621–1627.

28. Yoshida K, Gould KL. Quantitative relation of myocardial infarct size and myocardial viability by positron emission tomography to left ventricular ejection fraction and 3-year mortality with and without revascularization. *J Am Coll Cardiol* 1993;22:984–997.

29. DiCarli MF, Davidson M, Little R, et al. Value of metabolic imaging with positron emission tomography for evaluating prognosis in patients with coronary artery disease and left ventricular dysfunction. *Am J Cardiol* 1994;73:527–533.

30. Lee KS, Marwick TH, Cook SA, et al. Prognosis of patients with left ventricular dysfunction, with and without viable myocardium after myocardial infarction: relative efficacy of medical therapy and revascularization. *Circulation* 1994;90:2687–2694

31. Bax JJ, Wijns W, Cornel JH, Visser FC, Boersma E, Fioretti PM. Accuracy of currently available techniques for prediction of functional recovery after revascularization in patients with left ventricular dysfuncion due to chronic coronary artery disease: comparison of pooled data. *J Am Coll Cardiol* 1997;30:1451–1460.

13

Other Diseases of the Heart

Philipp A. Kaufmann

DILATED CARDIOMYOPATHY

Dilated cardiomyopathy represents a group of conditions with multiple etiologies primarily involving the heart muscle that are not secondary to myocardial ischemia or valvular disease. It leads to heart failure: the inability of the heart to deliver blood and therefore oxygen at a rate commensurate with the requirements of the metabolizing tissues at rest or during exercise. Several cellular and molecular alterations have been identified in the failing heart that support the concept of progressive myocardial overload contributing to a chronic energy deficit and setting up a vicious cycle. This has prompted interest in the evaluation of left ventricular (LV) performance in relation to myocardial oxygen consumption, so called mechanical efficiency. PET using acetate tagged with radioactive carbon (^{11}C-acetate) provides a unique noninvasive tool for the evaluation of myocardial oxygen consumption in conjunction with ventricular performance as assessed by angiography, echocardiography, or radionuclide angiography. The PET-derived ^{11}C-acetate kinetic approach has provided objective means for evaluating the effects of acute therapy on the metabolic and hemodynamic performance of the heart and may improve the ability to optimize therapy in patients with heart failure.

PRIMARY AND SECONDARY LEFT VENTRICULAR HYPERTROPHY

Recently, my colleagues and I found reduced epicardial coronary vasodilator capacity in patients with LV hypertrophy secondary to aortic stenosis (1). Accordingly, coronary flow reserve as assessed with PET has been found to be blunted in patients with primary and secondary LV hypertrophy. This has major clinical implications, since up to two-thirds of patients with hypertrophic cardiomyopathy die suddenly, most probably due to (subendocardial) ischemia. In fact, it was with PET that subendocardial hypoperfusion was first shown

P. A. Kaufmann: Nuclear Medicine and Cardiology, University Hospital, CH-8091 Zurich, Switzerland.

in patients with hypertrophic cardiomyopathy (2). Consequently, the specific beneficial role of calcium channel blockers in this setting was again first documented using PET (3). Surgical management of hypertrophic obstructive cardiomyopathy was introduced in the late 1950s by Cleland (4). The perioperative mortality rate varied between 1.3% and 17.6% in the elderly. Five- and 10-year survival rates, including perioperative mortality, of 96% and 84% were reported (5), and the tendency was toward fewer sudden cardiac deaths after surgery than with medical treatment. The mechanism of these favorable results is not clear. The postoperative decrease in systolic pressure gradient and LV end-diastolic pressure may be related to regression of secondary hypertrophy with less subendocardial ischemia after removal of the pressure burden. If improved myocardial perfusion and metabolism after surgical therapy could be observed, these findings would contribute essentially to risk stratification and therapeutic-strategy decision making, with a particular benefit for patients at high risk of sudden cardiac death. Recently, we documented a significantly better septal flow reserve after myectomy than with medical treatment (6). Thus, myectomy seems to have a beneficial effect on septal perfusion, suggesting that ischemia plays an important role in the pathogenesis of hypertrophic cardiomyopathy.

COMPLETE TRANSPOSITION OF THE GREAT ARTERIES

Complete transposition of the great arteries (TGA) is a common and potentially lethal form of heart disease in newborns and infants. It is characterized by the origin of the aorta arising from the morphologic right ventricle and that of the pulmonary artery from the morphologic LV. The development of arterial switch operations has greatly improved prognosis for infants with TGA. In this operation, both coronary arteries are transposed to the posterior artery; the aorta and pulmonary arteries are transected, contraposed, and anastomosed. Arterial-switch anatomic correction may be complicated by coronary ostial stenosis and postoperative granuloma obstructing the left main coronary artery at the orifice and requiring surgical removal.

EVALUATION OF CARDIAC RECEPTORS

Heart diseases can alter cardiac receptor density and distribution. This has mainly been demonstrated in samples collected by endomyocardial biopsy, during surgery, or at autopsy. PET now offers the possibility of *in vivo* determination of receptor density in humans. Measurements are based on the synthesis of a radioligand, usually a selective receptor antagonist labeled with a positron-emitting radioisotope. The use of [^{11}C]CGP 12177 for clinical investigation of beta-adrenergic receptors has been validated in patients with dilated cardiomyopathy in whom reduced receptor concentrations were found. Receptor downregulation was also shown in patients with hypertrophic cardiomyopathy and attributed to an impaired uptake mechanism and hence increased local catecholamine levels (7). Similarly, both presynaptic catecholamine reuptake and postsynaptic receptor density have been found to be reduced in patients with idiopathic right ventricular outflow tract tachycardia. Locally increased sympathetic activity may play a major role in the pathophysiology of this tachycardia (8).

REFERENCES

1. Vassalli G, Kaufmann P, Villari B, et al. Reduced epicardial coronary vasodilator capacity in patients with left ventricular hypertrophy. *Circulation* 1995;91:2916–2923.
2. Camici PG, Cecchi RG, Montereggi A, Salvadori PA, Dolara A, L'Abbate A. Dipyridamole-induced subendocardial underperfusion in hypertrophic cardiomyopathy assessed by positron-emission tomography. *Coron Artery Dis* 1991;2:837–841.
3. Gistri R, Cecchi F, Choudhury L, et al. Effect of verapamil on absolute myocardial blood flow in hypertrophic cardiomyopathy. *Am J Cardiol* 1994;74:363–368.

4. Cleland WP. The surgical management of obstructive cardiomyopathy. *J Cardiovasc Surg* 1963;4:4889–4891.
5. Seiler C, Hess OM, Schoenbeck M, et al. Long-term follow-up of medical versus surgical therapy for hypertrophic cardiomyopathy: a retrospective study. *J Am Coll Cardiol* 1991;17:634–642.
6. Ciopor M, Kaufmann P, Turina J, et al. Regional myocardial ischemia in hypertrophic cardiomyopathy: influence of myectomy. *Circulation* 1998;98:I-581[abst].
7. Schafers M, Dutka D, Rhodes CG, et al. Myocardial presynaptic and postsynaptic autonomic dysfunction in hypertrophic cardiomyopathy. *Circ Res* 1998;82:57–62.
8. Schafers M, Lerch H, Wichter T, et al. Cardiac sympathetic innervation in patients with idiopathic right ventricular outflow tract tachycardia. *J Am Coll Cardiol* 1998;32:181–186.

PART IV

Clinical PET Imaging in Body Oncology

14

Head and Neck Cancer and Thyroid Cancer

Hans Ch. Steinert, Georg Kacl, and Gustav K. von Schulthess

HEAD AND NECK TUMORS

Patients with head and neck carcinomas have a poor prognosis, especially with advanced disease. Prognosis depends on local tumor invasion and lymph node involvement. The presence of lymph node metastases, especially on the contralateral side, determines the type of therapy (Fig. 14-1). Accurate preoperative assessment of tumor extent and lymph node involvement is mandatory for planning of therapy in patients with head and neck cancer. The majority of these tumors are squamous cell carcinomas originating in mucosal structures. Endoscopy with multiple biopsies is the key examination for determining the nature and the superficial spread of the disease. Ultrasound (US), computed tomography (CT) and magnetic resonance (MR) imaging provide essential information about tumor localization, size, and locoregional extent.

Positron emission tomography (PET) using fluorodeoxyglucose tagged with fluorine 18 ([18F]FDG) can be used clinically for evaluating patients with an unknown primary, staging lymph node metastases, and detecting recurrent tumors. In the case of an unknown primary and biopsy-proven cervical lymph node metastasis, endoscopy with multiple biopsies will be performed. If no tumor can be detected, imaging is used to search for the primary. Rege et al. (1) and Laubenbacher et al. (2) showed that [18F]FDG PET is superior to MR imaging in the detection of an unknown primary head and neck cancer.

Clinical examination and US are the standard methods for assessing lymph node involvement. CT and MR imaging are also used to evaluate lymph node involvement. Identification of lymph node involvement using these methods is based on lymph node size. This criterion has limited accuracy because small nodes may be malignant and large nodes

H. Ch. Steinert and G. K. von Schulthess: Nuclear Medicine, University Hospital, CH-8091 Zurich, Switzerland.

G. Kacl: Diagnostic Radiology and Nuclear Medicine, Spital Limmattal, CH-8902 Urdorf, Switzerland.

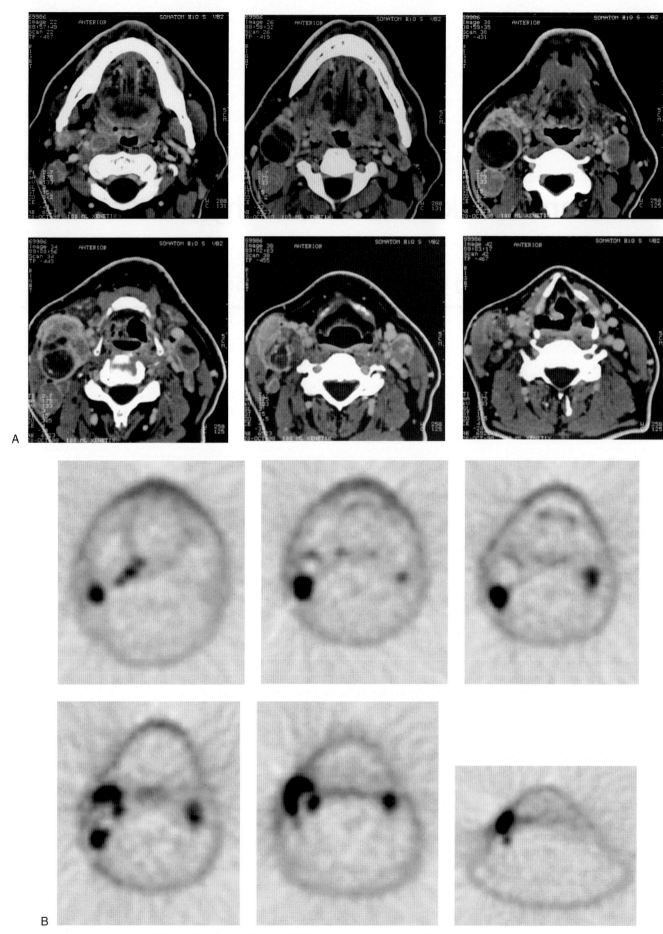

Figure 14-1. A: Corresponding axial CT scans show the centrally necrotic tumor on the right and the left-sided metastasis.

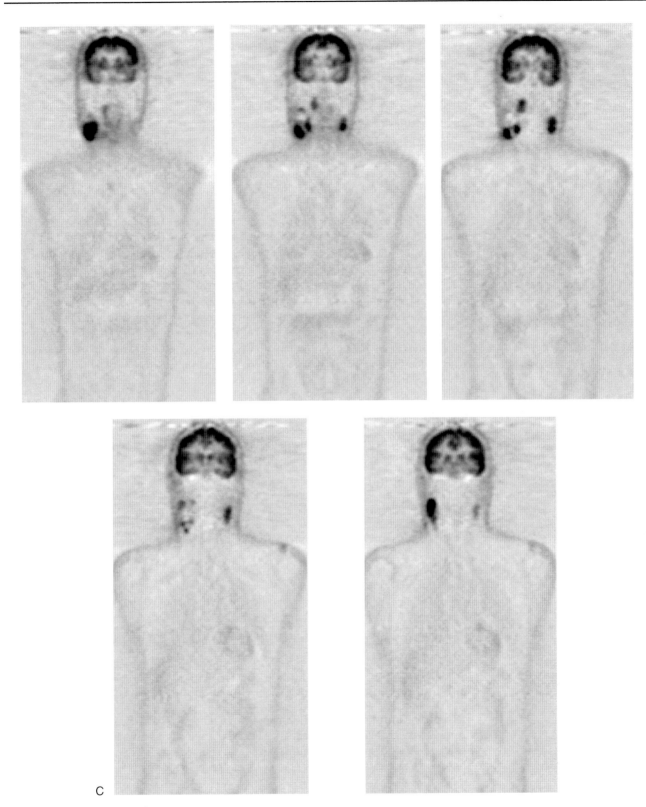

C

Figure 14-1. *(Continued)* A 48-year-old man with biopsy-proven carcinoma of the tonsils on the right and lymph node metastases on both sides, T2N3M0. Axial **(B)** and coronal **(C)** [^{18}F]FDG PET scans demonstrate markedly increased tracer uptake in the primary tumor of the right tonsil and multiple lymph node metastases on both sides.

may be benign. Correct staging is particularly important in these patients because the therapy changes depending on the metastatic spread of the disease. Identification of contralateral lymph node metastases may change the therapeutic regimen. Several studies have shown that [18F]FDG PET is an excellent imaging modality for screening for metastases in patients with head and neck cancer (1–5). Unfortunately, [18F]FDG PET has a significant number of false-positive results due to inflammatory reactions. The main advantage of PET is the detection of unknown contralateral metastases.

A difficult problem in the management of patients with head and neck cancer is the diagnosis of residual or recurrent tumor after therapy. When a suspicious lesion is identified by means of physical examination and confirmed to be malignant with biopsy, the role of imaging is limited. In recurrent tumors presenting as masses, anatomic imaging with CT and MR imaging is used to evaluate deep tumor extension. [18F]FDG PET seems to be most effective in detecting recurrence when no lesion is identified by means of the physical examination. In this situation, MR imaging and CT are limited because of tissue edema and fibrosis after surgical resection or irradiation. In comparison with anatomic methods, [18F]FDG PET has an improved diagnostic accuracy for recurrent head and neck cancers (1,2,6). When [18F]FDG PET imaging is suspicious for a recurrence, biopsy and anatomic imaging must be performed for therapeutic planning. When [18F]FDG PET is negative, the patient might be clinically followed without obtaining MR imaging or CT.

The question is whether an increased [18F]FDG uptake might be seen in a previously irradiated field, thus making differentiation between recurrent disease and postirradiation changes questionable. Greven et al. (7) reported that increased [18F]FDG uptake 1 month after irradiation strongly correlates with persistent tumor.

Imaging Protocol

Patient Preparation. Overnight fasting with no breakfast or fasting for at least 4 hours is required before [18F]FDG application.

Data Acquisition

After a 45-minute postinjection uptake phase, the patient is placed in the camera with hands down.

Partial whole-body two-dimensional (2D) acquisition is carried out step by step from pelvis to head.

Acquisition time is 4 minutes per bed position (axial field at view approximately 15 cm) for the emission scan.

With the same position of the patient, transmission scanning with 4-minute acquisition is performed for each bed position.

Image Fusion. Image fusion is usually performed for lesions less than 0.8 cm, if required for surgical resection.

Appraisal of Clinical Relevance of PET in Head and Neck Tumors (Table 14-1)

Primary Tumor. Biopsy will remain the reference standard for verifying malignancy in suspected head and neck cancers. PET can be clinically useful in patients with lymph node metastases of an unknown primary of head and neck cancers.

TABLE 14-1. *Appraisal/reimbursement status of PET in head and neck tumors*

Disease	German consensus classification	USZ classification	Replacement potential	US reimbursement status: Medicare/BC-BS	Swiss reimbursement status
Head/neck cancer: unknown primary	1a	2	2	no/no	no
Head/neck cancer: staging (II or more)	1b	3	3	no/no	no
Head/neck cancer: local recurrence	2a	4	3	no/no	no

See page 8 for abbreviations and appraisal scheme explanations.

Secondary Manifestations. Accurate early staging is essential for treatment planning. Patients considered for curable surgical resection may benefit from PET's defining the full extent of disease—or ruling out surgery if contralateral lymph node metastases are detected.

Tertiary Manifestations. Patients with distant metastases are not candidates for curable surgical resection.

Expected Clinical Consequences from PET Findings. Curable surgical resection is possible for patients without contralateral or distant disease. If the disease is not resectable, chemo- or radiotherapy is considered.

Exceptions. The detection of microscopic foci of metastases is not possible with any imaging method. Possibly false-positive results are caused by infection or inflammation.

THYROID CANCER

Differentiated papillary and follicular thyroid cancer is the most common type of thyroid malignancy and is associated with an excellent overall survival prognosis. The standard treatment for differentiated thyroid cancer is widely established and involves total thyroidectomy, radioiodine treatment, and thyroid-stimulating hormone–suppressive therapy with levothyroxine. The measurement of thyroglobulin (TG) levels is used to follow up the early diagnosis of local recurrence and lymph node or distant metastases. Iodine 131 whole-body scanning is a very specific imaging procedure for identifying local recurrences and metastases. However, not all metastases take up iodine, and awareness of this fact is important for patient management, because metastases can be removed surgically in most instances. It has been suggested that metastases that do not take up radioiodine are less differentiated and therefore unable to concentrate the radionuclide.

$[^{18}\text{F}]$FDG PET is clinically useful in the follow-up of patients with differentiated thyroid carcinoma when there is an increased TG level with a negative $[^{131}\text{I}]$ whole-body scan. $[^{18}\text{F}]$FDG PET seems to be particularly important in patients with oncocytic thyroid carcinoma and with high primary tumor stages (pT3 or pT4). Patients with differentiated thyroid cancer who have undergone thyroidectomy and ablative radioiodine therapy and present with a rising TG level have a very high likelihood of recurrent disease. It is important to localize all tumor manifestations to determine whether the metastases are resectable. In this situation, whole-body scintigraphy with $[^{131}\text{I}]$ is widely used to detect local recurrence or metastases. If radioiodine scans are negative, scintigrams with thallium 201 chloride, technetium 99m sestamibi and indium 111 octreotide are used to obtain the necessary information. Due to low spatial resolution and limited sensitivity, metastases smaller than 1 cm are difficult to detect with these methods.

Several investigators have reported substantial differences in imaging results between $[^{131}\text{I}]$ scintigraphy and $[^{18}\text{F}]$FDG PET. In a study with 41 patients, Feine et al. (8) found alternating uptake ("flip-flop") of $[^{131}\text{I}]$ and $[^{18}\text{F}]$FDG in 30 patients. In patients with elevated TG and negative $[^{131}\text{I}]$ scans, $[^{18}\text{F}]$FDG PET detected metastases with a sensitivity of 94%. Grünwald et al. (9) recommended the clinical use of $[^{18}\text{F}]$FDG PET in all patients with suspected or proven recurrence and/or metastases of differentiated thyroid cancer. If metastases are detected with $[^{131}\text{I}]$, $[^{18}\text{F}]$FDG PET enables detection of coexisting $[^{131}\text{I}]$-negative metastases, particularly in poorly differentiated tumors (Figs. 14-2, 14-3, and 14-4).

Imaging Protocol

Patient preparation, data acquisition, and image fusion are carried out in the same manner as described for head and neck cancers (see "Imaging Protocol" above).

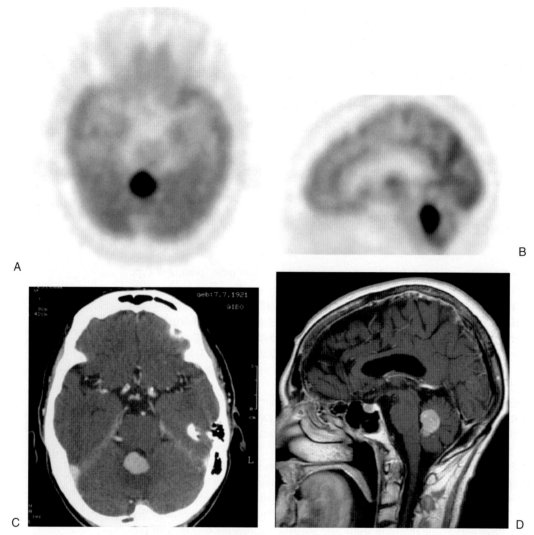

Figure 14-2. A 74-year-old woman with follicular thyroid carcinoma and brain metastases. TG levels were elevated; ^{131}I whole-body scan was negative. Axial **(A)** and sagittal **(B)** [18F]FDG PET scans of the brain demonstrate increased tracer uptake due to a metastasis in the vermis. **C:** Contrast-enhanced axial CT of the posterior fossa shows an oval lesion in the vermis with significant homogeneous contrast enhancement. **D:** Gd-DOTA-enhanced sagittal T1-weighted MR image shows an oval lesion with a maximum diameter of 2 cm in the vermis. There is important contrast enhancement in this lesion, highly suspicious for metastatic disease.

Appraisal of Clinical Relevance of PET in Thyroid Cancer (Table 14-2)

Primary Tumor. PET is not indicated. US, scintigraphy, and biopsy are well established tests for the initial diagnosis of thyroid cancer.

Secondary and Tertiary Manifestations. [18F]FDG PET is relevant in the follow-up of patients with differentiated thyroid carcinoma with an increased TG level and a negative [131I] whole-body scan.

Expected Clinical Consequences from PET Findings. Patients with [131I]-negative but [18F]FDG-positive metastases are probably candidates for surgery or radiotherapy. PET is important developing a more evidence-based treatment strategy.

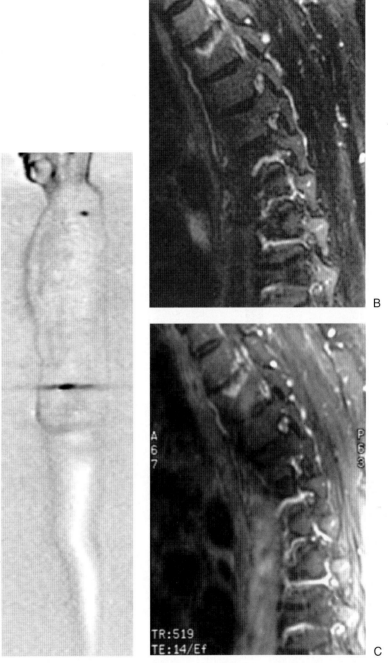

Figure 14-3. A 59-year-old man with papillary thyroid cancer. TG levels were elevated; ^{131}I whole-body scan was negative. **A:** Sagittal [^{18}F]FDG PET scan shows increased tracer uptake into a bone metastasis of the upper thoracic vertebral column. **B:** T2-weighted, fast spin-echo (SE) sagittal spinal MR image (TR 3500 ms/TE 108 ms) demonstrates a rim-like hyperintense lesion in the third thoracic vertebral body. **C:** T1-weighted, fat-saturated SE sagittal MR image (TR 519 ms/TE 14 ms) after Gd-DOTA administration shows rim-like contrast uptake of the vertebral lesion.

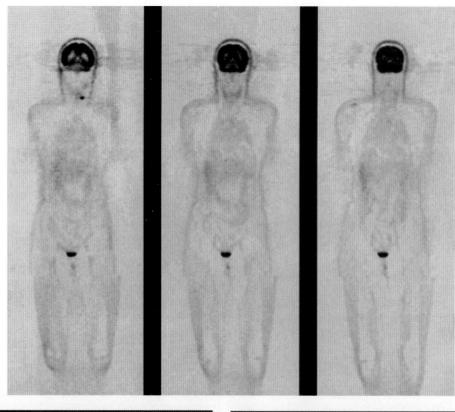

A

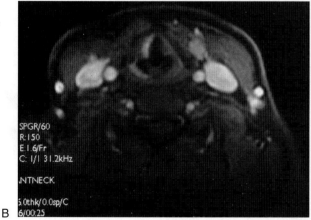

B

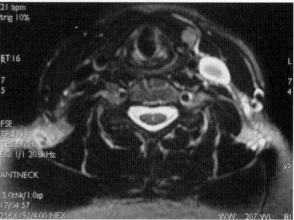

C

Figure 14-4. A 50-year-old woman with follicular-oncocytic thyroid cancer, renewed elevation of TG levels 10 years after initial diagnosis and therapy, and negative ^{131}I whole-body scan (not shown). **A:** Coronal [^{18}F]FDG PET scans show increased tracer uptake into a right paratracheal lymph node. **B:** Gd-DOTA-enhanced T1-weighted transaxial MR image (TR 150 ms/TE 10 ms, flip 60 degrees). **C:** T2-weighted, fat-saturated fast SE transaxial MR image, (TR 5714 ms/TE 96 ms) shows a lesion that was prospectively overlooked on MR imaging.

TABLE 14-2. *Appraisal/reimbursement status of PET in staging thyroid cancer*

Disease	German consensus classification	USZ classification	Replacement potential	US reimbursement status: Medicare/BC-BS	Swiss reimbursement status
Diff. thyroid cancer, neg I-131, el. TG	1a	4	3	no/no	no

See page 8 for abbreviations and appraisal scheme explanation.

REFERENCES

1. Rege S, Maass A, Chaiken L, et al. Use of positron emission tomography with fluorodeoxyglucose in patients with extracranial head and neck cancers. *Cancer* 1994;73:3047–3058.
2. Laubenbacher C, Saumweber D, Wagner-Manslau C, et al. Comparison of fluorine-18-fluorodeoxyglucose PET, MRI, and endoscopy for staging head and neck squamous-cell carcinomas. *J Nucl Med* 1995;36:1747–1757.
3. Jabour BA, Choi Y, Hoh CK, et al. Extracranial head and neck: PET imaging with 2-(F-18)-fluoro-2-deoxy-d-glucose and MR imaging correlation. *Radiology* 1993;186:27–35.
4. Braams JW, Pruim J, Freling NJL, et al. Detection of lymph node metastases of squamous cell cancer of the head and neck with FDG-PET and MRI. *J Nucl Med* 1995;36:211–216.
5. Minn H, Lapela M, Klemi PJ, et al. Prediction of survival with fluorine-18-fluorodeoxyglucose and PET in head and neck cancer. *J Nucl Med* 1997;38:1907–1911.
6. Anzai Y, Carroll WR, Quint, et al. Recurrence of head and neck cancer after surgery or irradiation: prospective comparison of 2-deoxy-2-(F-18)fluoro-d-glucose PET and MR imaging diagnoses. *Radiology* 1996;200:135–141.
7. Greven KE, Williams DW, Keyes JW, et al. Positron emission tomography of patients with head and neck carcinoma before and after high-dose irradiation. *Cancer* 1994;74:1355–1359.
8. Feine U, Lietzenmayer R, Hanke JP, Held J, Wöhrle H, Müller-Schauenburg W. Fluorine-18-FDG and iodine-131-iodide uptake in thyroid cancer. *J Nucl Med* 1996;37:1468–1472.
9. Grünwald F, Schomburg A, Bender H, et al. Fluorine-18 fluorodeoxyglucose positron emission tomography in the follow-up of differentiated thyroid cancer. *Eur J Nucl Med* 1996;23:312–319.

15

Tumors of the Chest

Hans Ch. Steinert and Georg Kacl

LUNG CARCINOMA

Lung carcinoma is one of the leading causes of death from cancer in all parts of the world. The frequency of this tumor is increasing. In the United States, death in women from lung cancer now exceeds death from breast carcinoma. The prognosis depends mainly on the histologic type and tumor stage at initial diagnosis.

Positron emission tomography (PET) using fluorodeoxyglucose tagged with fluorine 18 ([18F]FDG) is clinically used to differentiate benign from malignant focal pulmonary abnormalities, to stage mediastinal and extrathoracic metastases, and to identify recurrence.

Focal Pulmonary Abnormalities

Lung masses have traditionally been evaluated with plain chest x-rays, computed tomography (CT), and, more recently, magnetic resonance (MR) imaging. Some radiographic parameters, such as calcifications and smooth margins, may indicate a higher likelihood that a solitary nodule is benign, although a substantial portion remains radiographically indeterminate. Factors increasing the probability of malignancy include size, absence of calcification, and irregular margins (Fig. 15-1). Unchanged radiographic findings at follow-up examinations over a 2-year period imply that a lesion is benign. Definite diagnoses are established with invasive techniques such as bronchoscopy, mediastinoscopy, and biopsy. If the lesion is benign, nondiagnostic biopsy results are not uncommon.

The ability of PET to distinguish between benign and malignant lesions is high, but not perfect. For benign lesions, Patz et al. (1) demonstrated a very high specificity of [18F]FDG PET. Gupta et al. (2) showed that [18F]FDG PET is highly accurate in differentiating ma-

H. Ch. Steinert: Nuclear Medicine, University Hospital, CH-8091 Zurich, Switzerland.

G. Kacl: Diagnostic Radiology and Nuclear Medicine, Spital Limmattal, CH-8902 Urdorf, Switzerland.

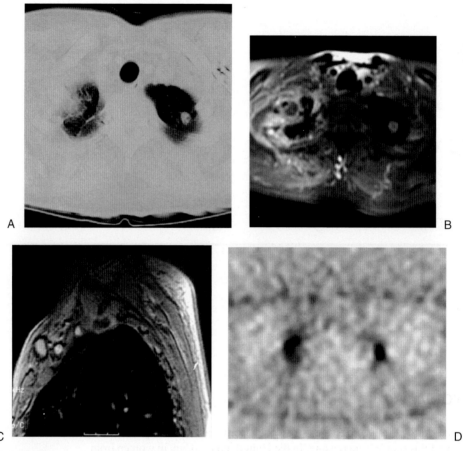

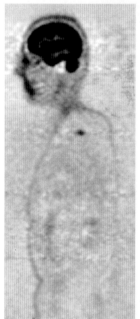

Figure 15-1. Surgically proved recurrence of a right-sided Pancoast's tumor with a contralateral intrapulmonary metastasis in the upper lobe in a 44-year-old man. **A:** Apical axial CT scan of the chest, lung window: irregular, scarred, 2-cm-diameter lesion in the right apex after resection of a Pancoast's tumor. There is a contralateral rounded 1-cm-diameter subpleural lesion in the apicoposterior segment. **B:** Corresponding Gd-DOTA-enhanced, T1-weighted spin-echo fat-saturation apical axial MR image (TR, 480 ms/TE 20 ms): inhomogeneous contrast uptake in the pleura and the adjacent soft tissues of the right apex. A contralateral apical round lesion shows similar contrast enhancement. **C:** Gd-DOTA-enhanced, T1-weighted gradient-echo dynamic sagittal MR of the right apex (TR 150 ms/TE 1.7 ms, flip angle 60 degrees): 2-cm-diameter, lobulated mass with peripheral contrast enhancement located in the apical soft tissues of the thoracic dome, typical for a recurrent Pancoast's tumor. Corresponding axial **(D)** and sagittal **(E)** [^{18}F]FDG PET scans demonstrate markedly increased tracer uptake in both upper lobes.

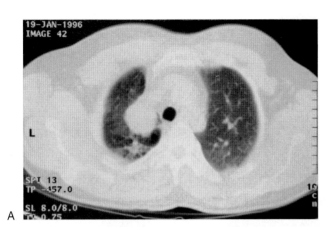

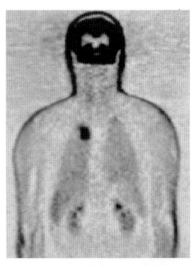

Figure 15-2. Surgically proved NSCLC in a 55-year-old woman with a history of tuberculosis. **A:** Axial CT scan of the upper chest, lung window: 4-cm-diameter, irregular right apical tumor close to the innominate vein and the trachea. There is posterior stellate subpleural scarring in the vicinity of the tumor. Differentiation between tumor spread and old tuberculous remnants is not possible. **B:** Coronal [18F]FDG PET scan demonstrates markedly increased [18F]FDG uptake in the right upper lobe. No other lesions with increased uptake are detected.

lignant from benign solitary pulmonary nodules (0.6 to 3 cm) when radiographic findings were indeterminate. In a series of 61 patients, [18F]FDG PET had a sensitivity of 93% and a specificity of 88% for detecting malignancy. [18F]FDG PET is also effective in detecting recurrence after previous lung resection or irradiation (3). It must be kept in mind that [18F]FDG PET may show negative results for bronchioloalveolar lung carcinoma (4).

[18F]FDG PET is clinically useful in patients with a solitary pulmonary nodule less than 3 cm in diameter, especially when biopsy may be risky or the patient has a low risk for malignancy based on the history or radiographic findings. Lesions with low [18F]FDG uptake can be considered benign and monitored with chest radiographs. Lesions with increased [18F]FDG uptake should be considered malignant, although false-positive results have been reported in cases of inflammatory and infectious processes, such as histoplasmosis, aspergillosis, or active tuberculosis (Figs. 15-2, 15-3, 15-4, and 15-5).

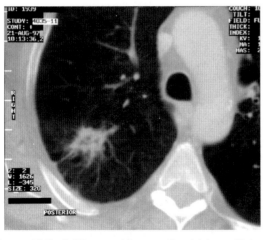

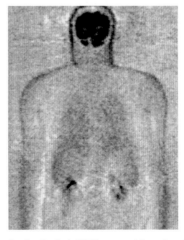

Figure 15-3. A 58-year-old man with a history of tuberculosis. **A:** Axial CT scan of the chest, lung window: 2-cm-diameter, irregular, spiculated lesion located in the posterior segment of the right upper lobe. Pleural scarring is associated with the lesion, which was considered to be malignant. **B:** Sagittal [18F]FDG PET scan demonstrates physiologic [18F]FDG distribution. Biopsy confirmed old tuberculous remnants.

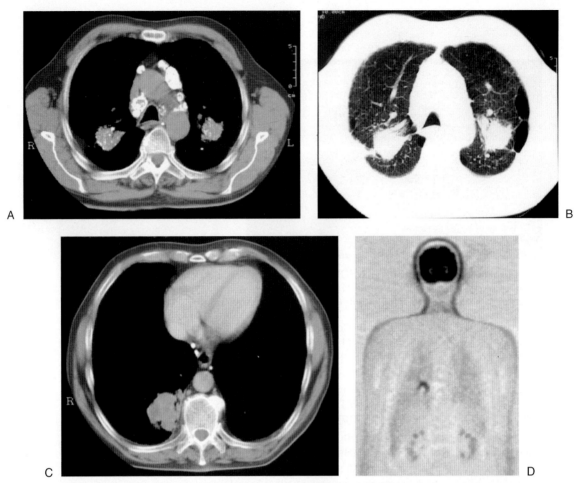

Figure 15-4. Surgically proved NSCLC in the right lower lobe and silicosis in both upper lobes in 72-year-old patient. **A:** Axial CT scan of the aortopulmonary region, soft tissue window: bilateral inhomogeneous, partly calcified pseudotumors in the upper lobes. The right pseudotumor is connected to a pleural thickening with a scar. Multiple bilateral calcified mediastinal lymph nodes are present. **B:** Axial CT scan of the same region, lung window: extensive scarring of the lung parenchyma with subpleural emphysema. There is shrinking of the lung parenchyma around the bilateral spiculated pseudotumors. **C:** Axial CT scan of the basal lung segments, soft issue window: inhomogeneous, irregular-shaped mass with necrotic areas and peripheral contrast enhancement. The 4.5-cm-diameter lesion lies in the right basal lower lobe segment and thickens the pleura. In contradistinction to the pseudotumors of the upper lobes, this lesion is highly suspicious of peripheral bronchial carcinoma. **D:** Sagittal [^{18}F]FDG PET scan demonstrates a circular increased uptake with a central cold spot in the lesion. No increased uptake is seen in the upper lobes.

Staging of Mediastinal Nodes

Accurate mediastinal staging is essential for lung cancer management. Surgical resection is the treatment of choice for early stages of non–small cell lung carcinoma (NSCLC). Due to its rapid dissemination, small cell lung cancer is commonly treated by chemotherapy or irradiation. In NSCLC, patients with ipsilateral mediastinal lymph node metastases (N2 disease) are considered to have potentially resectable disease. If contralateral mediastinal lymph node metastases (N3) exist, surgery is generally not indicated. CT and MR imaging have substantial limitations in depicting mediastinal lymph node metastases. The only CT and MR imaging criteria for tumor involvement are morphologic; that is, the criteria rely on the size and shape of the lymph nodes. However, normal-sized regional lymph nodes may prove to have metastases at histologic examination, and nodal enlargement can be due to reactive hyperplasia or other nonmalignant

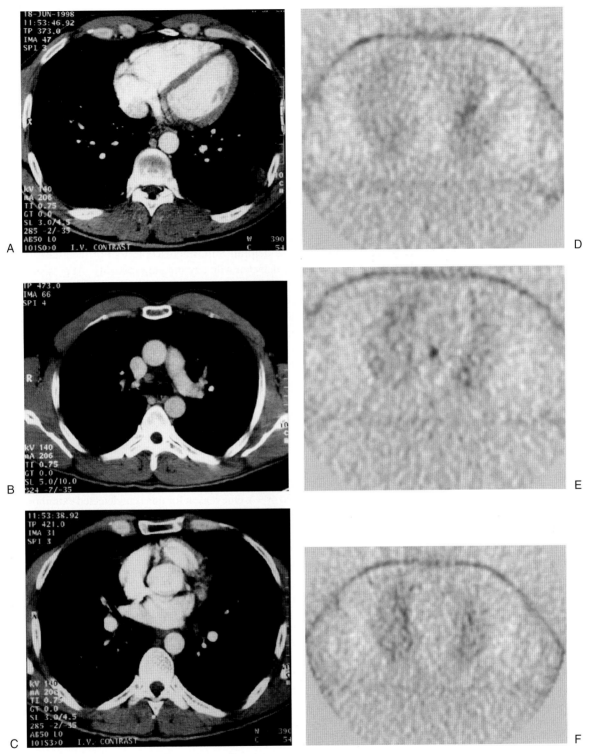

Figure 15-5. Surgically proved histiocytosis in a 39-year-old man. **A:** Axial CT scan of the chest, soft tissue window: 2-cm-diameter subpleural lesion in the left lateral lower lobe segment. The lesion is broadly based on the pleura and shows peripheral contrast enhancement. **B:** Axial CT scan of the mediastinum, soft tissue window: multiple inhomogeneous lymph nodes up to 2 cm in the pretracheal aortopulmonary window. **C:** Axial CT scan of the chest, soft tissue window: 1-cm-diameter oval lesion located subpleurally in the middle lobe segment. All lesions were considered to be malignant. Corresponding axial [^{18}F]FDG PET scans of the lower lobe **(D)**, the aortopulmonary window **(E)**, and the middle lobe segment **(F)**. Only a mediastinal lesion with a slightly increased uptake is seen. No typical [^{18}F]FDG pattern of a lung carcinoma was found.

conditions. The sensitivity and specificity of CT for determining lymph node metastases in NSCLC is 60% to 70% (5,6). Thus, in 30% to 40% of patients, CT will erroneously suggest the presence of mediastinal lymph node metastases and will miss lymph node metastases in 30% to 40% of cases.

In a recent study in which correlative lymph node mapping and extensive nodal sampling were performed, our colleagues and we (7) found that [18F]FDG PET was significantly more accurate than CT in determining nodal status. In a series of 47 patients, [18F]FDG PET assigned the correct N stage in 96% of patients, whereas CT was correct in 79%. Sensitivity was 89% for [18F]FDG PET and 57% for CT for staging of N2 or N3 disease in mediastinal nodes. For exact localization of lymph node metastases, emission and transmission-corrected PET scans were needed, especially in the aortopulmonary and paraaortic node stations. A study by Wahl et al. (8) also found that [18F]FDG PET was significantly more accurate than CT in staging mediastinal lymph node disease.

[18F]FDG PET appears to be superior to CT for mediastinal staging of NSCLC; however, PET is not without limitations. For exact localization of mediastinal lymph nodes, image fusion of PET and CT can be helpful. Still, microscopic foci of metastases within very small lymph nodes cannot be detected with any imaging modality. At present, an imaging strategy that includes both [18F]FDG PET and CT appears to be the best noninvasive means of mediastinal staging in patients with NSCLC (Fig. 15-6). Gambhir et al. (9) showed that this combined strategy resulted in cost savings of $1,154 per patient without a loss of life expectancy, compared to the alternate strategy of CT alone. These effects were the result of improved staging of NSCLC prior to the decision of surgery. An analysis of data presented recently by Dwamena et al. (10) suggested that in the future a strategy involving PET initially may be appropriate when initial imaging using chest x-ray and cytology diagnose NSCLC.

Staging of Extrathoracic Metastases

Despite radical surgical treatment of potentially curable NSCLC, the overall 5-year survival rate remains low (20% to 40%). One reason for this is undetected extrathoracic metastases, which cause underestimation of tumor stage. The most common sites of distant metastases are liver, adrenal glands, bone, and brain. Although the incidence of metastatic disease in NSCLC is high, routine staging of all patients with bone scintigraphy and CT or MR imaging of the head and abdomen is not routinely performed, because the likelihood of a true-positive finding in bone scintigraphy and a CT or MR scan in an asymptomatic patient is small. Using bone scintigraphy as a routine diagnostic method, only 14% of positive focal findings in patients with cancer were caused by a metastasis of the known tumor. In addition, a metaanalysis by Silvestri et al. (11) demonstrated that the negative predictive value for detecting metastatic disease in CT scans in patients with NSCLC is not higher than the clinical evaluation.

Whole-body [18F]FDG PET is a promising tool for screening for distant metastases. In a recent study in which all PET findings were confirmed histologically and/or radiologically, Weder et al. (12) found that whole-body [18F]FDG PET is an accurate imaging modality in detecting previously unknown and unsuspected extrathoracic metastases. A series of 100 patients was studied. Of the 69 patients conventionally staged as N0/N1, six (9%) were classified stage M1 with PET. Seven (28%) of the 25 patients with stage N2 and six of six patients with stage N3 were positive for extrathoracic metastases. No false-positive findings were found. In a series of 99 patients, Valk et al. (13) reported detecting previously unsuspected distant metastases in 11 patients. Previous studies comparing the sensitivity and specificity of [18F]FDG PET and CT scans in the evaluation of metastases of the adrenal gland demonstrated that [18F]FDG PET is more sensitive and specific than CT (14,15). Lewis et al. (16) reported that whole-body [18F]FDG PET changed management to nonsurgical therapy in 18% of patients with NSCLC.

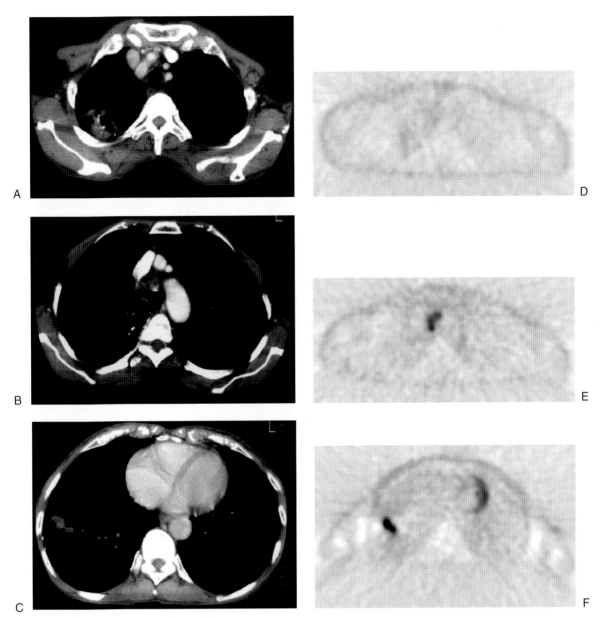

Figure 15-6. Surgically proven NSCLC in the right lower lobe, ipsilateral mediastinal lymph node metastases, and old tuberculous remnants in the right upper lobe in a 67-year-old man. **A:** Apical thoracic axial CT scan, soft tissue window: inhomogeneous, 4.5-cm-diameter, stellate lesion with calcifications in the posterior segment of the upper lobe. The size and shape are suspicious for malignancy, although calcifications signal benign disease. **B:** Axial mediastinal CT scan, soft tissue window: irregular, partly hypodense retrocaval and azygos lymph node cluster with a diameter of 3 cm. **C:** Axial CT scan of the lung base, soft tissue window: 3.5-cm-diameter lobulated subpleural mass located in the right lateral lower lobe segment and extending toward the right hilus. The findings were consistent with peripheral bronchial carcinoma and mediastinal lymph node involvement. Corresponding axial [^{18}F]FDG PET scans of the apical thorax **(D)**, mediastinum **(E)**, and lung base **(F)** show a markedly increased [^{18}F]FDG uptake in the primary tumor in the right lateral lower lobe and in mediastinal lymph node metastases. No significant uptake is seen in the lesion of the upper lobe, characterizing the lesion as benign.

It has been demonstrated that whole-body [^{18}F]FDG PET is an accurate method of screening for mediastinal and distant metastases in patients with newly diagnosed NSCLC. Current imaging methods are inadequate for accurate M-staging of patients, as demonstrated by 10% to 20% of patients upstaged by [^{18}F]FDG PET scanning.

Imaging Protocol

Patient Preparation. Overnight fasting with no breakfast or fasting for at least 4 hours is required before [^{18}F]FDG application.

Data Acquisition

After a 45-minute postinjection uptake phase, the patient is placed in the camera with hands down.

Partial whole-body two-dimensional (2D) acquisition is carried out step by step from pelvis to head.

Acquisition time is 4 minutes per bed position (AFOW approximately 15 cm) for the emission scan.

With the same position of the patient, transmission scanning with 4-minute acquisition is performed for each bed position.

Image Fusion. Image fusion is usually performed for lesions less than 0.8 cm, if required for surgical resection.

Appraisal of Clinical Relevance of PET in Lung Cancer (Table 15-1)

Primary Tumor. [^{18}F]FDG PET has a sensitivity and specificity of 80% to 90% in differentiating between benign and malignant focal pulmonary abnormalities (0.6 to 3 cm) when radiographic findings are indeterminate.

Secondary Manifestations. The indication for [^{18}F]FDG PET is very strong, as it is the best noninvasive means of detecting mediastinal lymph node metastases.

Tertiary Manifestations. The indication for [^{18}F]FDG PET is very strong, as it is the best single test for detecting distant metastases of lung carcinoma (bone, liver, adrenal gland, supraclavicular nodes, brain).

Expected Clinical Consequences from PET Findings. Curable surgical resection is possible for the early stages of NSCLC (stage IIIa or lower, stage T3N2M0 or lower). Patients with contralateral mediastinal lymph node metastases or distant metastases are referred for chemo- or radiotherapy.

Exceptions. [^{18}F]FDG PET has a high sensitivity for detecting metastases. However, the detection of microscopic foci of metastases is not possible with any imaging method. Possibly false-positive results are caused by infection and inflammation.

TABLE 15-1. *Appraisal/reimbursement status of PET in lung cancer*

Disease	German consensus classification	USZ classification	Replacement potential	US reimbursement status: Medicare/BC-BS	Swiss reimbursement status
Nonsmall cell lung cancer NSCLC					
NSCLC, mediastasis lymph node staging	1a	4	3	yes/yes	yes
NSCLC, recurrence	1a	4	4	yes/yes	yes
NSCLC, distant metastases	2b	4	4	yes/yes	yes
Therapy control NSCLC	2a	4	4	yes/yes	yes
Solitary pulmonary nodule (high risk)	1a	3	3	yes/yes	yes

See page 8 for abbreviations and appraisal scheme explanations.

ESOPHAGEAL CANCER

Esophageal cancer has one of the most unfavorable prognoses in digestive malignancies. Most patients have advanced disease at the time of initial diagnosis. Depending on the disease stage and tumor resectabilty, local therapy (surgical resection and/or radiation) or systemic therapy (chemotherapy) is performed. Accurate staging is important for selecting appropriate treatment and for prognostic information. Conventional radiologic imaging (CT, endoscopic ultrasonography, and MR imaging) is inaccurate in detecting locoregional and distant metastases in 30% to 40% of patients. The poor long-term survival of patients after complete tumor resection is in part due to unknown distant metastases at the time of surgery.

[^{18}F]FDG PET

Study results reveal that [^{18}F]FDG PET is more accurate than conventional imaging modalities in staging patients with esophageal cancer. As a rule esophageal carcinomas can be identified by increased tracer accumulation (17) (Fig. 15-7). Flanagan et al. (18) per-

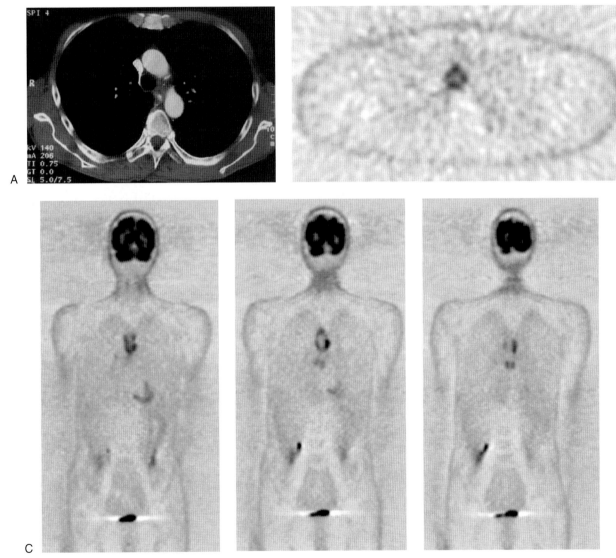

Figure 15-7. Biopsy-proved esophageal carcinoma in a 53-year-old man. **A:** Axial CT scan, soft tissue window: wall thickening of the esophagus with adjacent enlarged lymph nodes. **B:** Corresponding axial [^{18}F]FDG PET scan demonstrates an increased inhomogeneous circular uptake. **C:** Coronal [^{18}F]FDG PET scans shows the extent of the increased uptake in the esophagus.

TABLE 15-2. *Appraisal/reimbursement status of PET in esophageal cancer*

Disease	German consensus classification	USZ classification	Replacement potential	US reimbursement status: Medicare/BC-BS	Swiss reimbursement status
Esophageal cancer	—	3	3	no/no	no

See page 8 for abbreviations and appraisal scheme explanations.

formed whole-body [^{18}F]FDG PET in 35 patients with potentially resectable esophageal cancer. PET detected nine sites of distant metastases missed by conventional scanning. There were 11 false-negative PET scans for small (<1 cm) locoregional nodal metastases. For distant metastases, sensitivity was 88%, specificity 93%, and accuracy 91%. For locoregional nodal metastases, sensitivity was 45%, specificity 100%, and accuracy 48%. The authors concluded that early use of PET in the staging of patients with esophageal cancer could improve treatment planning by identifying previously unknown distant metastases. Block et al. (19) also found that [^{18}F]FDG PET is more sensitive than CT for revealing distant metastases in patients with esophageal cancer.

Imaging Protocol

Patient preparation and data acquisition are carried out in the same manner as described for lung cancer (see "Imaging Protocol" above).

Appraisal of Clinical Relevance of PET in Esophageal Cancer (Table 15-2)

Primary Tumor. [^{18}F]FDG PET has a limited role in identifying the primary tumor.

Secondary Manifestations. There is a possible role for [^{18}F]FDG PET, but small lymph node metastases adjacent to the tumor can be missed.

Tertiary Manifestations. The indication for [^{18}F]FDG PET is strong, as it is probably best single test for detecting distant metastases.

Expected Clinical Consequences from PET Findings. Curable surgical resection is only possible for early stages of esophageal cancer. Patients with distant metastases are referred for chemo- or radiotherapy.

Exceptions. [^{18}F]FDG PET has a high sensitivity for detecting metastases. However, the detection of microscopic metastatic foci is not possible with any imaging method. Possibly false-positive results are caused by infection or inflammation.

REFERENCES

1. Patz EF, Lowe JM, Hoffman JM, et al. Focal pulmonary abnormalities: evaluation with F-18 fluorodeoxyglucose PET scanning. *Radiology* 1993;188:487–490.
2. Gupta NC, Maloof J, Gunel E. Probability of malignancy in solitary pulmonary nodules using flurine-18-FDF and PET. *J Nucl Med* 1996;37:943–948.
3. Inoue, T. Kim EE, Komaki R, et al. Detecting recurrent or residual lung cancer with FDG-PET. *J Nucl Med* 1995;36:788–793.
4. Higashi K, Ueda Y, Seki H, et al. Fluorine-18-FDG imaging is negative in bronchioloalveolar lung carcinoma. *J Nucl Med* 1998;39:1016–1020.
5. Webb WR, Gatsonis C, Zerhouni A, et al. CT and MR imaging in staging non-smal cell bronchogenic carcinoma. Report of the radiologic diagnostic oncology group. *Radiology* 1991;178:705–713.
6. McLoud TC, Bourgouin R, Greenberg RW, et al. Bronchogenic carcinoma: Analysis of staging in the mediastinum with CT by correlative lymph node mapping and sampling. *Radiology* 1992;182:319–323.
7. Steinert HC, Hauser M, Allemann F, et al. Non-small cell lung cancer: Nodal staging with FDG-PET versus CT with correlative lymph node mapping and sampling. *Radiology* 1997;202:441–446.
8. Wahl RL, Quint LE, Greenough RL, Meyer CR, White RI, Orringer MB. Staging of mediastinal non-small cell lung cancer with FDG-PET, CT, and fusion images: Preliminary prospective evaluation. *Radiology* 1994;191:371–377.
9. Gambhir SS, Hoh CK, Phelps ME, Madar I, Maddaahi J. Decision tree analysis for cost-effectiveness of FDG-PET in the staging and management of non-small-cell lung carcinoma. *J Nucl Med* 1996;37:1428–1436.

10. Dwamena BA, Fendrick AM, Wahl RL. Should FDG-PET replace CT or be used complementary to CT in the mediastinal staging of NSCLC: Clinical and economic considerations. *Radiology* 1998;209 (P):290.
11. Silvestri GA, Littenberg B, Colice GL. The clinical evaluation for detecting metastatic lung cancer: A meta-analysis. *Am J Respir Crit Care Med* 1995;152:225–230.
12. Weder W, Schmid R, Bruchhaus H, Hillinger S, von Schulthess GK, Steinert HC. Detection of extrathoracic metastases by positron emission tomography in lung cancer. *Ann Thorac Surg* 1998;66:886–893.
13. Valk PE, Pounds TR, Hopkins DM, et al. Staging non-small cell lung cancer by whole-body positron emission tomographic imaging. *Ann Thorac Surg* 1995;60:1573–1582.
14. Lamki LM. Positron emission tomography, bronchogenic carcinoma, and the adrenals. *AJR* 1997; 168:1361–1362.
15. Erasmus JJ, Patz EF, Mc Adams HP, et al. Evaluation of adrenal masses in patients with bronchogenic carcinoma using 18F-fluorodeoxyglucose positron emission tomography. *AJR* 1997;168:1357–1362.
16. Lewis P, Griffin S, Marsden P, et al. Whole-body 18-F-fluorodeoxyglucose positron emission tomography in preoperative evaluation of lung cancer. *Lancet* 1994;5:1265–1266.
17. Fukunaga T, Okazumi S, Koide Y, Isono K, Imazeki K. Evaluation of esophageal cancers using fluorine-18-fluorodeoxyglucose PET. *J Nucl Med* 1998;39:1002–1007.
18. Flanagan FL, Dehdashti F, Siegel BA, et al. Staging of esophageal cancer with 18F-fluorodeoxyglucose positron emission tomography. *Am J Roentgenol* 1997;168:417–424.
19. Block MI, Patterson GA, Sundaresan RS, et al. Improvement in staging of esophageal cancer with the addition of positron emission tomography. *Ann Thorac Surg* 1997;64:770–777.

16

Breast Carcinoma

Hans Ch. Steinert, Rahel Kubik-Huch, and Gustav K. von Schulthess

Breast carcinoma is the most frequently diagnosed cancer in women in the United States. Currently, in about 50% of patients with breast cancer, recurrence will not be expected, and one-third will die of their disease. The number of axillary lymph node metastases has been identified as the most important prognostic factor. The axillary nodes are considered a filter before cancer cells spread to distant sites. Therefore, axillary lymph node dissection is the standard diagnostic procedure in breast cancer patients. In general, patients with axillary lymph node metastases will receive adjuvant therapy. Another valuable prognostic factor is tumor size, which correlates with the number of positive nodes. The time to the development of metastases becomes shorter as tumor size increases.

The clinical role of positron emission tomography (PET) in patients with breast carcinoma is not yet fully established. PET using fluorodeoxyglucose tagged with fluorine 18 ([18F]FDG) is considered clinically useful in the detection of axillary lymph node metastases in patients with primary tumors larger than 2 cm in diameter (stage pT2) and in the detection of distant metastases in patients with advanced breast cancer.

EVALUATION OF PRIMARY BREAST CARCINOMA

[18F]FDG PET has been used by several investigators to image patients with breast cancer. Wahl et al. (1) reported visualizing all 10 primary breast cancers in patients with known advanced breast carcinomas. The smallest tumor studied was 3.2 cm in diameter. In a study by Nieweg et al. (2), 10 of 11 primary breast cancers were clearly visualized with [18F]FDG PET. However, the smallest tumor detected by PET in this study was 1.8 cm in diameter. Adler et al. (3) undertook a study to evaluate the ability of [18F]FDG PET to discriminate between benign and malignant breast lesions. [18F]FDG PET allowed discrimination of eight benign and 28 malignant breast masses, with a sensitivity of 96% and a specificity of

H. Ch. Steinert and G. K. von Schulthess: Nuclear Medicine, University Hospital, CH-8091 Zurich, Switzerland.

R. Kubik-Huch: Diagnostic Radiology, University Hospital, CH-8091 Zurich, Switzerland.

100%. Due to the low number of benign lesions and the absence of fibroadenomas, hamartomas, and adenomas, the high specificity of this study cannot be generalized. The smallest malignant tumor studied was 1.2×1.5 cm in diameter.

Overall, the role of [^{18}F]FDG PET in the evaluation of primary breast carcinoma is limited. Examination and mammography will continue to be the primary means of detecting breast masses and identifying those suspicious for malignancy. Biopsy is the logical course in verifying malignancy. In patients in whom mammography has limited diagnostic value (e.g., patients with radiodense breasts or implants), [^{18}F]FDG PET may be useful in distinguishing benign from malignant processes.

STAGING OF LOCOREGIONAL LYMPH NODE METASTASES

No imaging modality is currently available for accurate evaluation of axillary lymph node metastases. Computed tomography (CT), ultrasonography, scintigraphy with monoclonal antibodies, and technetium Tc 99m sestamibi have been used for staging axillary lymph node metastases, but none of these techniques shows sufficient sensitivity. Therefore, axillary lymph node dissection is performed as a necessary diagnostic procedure. To avoid misclassifications, at least 8 to 10 nodes must be removed from the lower axilla (levels I and II). The axillary node stations are divided in three levels:

Level I: lymph nodes lateral to the border of the pectoralis minor muscle;
Level II: lymph nodes behind the pectoralis minor muscle;
Level III: lymph nodes medial to the border of the pectoralis minor muscle.

In general, axillary lymph node dissection is well tolerated. Nevertheless, complications are common, including postoperative seroma, edema of the arm and breast, shoulder dysfunction, and nerve injuries. Less aggressive diagnostic procedures providing accurate staging of the axilla would be extremely helpful. The sentinel lymph node biopsy is a promising minimally invasive technique for staging of the axilla without complete axillary dissection (4).

In a study involving 51 women, Avril et al. (5) found that [^{18}F]FDG PET is accurate in detecting axillary lymph node metastases in patients with stage pT2 (tumor size >2 cm) breast cancer and higher. PET was especially valuable in detecting tumor involvement in the upper axilla (level III) and spread to supraclavicular or internal mammary lymph nodes (Fig. 16-1). In 29% of patients, axillary PET imaging provided additional diagnostic information with regard to tumor extension to other sites. However, the sensitivity of [^{18}F]FDG PET imaging of axillary lymph nodes depended on the extent of lymph node involvement and the size of lymph node metastases. If only one lymph node was affected, the sensitivity of PET was 25%. None of the patients with micrometastases was identified. The investigators concluded that axillary [^{18}F]FDG PET could not substitute for histopathologic analysis of axillary lymph nodes in breast cancer patients.

In a recent study, Adler et al. (6) proposed performing high-dose (740 MBq) [^{18}F]FDG PET of the axilla to screen for metastases. In comparison with axillary lymph node dissection findings, PET had a sensitivity of 95%, negative predictive value of 95%, specificity of 66%, and accuracy of 77%. False-positive findings were seen in lymph nodes with extensive sinus histiocytosis, plasmacytosis, and macrophages. It was difficult with PET to exactly determine the number of metastatic lymph nodes, which is an important prognostic factor. Therefore, patients with positive PET findings still require axillary lymph node dissection.

STAGING FOR DISTANT METASTASES

The extent of preoperative screening for metastatic disease depends on the clinical stage of the tumor and the patient's symptoms. The incidence of occult bone metastases detected by

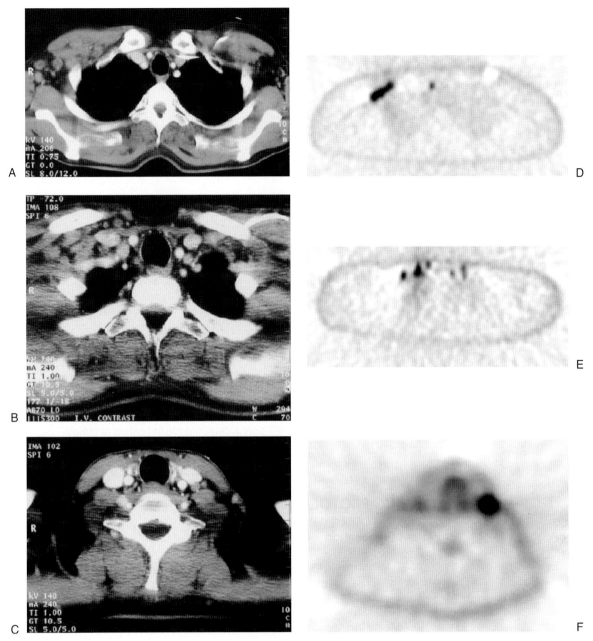

Figure 16-1. Biopsy-proved breast carcinoma on the right and extensive lymph node metastases in a 50-year-old woman. **A:** Thoracic axial CT scan, soft tissue window: enlarged lymph nodes in the right axilla. **B:** Apical axial CT scan of the chest, soft tissue window: multiple normal-sized lymph nodes in a retroclavicular location on the right. **C:** Axial CT scan of the neck demonstrates normal-sized lymph nodes on the left. Corresponding axial [18F]FDG PET scans of the axilla **(D)**, the apical chest **(E)**, and the neck **(F)** demonstrate multiple lymph node metastases in the right axilla, the retro- and supraclavicular region ipsi- and contralaterally, and the cervical region on the left.

scintigraphy is low in patients with early stages. In contrast, bone metastases are found in 25% of asymptomatic patients with stage III disease (T3,N2) using bone scintigraphy. Recently, Cook et al. (7) reported that [18F]FDG PET is superior to bone scintigraphy in detecting osteolytic breast cancer metastases. The value of whole-body PET in the staging of breast cancer patients is still under investigation. Even though whole-body [18F]FDG PET has a large potential to detect distant metastases, the effectiveness of whole-body PET and the selection of specific patient groups must be evaluated in patients with breast cancer.

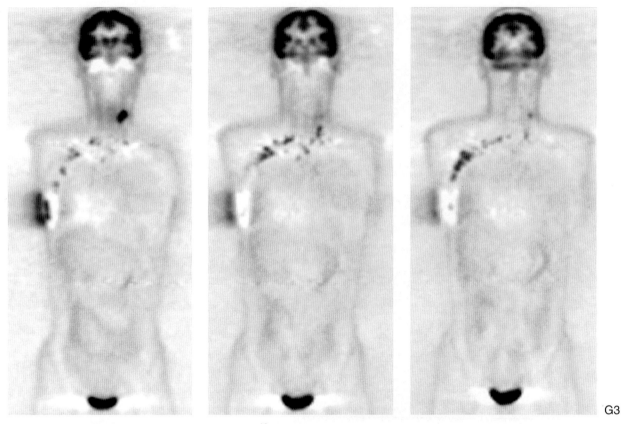

G1, G2   G3

Figure 16-1. *(continued)* **G:** Coronal [^{18}F]FDG PET scans demonstrate the extent of metastases to better advantage.

IMAGING PROTOCOL

Patient Preparation

Overnight fasting with no breakfast or fasting for at least 4 hours is required before [^{18}F]FDG application.

Data Acquisition

Administration of 740 MBq of [^{18}F]FDG through a contralateral arm vein or a foot vein.

After a 45-minute postinjection uptake phase, the patient is placed in the camera with hands down.

Partial whole-body two-dimensional (2D) acquisition is carried out step by step from pelvis to head.

Acquisition time is 4 minutes per bed position (axial field at view approximately 15 cm) for the emission scan.

With the patient in prone and with hands above the head (if possible), 2D acquisition of the axillae and mammae is carried out with an acquisition time of 10 minutes per bed position.

Image Fusion

Image fusion is usually performed for lesions less than 0.8 cm, if required for surgical resection.

TABLE 16-1. *Appraisal/reimbursement status of PET in breast cancer*

Disease	German consensus classification	USZ classification	Replacement potential	US reimbursement status: Medicare/BC-BS	Swiss reimbursement status
Breast cancer: local recurrence	2a	3	4	no/no	yes
Breast cancer: lymph node staging	2a	3	2	no/no	yes
Breast cancer: distant metastases	2a	3	3	no/no	yes
Breast cancer: therapy control	2a	3	3	no/no	yes

See page 8 for abbreviations and appraisal scheme explanations.

Appraisal of Clinical Relevance of PET in Breast Cancer (Table 16-1)

Primary Tumor. In patients in whom mammography has limited diagnostic value (e.g., patients with radiodense breasts or implants), [^{18}F]FDG PET may be useful in distinguishing benign from malignant processes.

Secondary Manifestations. There is a strong indication for PET as the best noninvasive test for detecting lymph node metastases in the axilla and spread to supraclavicular or internal mammary lymph nodes.

Tertiary Manifestations. There is a strong indication for PET in patients with advanced breast cancer.

Expected Clinical Consequences from PET Findings. Because of deficient sensitivity for detecting small axillary lymph node metastases, [^{18}F]FDG PET will not replace axillary lymph node dissection. PET may give clinically important information about the locoregional spread of metastases into the upper axilla or supraclavicular or internal mammary lymph nodes. Identification of these metastases might have implications for local treatment (i.e., surgery or local irradiation). PET is likely to lead to more individualized patient management.

Exceptions. A major clinical limitation of [^{18}F]FDG PET is the likelihood of overlooking micrometastatic foci in axillary lymph nodes.

REFERENCES

1. Wahl RL, Cody RL, Hutchins GD, Mudgett EE. Primary and metastatic breast carcinoma: initial clinical evaluation with PET with the radiolabeled glucose analogue 2-[F-18]-fluoro-2-deoxy-d-glucose. *Radiology* 1991;179:765–770.
2. Nieweg OE, Kim EE, Wong WH, et al. Positron emission tomography with fluorine-18-deoxyglucose in the detection and staging of breast cancer. *Cancer* 1993;71:3920–3925.
3. Adler LA, Crowe JP, Al-Kaisi NK, Sunshine JL. Evaluation of breast masses and axillary lymph nodes with [F-18]2-deoxy-2-fluoro-d-glucose PET. *Radiology* 1993;187:743–750.
4. Veronesi U, Paganelli G, Galimberti V, et al. Sentinel-node biopsy to avoid axillary dissection in breast cancer with clinically negative lymph nodes. *Lancet* 1997;349:1864–1867.
5. Avril N, Dose J, Jänicke F, et al. Assessment of axillary lymph node involvement in breast cancer patients with positron emission tomography using radiolabeled 2-(fluorine-18)-fluoro-2-deoxy-d-glucose. *J Natl Cancer Inst* 1966;88:1204–1209.
6. Adler LP, Faulhaber PF, Schnur KC, Al-Kasi NL, Shenk RR. Axillary lymph node metastases: screening with [F-18]2-deoxy-2-fluoroglucose (FDG) PET. *Radiology* 1997;203:323–327.
7. Cook GJ, Houston S, Rubens R, Maisey MN, Fogelman I. Detection of bone metastases in breast cancer by ^{18}FDG PET: differing metabolic activity in osteoblastic and osteolytic lesions. *J Clin Oncol* 1998;16:3375–3379.

17

Tumors of the Abdomen and Pelvis

Hans Ch. Steinert, Rahel Kubik-Huch, and Georg Kacl

COLORECTAL CANCER

Colorectal cancer is one of the most common cancers in the European Community and the United States. About 70% of patients have curable, resectable tumor at initial diagnosis. The most important factor for survival or recurrence after surgery is tumor stage, which is determined by the depth of penetration through the bowel wall and the number of positive lymph nodes. Recurrent disease develops in 35% of potentially curable patients, mostly within the first 2 years after operation. Typical findings are locoregional recurrence, liver and pulmonary metastases, or disseminated disease.

Positron emission tomography (PET) using fluorodeoxyglucose tagged with fluorine 18 ([^{18}F]FDG) is clinically used for staging colorectal tumors and detecting recurrence.

The major problem in patients with colorectal cancer lies in the follow-up after surgery for detection of locally recurrent disease, as well as distant metastases. Clinical symptoms are found only in advanced stages of local recurrent disease, especially when the tumor has already invaded surrounding structures. However, postoperative healing, postirradiation reaction, or scar formation may produce similar complaints. Even high serum levels of carcinoembryonic antigen (CEA) are not always reliable; only a progressive elevation is characteristic of a local recurrence, if distant metastases can be ruled out. With the morphologic imaging modalities, computed tomography (CT) and magnetic resonance (MR) imaging, differentiation of recurrence and scar can be difficult (1). In most cases, a suspicious mass will be demonstrated with these methods, resulting in further evaluation with CT-guided fine-needle aspiration biopsy. A positive biopsy result is highly predictive of recurrence. Because of sampling problems, a negative biopsy cannot rule out recurrence. In addition, metastases to the peritoneum, mesentery, and lymph nodes are often missed with CT. Despite a negative CT, 25% to 50% of patients will have nonresectable lesions at the time of exploratory laparotomy for recurrence.

H. C. Steinert: Nuclear Medicine, University Hospital, CH-8091 Zurich, Switzerland.

R. Kubik-Huch: Diagnostic Radiology, University Hospital, CH-8091 Zurich, Switzerland.

G. Kacl: Diagnostic Radiology and Nuclear Medicine, Spital Limmattal, CH-8902 Urdorf, Switzerland.

Primary Colorectal Carcinoma

In a recent study, the diagnostic usefulness of [18F]FDG PET in patients with primary colorectal carcinoma was evaluated (2). PET was highly sensitive in the detection of primary tumors, but false-positive findings in inflammatory bowel conditions (acute diverticulitis, abscess) were common. The ability of [18F]FDG PET to depict lymph node metastases had a sensitivity of 29%, which is rather low. [18F]FDG PET depicted liver metastases in seven of eight patients and was superior to CT, which demonstrated liver metastases in only three patients. In addition, in 11% of all patients, the disease was upstaged from localized to metastatic disease.

Detection of Locoregional Recurrence

Several studies have demonstrated that [18F]FDG PET is an excellent imaging modality for differentiating scar tissue from tumor recurrence (Fig. 17-1). In a series of 29 patients, Strauss et al. (3) reported an increased [18F]FDG uptake in all 21 patients with recurrent cancer. In one patient, quantification of tracer uptake led to a misclassification as benign disease. PET was negative in all eight patients without recurrence on biopsy or surgery. Similar results were found by Ito et al. (4) and Schiepers et al. (5). Even in proven recurrence, imaging methods must demonstrate the exact extent of the tumorous mass to allow further surgery planning. At present, metabolic imaging with PET and anatomic imaging with CT or MR should be considered complementary in this setting.

Detection of Distant Metastases

Delbeke et al. (6) reported that whole-body [18F]FDG PET is the most accurate noninvasive method for patients with recurrent metastatic colorectal carcinoma. In a series of 52 patients, [18F]FDG PET detected unsuspected metastases in 17 patients and altered surgical management in 28%. [18F]FDG PET was more accurate than CT in detecting liver metastases (92% versus 78%) and extrahepatic metastases (92% versus 71%). In a series of 76 patients, Schiepers et al. (5) described a high accuracy for PET, CT, and ultrasound (US) in detecting liver metastases. However, the number of lesions detected was higher with PET, directly affecting the therapeutic strategy (i.e., surgical resection or chemotherapy). Furthermore, unexpected extrahepatic metastases were detected by whole-body [18F]FDG PET in 14 locations in 10 (13%) patients.

The major advantage of [18F]FDG PET in patients with suspected recurrence of colorectal carcinoma is its whole-body information (see Fig. 17-1). PET cannot detect microscopic foci of tumor, but in general metabolically active tumors are detected before a morphologic change is present. The limitations of PET are its inability to detect small metastases (<1 cm) and possible false-positive findings due to normal gastrointestinal tract uptake and lesions containing white cells.

Imaging Protocol

Patient Preparation

Overnight fasting with no breakfast or fasting for at least 4 hours is required before [18F]FDG application.

Emptying of the bladder is required before PET acquisition; lavage of the bladder, if required, is performed via a urinary catheter with 2 L of 0.9% saline solution during PET acquisition in the pelvis.

Data Acquisition

After a 45-minute postinjection uptake phase, the patient is placed in the camera with hands down.

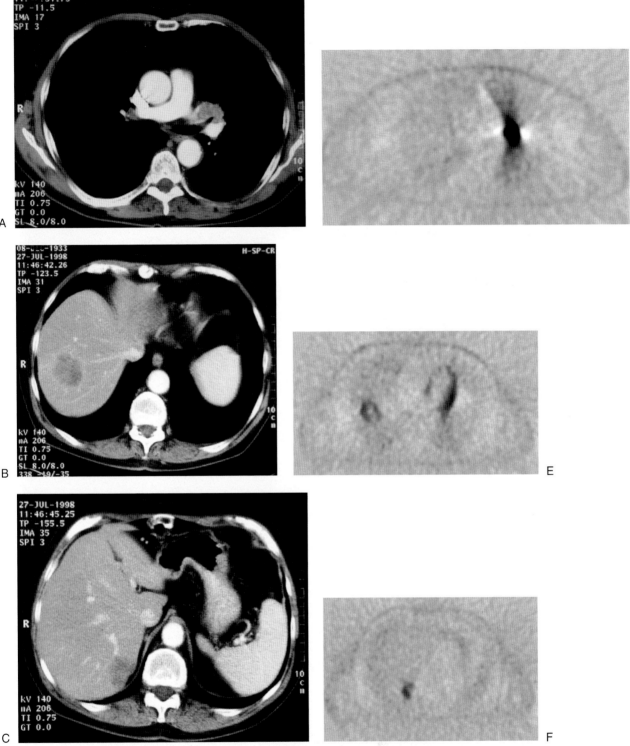

Figure 17-1. A 55-year-old man status postresection of a rectal carcinoma and recent elevation of the CEA level. **A:** Axial CT of the thorax, soft tissue window: left hilar tumor with a maximum diameter of 3 cm originating from and narrowing the left main stem bronchus, and a suspicious right hilar lymph node. **B:** Spiral CT of the upper abdomen, portal phase: 4.5-cm-diameter, ovaloid hypodense mass with peripheral contrast enhancement in segment VII of the liver, highly suspicious for liver metastasis. **C:** Spiral CT of the upper abdomen, portal phase: 3.5-cm-diameter, hypodense mass in segment V of the liver, highly suspicious for liver metastasis. **D:** Scan at the same level as **A** demonstrates increased [^{18}F]FDG uptake of the left peribronchial soft tissues but no accumulation in the right hilus, excluding tumorous involvement there. **E:** Scan at the same level as **B** shows increased uptake in the liver metastasis, as well as physiologic uptake in the heart. **F:** Scan at the same level as **C** shows increased uptake in the liver metastasis.

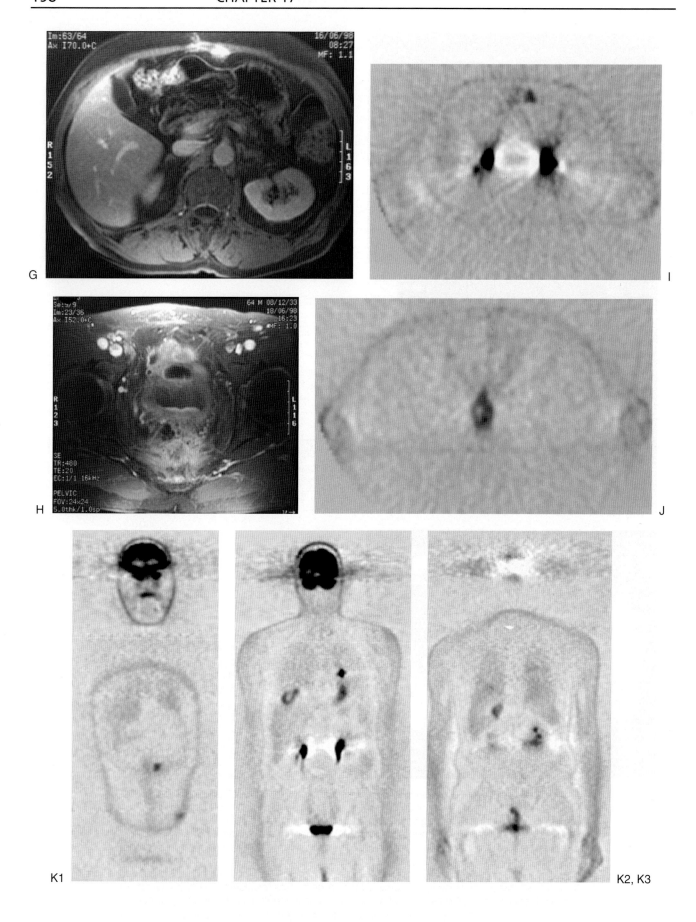

G

I

H

J

K1

K2, K3

TABLE 17-1. *Appraisal/reimbursement status of PET in colorectal cancer*

Disease	German consensus classification	USZ classification	Replacement potential	US reimbursement Medicare/BC-BS	Swiss reimbursement status
Colorectal cancer: staging, CEA>30	2b	—	—	yes/no	yes
Colorectal cancer: recurrence	1a	4	4	yes/no	yes
Colorectal cancer: therapy contr.	2a	—	—	yes/no	yes

See page 8 for abbreviations and appraisal scheme explanations.

Partial whole-body two-dimensional (2D) acquisition is carried out step by step from pelvis to head.

Acquisition time is 4 minutes per bed position (AFOW approximately 15 cm) for the emission scan.

With the same position of the patient, transmission scanning with 4-minute acquisition is performed for each bed position.

Image Fusion. Image fusion is usually performed for lesions less than 0.8 cm, if required for surgical resection.

Appraisal of Clinical Relevance of PET in Colorectal Cancer (Table 17-1)

Primary Tumor. [18F]FDG PET has a limited role in the evaluation of primary colorectal tumors.

Secondary Manifestations. [18F]FDG PET is primarily recommended for screening of distant metastases.

Tertiary Manifestations. There is a very strong indication for [18F]FDG PET as the best single test for detecting distant metastases (liver, lung).

Expected Clinical Consequences from PET Findings. Curable surgical resection is possible for early stages of colorectal cancer. Patients with distant metastases are referred for chemo- or radiotherapy.

Exceptions. [18F]FDG PET has a high sensitivity in detecting metastases. However, detection of microscopic foci of metastases is not possible with any imaging method. Possibly false-positive findings are due to normal gastrointestinal tract [18F]FDG uptake and to infection or inflammation.

CANCER OF THE PANCREAS

Cancer of the pancreas is a major unsolved health problem. Because of difficulties in diagnosis, the aggressiveness of pancreatic cancers, and the lack of effective therapies, fewer than 5% of patients with adenocarcinoma of the pancreas will be alive 5 years after diagnosis. Pancreatic cancer spreads early to regional lymph nodes, and liver metastases are present in most patients at the time of diagnosis. Patient survival depends on disease extent

---

Figure 17-1. *(continued)* **G:** Axial dynamic contrast-enhanced MR scan (gradient recall echo) of the abdomen: Thickening of the abdominal wall shows strong gadolinium (Gd)-enhancement in a 1-cm lesion, suggestive of tumorous spread (the lesion was missed during prospective MR reading). **H:** Axial T1-weighted spin-echo MR scan (TR 480 ms/TE 20 ms) after of Gd-DOTA and fat suppression shows inhomogeneous contrast uptake in the presacral space with infiltration of the gemelli muscles, highly suspicious of local recurrence. **D–F, I–K:** Corresponding transaxial [18F]FDG PET scans. **I:** Scan at the same level as **G** shows increased uptake in the metastasis of the abdominal wall (midline anterior). There is physiologic high uptake in both kidneys. **J:** Scan at the same level as **E** shows increased uptake in the presacral recurrence. **K(1–3):** Corresponding coronal [18F]FDG PET scans.

(resectable, locally advanced, or metastatic) at diagnosis. Local recurrence occurs in the majority of patients who undergo surgery alone. Liver metastases occur in 50% to 70% of patients after curative combined-modality treatment with chemoradiation and surgery. Patients with metastases have only a short survival. Therefore, early diagnosis is essential to refer patients for potentially curative surgery.

Some groups use [18F]FDG PET clinically to differentiate pancreatic adenocarcinoma from benign chronic pancreatitis and mass-forming pancreatitis. To minimize false-positive and false-negative PET results, adequate triage of patients before the examination is mandatory. Patients with signs of acute inflammation of the pancreas should be excluded from a PET examination, as well as those with hyperglycemia because of [18F]FDG PET's limited usefulness in hyperglycemic patients. The role of PET in the detection of metastases is not yet established.

Pancreatic carcinoma and pancreatitis have many pathologic features in common. Pancreatic enlargement, ductal dilatation, cyst formation, infiltration, and ascites can occur in cancer or pancreatitis. Currently, anatomic procedures such as US, endoscopic US, CT, and MR imaging are of limited value in establishing the differential diagnosis of chronic pancreatitis. These methods are used particularly to determine the resectability of pancreatic tumors. Zimny et al. (7) reported on their experience with [18F]FDG PET in the differential diagnosis of pancreatic carcinoma in 106 patients with unclear pancreatic masses. [18F]FDG PET using visual interpretation correctly identified 85% of pancreatic carcinomas and 84% of chronic pancreatitis cases. Typically, malignant pancreatic tumors showed a focally increased tracer uptake, whereas diffuse or absent uptake was seen in patients with chronic pancreatitis. However, the clinical application of [18F]FDG PET is limited by several factors:

1. Focal [18F]FDG uptake in the pancreas is not specific for carcinoma and can also occur in inflammatory pancreatic disease (8). To reduce false-positive PET results, appropriate patient selection is necessary. Patients with signs of acute pancreatitis should be excluded from a PET examination.
2. [18F]FDG uptake in pancreatic cancer may be suppressed by high serum glucose levels (7,9). Patients with pancreatic cancer or pancreatitis are likely to be hyperglycemic. It is mandatory that hyperglycemia is corrected before a PET examination.
3. The poor anatomic information available from PET makes it difficult to determine tumor resectability.

In conclusion, [18F]FDG PET is an accurate imaging modality for the differentiation of pancreatic carcinoma and should be the method of choice in patients with equivocal results using conventional anatomic imaging.

Another significant problem in the staging of pancreatic carcinoma is early detection of lymph node metastases and distant metastases. Zimny et al. (7) reported that lymph node involvement was correctly diagnosed by [18F] PET in 12 (46%) of 26 patients, and distant metastases were correctly diagnosed in 16 (52%) of 31 patients. Further studies need to be performed to examine the significance and problems of [18F]FDG PET in N- and M-staging of pancreatic cancer.

Appraisal of the clinical relevance of PET in pancreatic cancer appears in Table 17-2.

TABLE 17-2. *Appraisal/reimbursement status of PET in pancreatic cancer*

Disease	German consensus classification	USZ classification	Replacement potential	US reimbursement status: Medicare/BC-BS	Swiss reimbursement status
Pancreatic cancer: primary	1a	2	2	no/no	no
Pancreatic cancer: local recurrence	1b	—	—	no/no	no
Pancreatic cancer: NM staging	2b	—	—	no/no	no

See page 8 for abbreviations and appraisal scheme explanations.

OVARIAN CANCER

Early diagnosis and accurate staging in patients with ovarian cancer present a challenge. The majority of women with ovarian cancer are diagnosed late with unspecific signs and symptoms. More than 70% of women have extensive disease at the time of initial diagnosis. Due to its late diagnosis and poor prognosis, ovarian cancer is the leading cause of death from gynecologic tumors. Ovarian carcinoma metastasizes directly via peritoneal seeding and lymphatic paraaortic and peritoneal spread. Hematogenous metastases may occur but are uncommon.

Imaging does not yet have a clearly defined place in the management of ovarian cancer. In patients with suspected malignancy, imaging may help in preoperative planning by providing accurate information on tumor spread. Unfortunately, US, CT, and MR imaging lack sensitivity and specificity for accurate diagnosis and staging of primary and residual or recurrent disease.

Serum CA125 is the "gold standard" for tumor markers in the evaluation of pelvic masses. While rising values of serial CA125 assays are suggestive of an ovarian malignancy, CA125 is only elevated in approximately 50% of patients with early disease and in approximately 80% of patients with advanced disease.

At present, surgical exploration is the "gold standard" investigation in primary and recurrent ovarian carcinoma. Staging laparotomy is required for histologic confirmation of the diagnosis, identification of tumor spread, and debulking of tumor masses prior to chemotherapy. Chemotherapy is usually followed by second-look laparotomy to assess the response. Most patients with advanced disease undergo chemotherapy followed by a second-look laparotomy to assess the response or further debulk the lesions.

[18F]FDG PET can be clinically used for a more complete staging of patients with primary or recurrent ovarian cancer (Figs. 17-2 to 17-4). However, no imaging modality can replace staging laparatomy.

The largest series of [18F]FDG PET scans in ovarian cancer has been published by Hubner et al. (10). Fifty-one patients were evaluated with limited-field [18F]FDG PET and CT prior to laparotomy for suspected ovarian cancer. The sensitivity and specificity of PET for ovarian cancer was 93% and 82%, compared to 82% and 53% for CT, respectively. False-positive results were reported in benign serous cystadenoma, endometriosis, and endometrioma. False-positive [18F]FDG PET findings due to inflammatory processes are a recognized problem (7,11). At our institution, the accuracy of CT, MR imaging, and whole-body [18F]FDG PET was prospectively compared in 19 patients with primary and recurrent/metastatic ovarian carcinoma. In terms of primary diagnosis, the study found no difference in the abilities of the three methods of investigation to differentiate malignant from benign lesions. It confirmed earlier reports that whole-body [18F]FDG PET appears to be very sensitive in demonstrating metastatic disease (see Figs. 17-3 and 17-4). In patients with histologically confirmed recurrences, PET had the highest accuracy of 90%. The accuracy of CT and MR imaging was 43% and 89%, respectively. However, all imaging modalities were limited in the detection of microscopic peritoneal disease.

Appraisal of the clinical relevance of [18F]FDG PET in ovarian cancer is presented in Table 17-3.

GERM CELL CARCINOMAS

Germ cell tumors (GCTs) are the most common solid tumor in men between the ages of 20 and 35 years. GCTs are categorized histologically into two major subgroups: seminoma and nonseminoma. Seminoma represents 50% of all GCTs and is the most common tumor in the undescended testis. Elevated human chorionic gonadotropin (hCG) is present in 15% to 20% of patients with seminoma. The tumor is sensitive to radiation and chemotherapy. Nonseminomatous GCTs are mostly mixed cancers, consisting of two or more cell types. The presence of any nonseminomatous cell type is responsible for the prognosis and man-

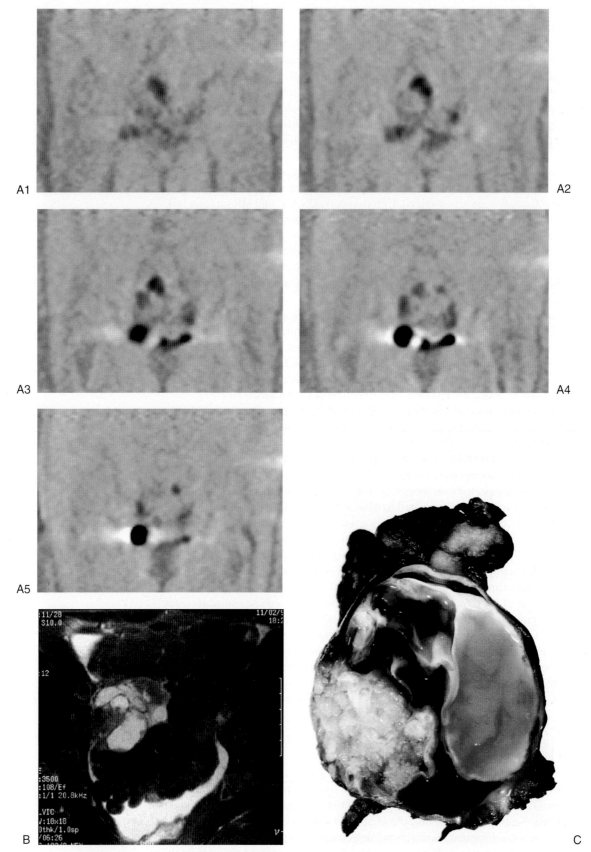

Figure 17-2. Histologically confirmed serous ovarian cancer in a 62-year-old woman. **A:** Coronal [^{18}F]FDG PET scans of the pelvis show circular increased uptake of the ovarian cancer. Lavage of the bladder via a urinary catheter was performed during PET acquisition. **B:** Corresponding T2-weighted fast spin-echo axial MR image demonstrates a large adnexal, mainly cystic lesion with solid nodules and ascites. **C:** Specimen of ovarian cancer.

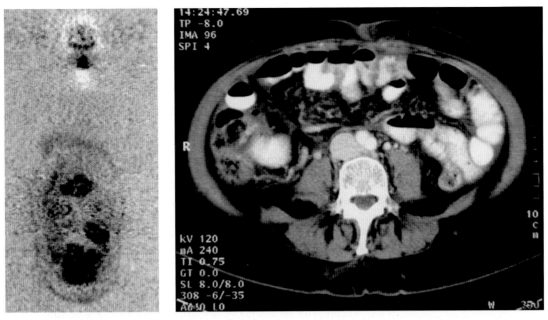

A

B

Figure 17-3. Surgically confirmed peritoneal carcinomatosis of ovarian cancer in a 63-year-old woman. **A:** Coronal [^{18}F]FDG PET scans demonstrated focally increased uptake in the entire abdomen. **B:** Axial CT scan shows no evidence of peritoneal carcinomatosis.

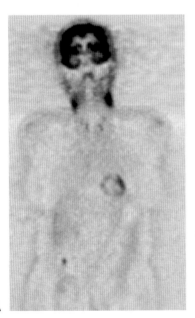

A

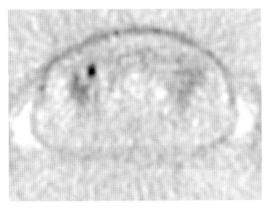

B

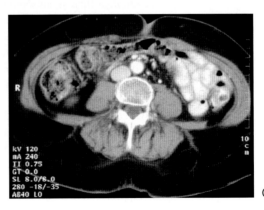

C

Figure 17-4. Surgically confirmed metastasis of an ovarian carcinoma in the ascending colon of a 62-year-old woman. Coronal **(A)** and axial **(B)** [^{18}F]FDG PET scans demonstrate a focus with an increased uptake in the left anterior abdomen. **C:** Axial CT scan shows no evidence of abdominal tumor.

TABLE 17-3. *Appraisal/reimbursement status of PET in ovarian cancer*

Disease	German consensus classification	USZ classification	Replacement potential	US reimbursement status: Medicare/BC-BS	Swiss reimbursement status
Ovarian cancer: recurrence	2a	2	2	no/no	no
Ovarian cancer: primary, dist. mets., therapy control	2b	2	2	no/no	no

See page 8 for abbreviations and appraisal scheme explanations.

agement decisions. Embryonal cell carcinoma is the most common component of mixed testicular tumors and the most aggressive GCT. Choriocarcinoma is usually associated with widespread hematogenous metastases and high levels of hCG. Teratoma consists of cell types from more than one germ cell layer (mature, immature, with malignant transformation). Although a mature teratoma may be histologically benign, it is derived from a totipotential, malignant precursor cell. Therefore, a teratoma in a postpubertal male must be considered to be a malignant GCT.

Treatment of GCT is based on surgery with additional radiotherapy and/or chemotherapy, depending on the type and stage of disease. Overall prognosis is good (survival rate 85%) for patients with seminoma or nonseminomatous GCT with low values of tumor markers (hCG, alpha-fetoprotein [AFP], lactate dehydrogenase) and no visceral metastases, while it is poor if high tumor marker levels and/or visceral metastases are present. A major therapeutic problem in GCT is the indication for surgical resection of residual masses after chemotherapy. Response to therapy can be assessed by a decrease in tumor mass on CT or normalization of tumor marker levels. Residual masses are common after chemotherapy for seminoma and malignant teratoma. Twenty percent of teratomas are malignant teratomas. Two-thirds of patients with bulky seminoma have a residual mass after chemotherapy, and 15% have residual malignant disease. For either histologic subtype of GCT, it is not possible with conventional imaging techniques to distinguish residual and recurrent malignant tissue from fibrosis, necrosis, or differentiated teratoma.

Indications for [18F]FDG PET in GCTs are classification of residual tumor masses after chemo- and/or radiotherapy and staging of recurrent GCT (Fig. 17-5).

Staging, as well as treatment control, is usually made by CT or US and elevated tumor markers. False-negative findings are common in CT-based staging. Tumor markers are highly specific, although not sensitive, since only a part of the tumors is positive. Due to the lack of sensitivity and specificity of the conventional diagnostic methods, surgical staging is necessary for the correct classification of residual masses. Histologic examination reveals necrosis/fibrosis in 40% to 50% and persistent viable malignancy in 20% to 40% of patients. Although teratomas should be resected because malignant transformation may occur, approximately 40% of patients with residual masses after chemotherapy would not need laparotomy if viable residual tumors could be excluded noninvasively.

Recently, Cremerius et al. (12) reported the results of 54 [18F]FDG PET studies in 33 patients with GCT. True-positive PET scans revealed significantly higher tracer uptake in seminomas than in nonseminomas. The lowest uptake was found in combined tumors. The diagnostic accuracy of [18F]FDG PET and CT in seminomas was 90% and 79%, respectively. The diagnostic accuracy of [18F]FDG PET and CT in nonseminomas was 81% and 52%, respectively. The advantage of PET over CT in nonseminomas was based mostly on its higher specificity (92% versus 50%). The authors discussed a transient suppression of metabolic activity in GCT shortly after chemotherapy regardless of the final therapy response. They concluded that PET scanning should not be performed earlier than 2 weeks after completion of therapy. Stephens et al. (13) also found a poor sensitivity of [18F]FDG PET for teratoma. In their study, 30 patients with postchemotherapy residual masses were evaluated. [18F]FDG PET did not differentiate necrotic/fibrous tissue from teratoma. However, it was able to differentiate viable GCT from residual necrotic/fibrous tissue or teratoma.

Appraisal of the clinical relevance of [18F]FDG PET in GCT is presented in Table 17-4.

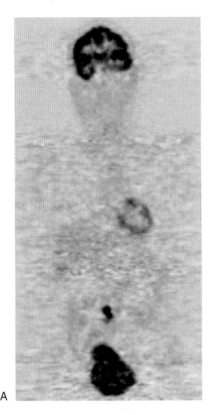

A

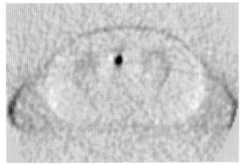

B

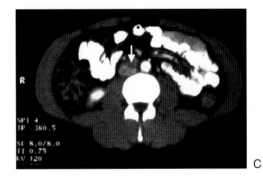

C

Figure 17-5. A 40-year-old man status postresection and postchemotherapy of an embryonal cell carcinoma and elevation of AFP level. **A:** Coronal [^{18}F]FDG PET scan with transmission correction shows a paraaortic lesion with a markedly increased tracer uptake, indicating a lymph node metastasis. **B:** Corresponding axial [^{18}F]FDG PET scan. **C:** Corresponding axial CT of the abdomen shows the paraaortic lymph node metastasis. Note that the lesion was prospectively overlooked on CT *(arrow).*

TABLE 17-4. *Appraisal/reimbursement status of PET in germ cell cancers*

Disease	German consensus classification	USZ classification	Replacement potential	US reimbursement status: Medicare/BC-BS	Swiss reimbursement status
Germ cell ca.: non-seminomatous Therapy control (exd. diff. Teratoma)	1b	3	3	no/no	yes
Germ cell ca.: non-seminomatous Lymph node- and restaging	2a	3	3	no/no	yes
Germ cell ca. non-seminomatous: teratoma	2b	2	2	no/no	yes
Germ cell ca. seminomatous	2b	2	2	no/no	no

See page 8 for abbreviations and appraisal scheme explanations.

REFERENCES

1. Krestin GP, Steinbrich W, Friedmann G. Recurrent rectal cancer: diagnosis with MR imaging versus CT. *Radiology* 1988;168:307–311.
2. Abdel-Nabi H, Doehr RJ, Lamonica M, et al. Staging of primary colorectal carcinomas with fluorine-18 fluoro-deoxy-glucose whole-body PET: correlation with histopathologic and CT findings. *Radiology* 1998;206:755–760.
3. Strauss LG, Corius JH, Schlag P, et al. Recurrence of colorectal tumors: PET evaluation. *Radiolgy* 1989;170:329–332.
4. Ito K, Kato T, Tadokoro M, et al. Recurrent rectal cancer and scar: differentiation with PET and MR imaging. *Radiology* 1992;182:549–552.
5. Schiepers C, Penninckx F, De Vadder, et al. Contribution of PET in the diagnosis of recurrent colorectal cancer: comparison with conventional imaging. *Eur J Surg Oncol* 1995;21:517–522.
6. Delbeke D, Vitola J, Sandler MP, et al. Staging recurrent metastatic colorectal carcinoma with PET. *J Nucl Med* 1997;38:1196–1201.
7. Zimny M, Bares R, Fass J, et al. Fluorine-18 fluorodeoxyglucose positron emission tomography in the differential diagnosis of pancreatic carcinoma: a report of 106 cases. *Eur J Nucl Med* 1997;24:678–682.
8. Shreve PD. Focal fluorine-18 fluorodeoxyglucose accumulation in inflammatory pancreatic disease. *Eur J Nucl Med* 1998;25:259–264.
9. Bares R, Klever P, Hauptmann S, et al. F-18 fluorodeoxyglucose PET *in vivo* evaluation of pancreatic glucose metabolism for detection of pancreatic cancer. *Radiology* 1994;192:79–86.
10. Hubner KF, McDonald TW, Niethammer JG, Smith GT, Gould HR, Buonocore E. Assessment of primary and metastatic ovarian cancer by positron emission tomography (PET) using 2-(18F)deoxyglucose (2-(¹⁸F)FDG). *Gynecol Oncol* 1993;51:197–204.
11. Römer W, Avril N, Dose J, et al. Metabolische Charakterisierung von Ovarialtumoren mit der Positronen-Emissions-Tomographie und F-18-fluorodeoxyglukose. *Rofo Fortschr Geb Rontgenstr Neuen Bildgeb Verfahr* 1997;166:62–68.
12. Cremerius U, Effert PJ, Adam G, et al. FDG PET for detection and therapy control of metastatic germ cell tumor. *J Nucl Med* 1998;39:815–822.
13. Stephens AW, Gonin R, Hutchins GD, Einhorn LH. Positron emission tomography evaluation of residual radiographic abnormalities in postchemotherapy germ cell tumor patients. *J Clin Oncol* 1996;14:1637–1641.

18

Lymphoma

Katrin D. M. Stumpe and Gustav K. von Schulthess

Lymphomas account for less than 8% of all malignant neoplasms. They are classified as Hodgkin disease (HD) or non-Hodgkin (NHL) lymphoma.

HODGKIN DISEASE

HD represents 25% of all malignant lymphomas and, at an early stage, is a localized lymph node disease. In advanced stages, it is a systemic disease that also manifests itself in extralymphatic organs. In 60% to 90% of patients, spread to contiguous lymph node stations takes place. In 85%, HD primarily involves intrathoracic disease extension that is limited to the upper mediastinum (prevascular, pretracheal) (1). A mediastinal mass is present in the anterior mediastinum in up to 70% of patients due to thymic involvement, and is frequently associated with other mediastinal lymphadenopathy. In one-third of patients with thoracic disease, unilateral or bilateral hilar lymphadenopathy is described. On the chest x-ray, hilar pathology is often obscured by bulky mediastinal disease. Masses from lymphoma mostly displace adjacent structures, rather than invading them. Lung involvement is seen in fewer than 10% of patients with mediastinal lymphoma (2,3).

The therapeutic approach to HD is not dependent on the histologic subtype but rather on the exact stage. The therapeutic standard for limited stage Ia disease without risk factors and without B-symptoms or mediastinal bulk is radiation therapy alone; in intermediate stages, combined chemo- and radiation therapy is used, and in advanced stages intensive chemotherapy is used alone, including radiation therapy to so-called bulk tumors. With this strategy, approximately 85% of all patients with HD can be cured.

NON-HODGKIN LYMPHOMA

Different classification schemes are used in NHL: the working formulation, the Kiel classification, and the revised European–American lymphoma classification distinguishing

K. D. M. Stumpe and G. K. von Schulthess: Nuclear Medicine, University Hospital, CH-8091 Zurich, Switzerland.

TABLE 18-1. *Ann Arbor classification of Hodgkin disease and non-Hodgkin lymphoma*

I.	Involvement of one nodal region (I/N) or one extranodal region
II.	Involvement of one or more nodal regions (II/N) or presence of localized extranodal lesions with one or more involved nodal regions on one side of the diaphragm
III.	Involvement of two or more nodal regions on both sides of the diaphragm (III/N) or presence of localized extranodal regions and lymph nodes on both sides of the diaphragm (III/E)
IV.	Disseminated involvement of one or more extranodal organs with or without lymph node involvement:
	A. Without general symptoms
	B. With fever (>38°C) and/or night sweats and/or weight loss (>10% in the last 6 mo)

between low-, intermediate-, and high-malignant subtypes. The Ann Arbor classification differentiates between four classes in HD and NHL (Table 18-1).

NHL is usually more extensive at presentation than HD and is often treated primarily with chemotherapy. In contrast to HD, spread is frequently noncontiguous and involves extranodal sites (4). Extranodal manifestations in NHL are predominantly in the gastrointestinal system (mostly B-cell lymphoma) or in the skin (T-cell lymphoma). At the time of presentation, intrathoracic lymph nodes, particularly superior mediastinal nodes, are involved in only 40% to 50% of patients. Hilar or posterior mediastinal lymphadenopathy, as well as lung involvement, is more common (4). Therapy of lymphomas of low malignancy depends in essence on disease stage. In early stages I and II, therapy currently consists of extended-field or total-nodal irradiation. In patients with advanced stages III to IV, the therapeutic approach is still under discussion, and intensive chemotherapy does not improve the disease-free survival. A conservative approach is therefore still justified. This consists of therapeutically intervening only when B symptoms appear or hematopoietic insufficiency is noted with progression of the lymphomatous involvement.

In the past 30 years with continued improvement in chemotherapy and radiation therapy strategies, HD and NHL have become two of the few malignancies that are potentially curable. Improved treatment outcomes depend on accurate staging. Lymphomas may be multifocal and widespread. Therefore, staging the entire body in a single imaging study is clinically valuable (see Table 18-1).

INDICATIONS FOR PET

General

A substantial body of literature suggests that positron emission tomography (PET) of the body manifestations of lymphoma is of substantial clinical relevance. This is the case for initial staging, as well as restaging, to assess the effects of therapy and recurrence. Published results indicate that PET using fluorodeoxyglucose tagged with fluorine 18 ([18F]FDG) may be equal or superior to computed tomography (CT) staging for the detection of nodal as well as extranodal involvement in HD (5–7), and superior to planar gallium Ga 67 citrate scintigraphy.

[18F]FDG imaging of lymphoma was first reported in 1987 by Paul (8) in Finland, who utilized planar imaging and compared [18F]FDG with gallium in a small number of patients. [18F]FDG was clearly superior in this small series. Several reports published since have compared [18F]FDG PET with other imaging modalities, notably CT, which is widely used as the method of choice in lymphoma staging (5–9). The feasibility of imaging lymphoma using [18F]FDG is of particular interest, as metabolic imaging does not face the difficulties of morphologic imaging modalities in defining the presence and extent of lymphomatous tumors (5,11).

Pitfalls

[18F]FDG physiologically accumulates in the saliva and in the oropharynx (Waldeyer's ring), and so it is important to rinse the buccal and pharyngeal activity before scanning (see also Chapter 7). In addition, it is necessary to encourage patients to relax during the examination and to place them comfortably in the scanner, as activity in the neck muscles due to increased muscle tension often obscures cervical lymph nodes. On scans, the distinguishing feature of such neck muscle activity is that the muscles usually appear as bilaterally accumulating linear, symmetric structures.

Other structures that may show physiologic [^{18}F]FDG accumulation that can be mistaken for lymphomatous involvement are activity in the bowel and the kidneys. If these structures are involved, a distinction between lymphoma and physiologic organ uptake may be difficult. After chemotherapy an increase in [^{18}F]FDG in the bone marrow may be seen (Fig. 7-13).

INITIAL STAGING

In the initial staging of lymphoma, it is critical to identify all sites of pathology. Therefore, a highly sensitive image method is highly desirable. However, since modern therapy of lymphomas, especially HD, differs only when stage IA rather than a higher-stage disease is present, PET imaging on diagnosis may be of limited importance for the initial therapeutic decision making process. Despite this limited clinical impact, PET is mandatory as a baseline for the assessment of therapeutic success.

Newman et al. (5) compared [^{18}F]FDG PET and CT in the same thoracoabdominal anatomic areas in 16 patients with lymphoma. PET was abnormal in all cases in which CT demonstrated abnormalities. Hoh et al. (6) found whole-body PET to be equal to conventional imaging in the staging of seven HD patients. In patients with NHL, the stage increased in three patients and decreased in one patient when whole-body PET was used.

Due to high [^{18}F]FDG uptake in PET, even small lymphoma manifestations can easily be visualized with modern cameras, potentially resulting in improved clinical staging of untreated patients. Manifestations of lymphoma can easily be recognized on PET scans, as only a few anatomic structures show physiologic [^{18}F]FDG uptake (Fig. 18-1). This fact has been recognized as a clear staging advantage in other malignant tumors (12).

In some studies, it was noted that increased [^{18}F]FDG uptake was proportional to the histologic grade, with the most malignant tumors accumulating the most [^{18}F]FDG (13–16). In other series, high- and low-grade NHL both showed prominent uptake at disease sites. Thus, this issue is still debated in the literature (5,7,13,14). Visualization of a central necrotic area not showing [^{18}F]FDG uptake is easier to distinguish in PET, with its functional characterization of tissues, than with imaging modalities providing morphologic information (Fig. 18-2).

The ability to exclude extranodal involvement and therefore a worse prognosis is of great importance, as a patient would be upstaged to stage III or IV (bone marrow) (17). A positive result, especially in patients without B symptoms, would change therapy management. Reported rates of bone marrow involvement in newly diagnosed lymphoma are 10% in HD and 25% in NHL (18,19).

PET is able to show discrete, clinically occult skeletal involvement (Fig. 18-3) and, due to its whole-body capabilities, generalized bone marrow involvement.

Reported rates of lymphomatous involvement in the liver and spleen are up to 3% and 23%, respectively, for HD and 15% and 22%, respectively, for NHL (18–20) (Fig. 18-4). In a study by Moog et al. (21), [^{18}F]FDG PET allowed not only detection of additional extranodal lesions compared to CT but also changes in staging in 16% of patients.

In suspected central nervous system (CNS) manifestations, [^{18}F]FDG PET proved to be helpful in differentiating lymphoma from inflammatory disease, particularly acquired immunodeficiency syndrome–related neurologic complications (22). Cerebral lymphoma is usually characterized by very high cerebral [^{18}F]FDG uptake, much exceeding that of normal brain tissue and often that of glioma. Hoffman et al. (22) found a significant difference in semiquantitatively determining [^{18}F]FDG uptake with the standard uptake value (SUV)

(text continues on page 214)

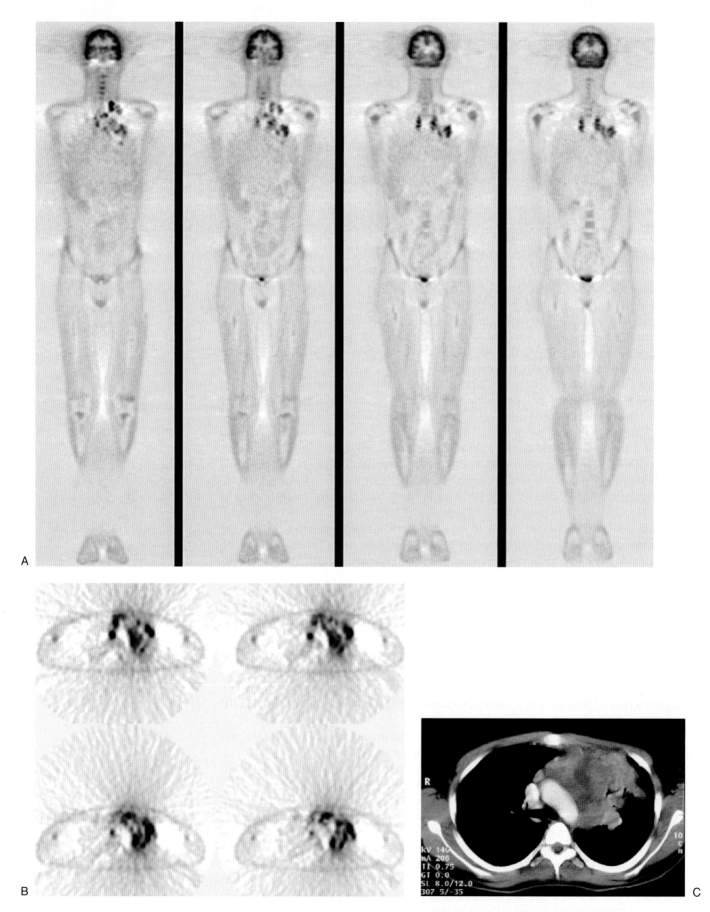

Figure 18-1. HD, nodular sclerosis type, stage IIB. **A:** Coronal [^{18}F]FDG PET sections demonstrate markedly increased uptake in the left supraclavicular lymph nodes, the mediastinum, and the left lung. **B:** Corresponding axial [^{18}F]FDG PET sections through the upper thorax. **C:** Axial CT section at the level of the aortic arch shows a large mass in the left lung and the mediastinum.

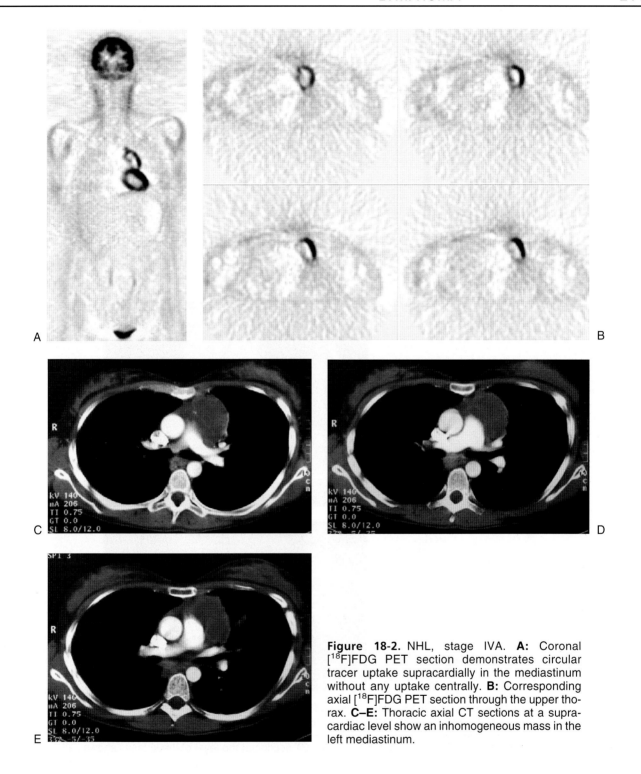

Figure 18-2. NHL, stage IVA. **A:** Coronal [^{18}F]FDG PET section demonstrates circular tracer uptake supracardially in the mediastinum without any uptake centrally. **B:** Corresponding axial [^{18}F]FDG PET section through the upper thorax. **C–E:** Thoracic axial CT sections at a supracardiac level show an inhomogeneous mass in the left mediastinum.

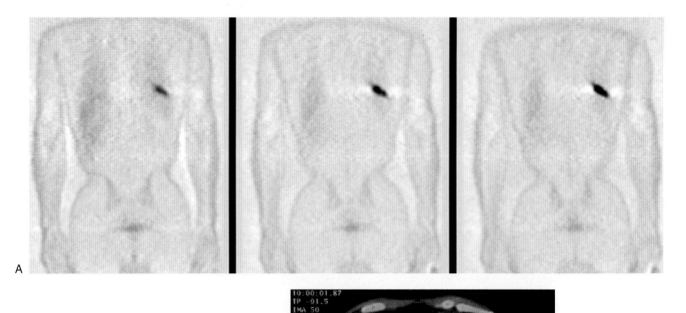

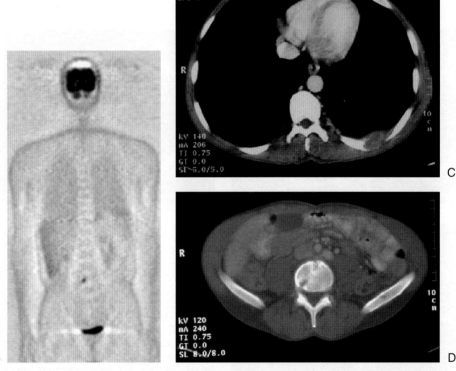

Figure 18-3. HD and osseous involvement of the chest wall and lumbar spine. **A:** Coronal [^{18}F]FDG PET sections demonstrate left rib involvement. **B:** Coronal [^{18}F]FDG PET shows focal tracer uptake of in the L-3 vertebra. **C:** Axial CT section through the lower thorax shows rib involvement posteriorly on the left. **D:** Axial CT section at the level of the kidneys shows the lumbar spine lesion.

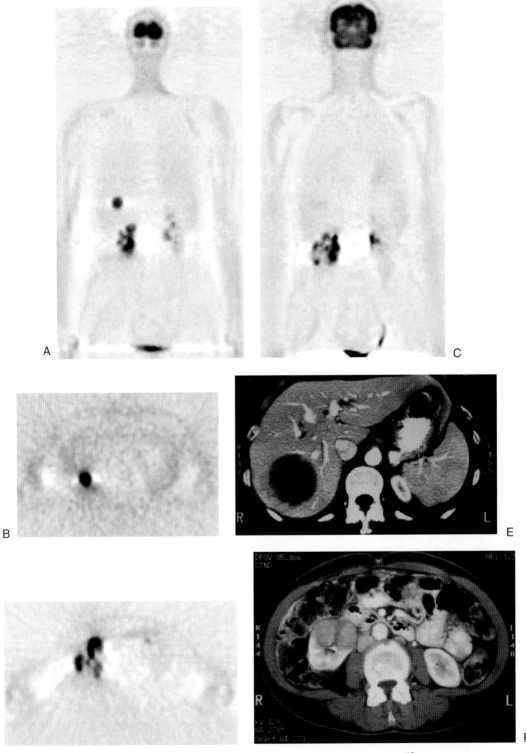

Figure 18-4. NHL in a human immunodeficiency virus–positive. **A:** Coronal [^{18}F]FDG PET section shows a focus of tracer uptake in the liver. **B:** Corresponding axial [^{18}F]FDG PET section at the liver level. Coronal **(C)** and corresponding axial **(D)** [^{18}F]FDG PET sections show lymphomatous multifocal tracer uptake in the parenchyma of the right kidney. **E:** Axial CT section through the upper abdomen shows a large mass in the right lobe of the liver. **F:** Axial CT section at the level of the kidney shows a mass in the right renal parenchyma.

between CNS lymphoma and inflammatory disease in patients with an immunodeficiency syndrome. Compared to other malignancies and inflammatory lesions, SUVs are high (median, 8.5) (11). Therefore, it is suggested that the visual interpretation for evaluating a focus with pathologic [^{18}F]FDG uptake is sufficient (21). Cerebral lymphoma is discussed in detail in Chapter 8.

FOLLOW-UP OF THERAPY AND DETECTION OF RECURRENCES

[^{18}F]FDG PET is successfully used to evaluate tumor viability after chemotherapy and irradiation. The most critical question in the assessment of therapy is whether viable tumor is absent or still present, and, if present, whether the tumor has regressed, remained stationary, or increased in size. While CT cannot distinguish viable tumor from involutional fibrosis, scar tissue, or necrosis, the accuracy of [^{18}F]FDG PET exceeds 90% regarding this question (7,23). Residual [^{18}F]FDG uptake on PET images in such masses is highly suggestive of residual tumor or recurrence, while absence of tracer uptake excludes persistent tumor with a high degree of accuracy (Fig. 18-5).

[^{18}F]FDG PET is probably so successful because changes in anatomic indicators are slow and lag behind the reduction in the number of viable tumor cells. It appears that fibrosis develops as a result of tumor necrosis, and initially enlarged tumor sites may remain permanently enlarged after effective treatment of the tumor. During treatment for malignant lymphoma, there is no satisfactory way of using morphologic imaging to identify patients at risk for relapse after chemotherapy (23,24), or those overtreated. PET appears ca-

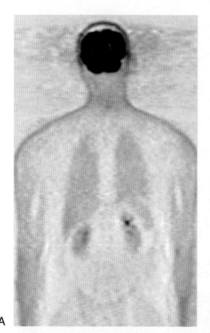

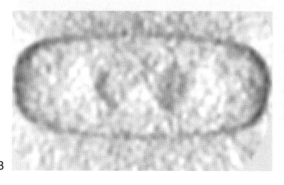

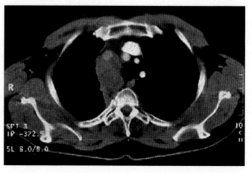

Figure 18-5. HD, nodular sclerosis, stage I, postirradiation. Coronal **(A)** and corresponding thoracic axial **(B)** [^{18}F]FDG PET scans show lack of tracer uptake in a mass in the right upper mediastinum. **C:** Corresponding axial CT section demonstrates a residual mass in the right upper mediastinum.

pable of distinguishing patients who respond to treatment from those who do not, and therefore may help guide the therapeutic management of lymphoma (25). Hoekstra et al. (26) found that [^{18}F]FDG uptake was decreased in lymphoma under therapy, with this decrease being more prominent than the volume reduction in morphologic imaging. Marked reduction or normalization of [^{18}F]FDG uptake was predictive of good response to therapy, while incomplete response to therapy was predicted by lesser reduction in [^{18}F]FDG uptake. It is notable that reduced [^{18}F]FDG uptake was seen within days of the start of chemotherapy, so that very early prospective assessment of a therapeutic effect appears possible. Restaging will only yield reliable results if it is known beforehand that the tumor had adequate [^{18}F]FDG uptake on diagnosis. Therefore, a baseline PET scan before therapy is advisable. In addition, PET can likely be used to select responders for highly toxic or very expensive treatment, and to enhance both the cost effectiveness of treatment and the quality of life in these patients.

OTHER TRACERS IN LYMPHOMA IMAGING

Methionine or thymidine labeled with carbon 11 have also been used in PET imaging (13). Although SUVs, as well as tumor/background ratios, were high, the use of both tracers has been limited until now to small pilot studies evaluating selected lymphoma manifestations. The short physical half-life of ^{11}C is a major drawback, confining its use to PET centers that comprise a cyclotron and a competent radiopharmacy division.

OTHER IMAGING MODALITIES

The initial diagnosis of lymphoma is made either clinically by palpation of neck masses or by noting pathologic masses on chest x-ray or abdominal ultrasound examinations. Since primary lymphoma in other sites, such as brain or bone, is rare, except in high-risk groups such as patients with a high sedimentation rate, a large mediastinal mass, spleen involvement, or involvement of more than three nodal regions, the disease is relatively rarely discovered with other imaging modalities. Excisional biopsy of the most accessible lesion ensues.

The conventional methods for staging lymphomas are chest radiography, CT or magnetic resonance (MR) imaging, sonography, bone scan, gallium scan, lymphangiography, and laparotomy. The most widely used methods, CT and MR imaging, rely mostly on anatomic criteria for diagnosis. This leads to significant shortcomings because identification of a mass by itself has relatively low specificity.

The role of other imaging is limited. Ultrasound is used for initial screening if abdominal disease is suspected. Conventional radiographs of bones are not primarily indicated, but on occasion bony structures involved by lymphoma may present with typical sclerosis (ebony vertebra). Bone scanning is a good staging modality when skeletal involvement by lymphoma is known or suspected.

CT versus [^{18}F]FDG PET: Detecting Nodal and Extranodal Involvement

The principal imaging modality for the staging of lymphoma is CT, which is typically done to cover the body regions from the base of the skull to the pelvic floor. If substantial suspicion persists of involvement of an organ in light of negative CT results, MR imaging may be used additionally. CT examinations are done using vascular as well as bowel contrast enhancement. While identification of bulky lesions is readily accomplished on CT and rarely poses a diagnostic problem, lymph nodes that are marginally enlarged often cannot be adequately classified as being involved. CT also shows residual masses after therapy but cannot differentiate between residual tumor/recurrence and involutional tissue.

CT has been shown to be a useful tool for detecting hilar, mediastinal, paraaortic, paracaval, and mesenteric lymph node involvement in patients with lymphoma. In the mediastinum, CT shows additional sites of disease that are obscured on the chest x-ray (e.g., subcarinal, cardiophrenic angle, posterior mediastinum, and paravertebral nodes). In the abdomen, the spleen is frequently the first and only site that is affected in patients with HD. CT is not a reliable method for excluding splenic involvement, and so laparotomy and splenectomy are still in use for staging HD. CT is a reliable indicator of splenic size, but in one-third of patients with HD and NHL, the spleen will be normal in size but still harbor lymphoma. Ahmann et al. (27) reported a sensitivity of 38% and a specificity of 61% for CT in detecting splenic lymphoma on the basis of organ enlargement.

Small or borderline enlarged lymph nodes, as well as microscopic infiltrates in the solid organs, that may harbor active disease may be diagnosed as normal on CT. Intranodal architecture is not discernible on CT. In patients with lymphadenopathy due to reactive hyperplasia or benign disease, CT will be unable to exclude malignancy as a cause for lymph node enlargement. The accuracy of CT in detecting intraabdominal and pelvic lymphadenopathy in patients of lymphoma ranges from 68% to 100%, with a false-positive rate varying from 0% to 25% (28,29). False-positive diagnoses result from a misinterpretation of lymphadenopathy secondary to inflammatory processes, unopacified bowel loops, or normal vascular structures.

MR Imaging versus [^{18}F]FDG PET

MR imaging is an another technique for staging lymphoma, but again lymph nodes are identified on the basis of enlargement rather than any characteristic signal intensity (30). MR imaging is equal or superior to CT in the evaluation of the mediastinum, the hila, the chest wall, and the supraclavicular, paracardiac, and diaphragmatic regions. In addition, detection of lymphomatous involvement of the bone marrow is the domain of MR imaging (31,32). MR imaging is able to show early involvement. On the other hand, many diffuse infiltrations escape detection. Tesoro-Tess et al. (33) described a sensitivity and a positive predictive value for MR imaging of only 55% and 38.5%, respectively.

Bipedal Lymphadenopathy

Bipedal lymphangiography has been the technique employed in the past to investigate possible retroperitoneal lymph node abnormalities. However, the method is time-consuming, occasionally difficult to perform, invasive, uncomfortable for the patient, and difficult to interpret. Lymphangiography is also unable to evaluate mesenteric, high paraaortic, and internal iliac nodal chains.

Gallium Scintigraphy

Gallium scanning for lymphoma staging is still of importance in North America. In Europe, the use of Ga 67 for staging is quite limited because of the high radiation dose of (5 to 10 mCi [185 to 370 MBq]), low spatial resolution, relatively low specificity, and the difficulty in uptake quantification (13–15,34). It is known to be highly sensitive, but lymphomas not taking up Ga 67 are known to exist. Tumeh et al. (35) evaluated seven patients with NHL presenting with disease in the chest or abdomen. Sensitivity in detecting lymphoma in the chest was 66% and 96% for planar and single photon emission computed tomography, respectively; specificity was 66% and 100%, respectively. In the abdomen, sensitivity was reported to be 69% and 85%, respectively, and the specificity, 87% and 100%, respectively. The usefulness of Ga 67 is particularly limited in the evaluation of the abdomen owing to hepatic uptake and excretion into the bowel.

Staging Laparotomy

Staging laparotomy is still considered the standard of reference for detection of occult abdominal disease. Positive findings are still obtained in up to 30% of patients, with up to 90% of these patients showing involvement of the spleen (5,20). However, because of potential surgical complications and the immunologic consequences of splenectomy, use of this invasive method is no longer very popular.

PATIENT PREPARATION AND IMAGING PROTOCOL

Patients must fast for at least 4 hours to suppress [18F]FDG uptake in the myocardium. A dose of 6 to 10 mCi (240 to 400 MBq) of [18F]FDG is injected antecubitally, and there is a 30- to 40-minute waiting period to allow the tracer to accumulate in the tissues. No special precautions are necessary to control cerebral uptake. Good hydration is useful on injection of [18F]FDG, because this will help wash out activity in the renal collecting system. Before scanning, the patient is asked to void to minimize bladder activity. Rinsing of the oral cavity before scanning is also useful to minimize buccal and pharyngeal activity. This is particularly relevant in neck involvement by tumor.

The area covered in PET imaging is that also covered by CT (i.e., from the base of the skull to the pelvic floor). With a 15-cm axial field of view, this typically requires four to six cradle positions. Scanning per cradle position is 4 to 5 minutes with the scanner at our institution. Transmission correction is useful, particularly for chest involvement. With this, total imaging time is on the order of 1 hour (emission and transmission, 2 × 5 cradle positions × 5 minutes = 50 minutes). Image fusion with CT scans is of limited use, as long as systemic therapy is planned. It may be quite relevant when radiation therapy or surgery is planned.

On the basis of current evidence, staging and restaging of lymphoma are excellent indications for PET scanning (Table 18-2). While CT is the current modality of choice for the staging of lymphoma, it is conceivable that with the accumulation of further clinical data, PET may replace CT for staging and restaging in the future. If this indeed happens, the role of cross-sectional morphologic imaging with CT and MR imaging will be in nonsystemic treatment planning (i.e., the definition of a radiation-therapy field or preparation for surgery). While PET is an expensive examination, extended field-of-view imaging with CT and MR imaging is also quite expensive. Often, these modalities are charged for the body regions imaged, and lymphoma staging from skull base to pelvic floor involves four body regions (neck, thorax, abdomen, and pelvis), generating four times a base charge. Thus, PET may well be cost effective. Clinically, PET appears to be able to characterize and distinguish residual tumor from involutional tissue. This may result in a reduction in follow-up examinations for the purpose of unambiguously defining the origin of a residual mass. As the issues of cost-effectiveness assessment of PET imaging in lymphoma are multifaceted, involve the cost of other imaging modalities and staging protocols, and possibly affect chemotherapy regimens, no firm conclusions on this subject can currently be reached.

TABLE 18-2. *Appraisal/reimbursement status of PET in lymphoma*

Disease	German consensus classification	USZ classification	Replacement potential	US reimbursement status: Medicare/BC-BS	Swiss reimbursement status
Malignant lymphoma, initial staging	1b	3	2	yes/no	yes
Malignant lymphoma, residual tumor	1b	4	4	yes/no	yes
Malignant lymphoma, restag./recur.	2a	4	4	yes/no	yes
Malignant lymphoma, therapy response	2b	3	3	yes/no	yes

See page 8 for abbreviations and appraisal scheme explanations.

REFERENCES

1. Castellino RA. Hodgkin disease: practical concepts for the diagnostic radiologist. *Radiology* 1986; 159:305–310.
2. Castellino RA, Blank N, Hoppe RT et al. Hodgkin disease: contributions of chest CT in the initial staging evaluation. *Radiology* 1986;160:603–605.
3. Diehl LF, Hopper KD, Giguere J, et al. The pattern of intrathoracic Hodgkin disease assessed by computed tomography. *J Clin Oncol* 1991;9:438–443.
4. Castellino RA. The non-Hodgkin lymphomas: practical concepts for the diagnostic radiologist. *Radiology* 1991;178:315–321.
5. Newman JS, Francis IR, Kaminiski MS, Wahl RL. Imaging of lymphoma with PET with [^{18}F]-FDG: correlation with CT. *Radiology* 1994;190:111–116.
6. Hoh CK, Glaspy J, Rosen P, et al. Whole-body FDG-PET imaging for staging of Hodgkin's disease and lymphoma. *J Nucl Med* 1997;38:343–348.
7. Stumpe KDM, Urbinelli M, Steinert HC, et al. Whole-body positron emission tomography using fluorodeoxyglucose for staging of lymphoma: effectiveness and comparison with computed tomography. *Eur J Nucl Med* 1998;25:721–728.
8. Paul R. Comparison of fluorine-18-2-fluorodeoxyglucose and gallium-67 citrate imaging for detection of lymphoma. *J Nucl Med* 1987;28:288–292.
9. Moog F, Bangerter M, Diederichs CD, et al. Lymphoma: role of whole-body-FDG-PET in nodal staging. *Radiology* 1997;203:795–800.
10. Jochelson M, Mauch P, Balikian J, Rosenthal D, Canellos G. The significance of the residual mediastinal mass in treated Hodgkin's disease. *J Clin Oncol* 1985;5:637–640.
11. Lapela L, Leskinen S, Minn HR, et al. Increased glucose metabolism in untreated non-Hodgkin lymphoma: a study with positron emission tomography and fluorine-18-fluorodeoxyglucose. *Blood* 1995;86:3522–3527.
12. Steinert HC, Hauser M, Allemann F, et al. Non-small cell lung cancer: nodal staging with FDG PET versus CT with correlative lymph node mapping and sampling. *Radiology* 1997;202:441–446.
13. Leskinen-Kallio S, Ruotsalainen U, Nagren K, Terâs M, Joensuu H. Uptake of carbon-11-methionine and fluorodeoxyglucose in non-Hodgkin's lymphoma: a PET study. *J Nucl Med* 1991;32:1211–1218.
14. Okada J, Yoshikawa K, Itami M, et al. Positron emission tomography using fluorine-18-fluorodeoxyglucose in malignant lymphoma: a comparison with proliferative activity. *J Nucl Med* 1992;33:325–329.
15. Okada J, Yoshikawa K, Imazeki K, et al. The use of FDG-PET in the detection and management of malignant lymphoma: correlation and uptake with prognosis. *J Nucl Med* 1991;32:686–691.
16. Rodriguez M, Rehn S, Ahlstrom H, et al. Predicting malignancy grade with PET in non-Hodgkin's lymphoma. *J Nucl Med* 1995;36:1790–1796.
17. Moog F, Bangerter ST, Kotzerke J, et al. F-18 fluorodeoxy-glucose positron emission tomography as a new approach to detect lymphomatous bone marrow. *J. Clin. Oncol* 1998;16:603–609.
18. Kaplan HS, Anderson KC, Leonhard RC. Staging laparotomy and splenectomy in Hodgkin's disease: analysis of indications and patterns of involvement in 285 consecutive, unselected patients. *Natl Cancer Inst Monogr* 1973;36:291–198.
19. Rosenberg SA; Berard CW, Brown BW, et al. National Cancer Institute sponsored study of classification of non-Hodgkin's lymphomas: summary and description of a working formulation for clinical use. *Cancer* 1982;49:2112–2135.
20. Shirkoda A. Lymphoma of the solid abdominal viscera. *Radiol Clin North Am* 1990;28:785–799.
21. Moog F, Bangerter M, Diederichs CG, et al. Extranodal malignant lymphoma: detection with FDG PET versus CT. *Radiology* 1998;206:475–481.
22. Hoffmann JM, Waskin HA, Schifter T, et al. FDG-PET in differentiating lymphoma from non-malignant central nervous system lesions in patients with AIDS. *J Nucl Med* 1993;34:567–575.
23. Bares R, Altehoefer C, Cremerius U, et al. FDG-PET for metabolic classification of residual lymphoma masses after chemotherapy. *J Nucl Med* 1994;35:131[abst].
24. Urba WJ, Longo DL. Hodgkin's disease. *N Engl J Med* 1992;326:678–687.
25. Jerusalem G, Fassotte MF, Paulus P, et al. Whole-body positron emission tomography for staging, response evaluation and follow-up of Hodgkin's disease and non-Hodgkin lymphoma. *Blood* 1995;86(suppl 1):534a [abst.].
26. Hoekstra OS, Ossenkoppele GJ, Golding R, et al. Early treatment response in malignant lymphoma, as determined by planar fluorine-18-fluorodeoxyglucose scintigraphy. *J Nucl Med* 1993;34:1706–1710.
27. Ahmann DL, Kiely JM, Harrison EG, et al. Malignant lymphoma of the spleen: a review of 49 cases in which the diagnosis was made at splenectomy. *Cancer* 1966;19:461–469.
28. Lee JKT, Stanley RJ, Sagel SS, et al. Accuracy of computed tomography in detecting intra-abdominal and pelvic adenopathy in lymphoma. *Am J Roentgenol* 1978;131:675–679.
29. Castellino RA, Hoppe RT, Blank N, et al. Computed tomography, lymphography, and staging laparotomy: correlations in initial staging of Hodgkin's disease. *Am J Roentgenol* 1984;143:37–41.
30. Lee JKT, Heiken JP, Ling D, et al. Magnetic resonance imaging of abdominal and pelvic lymphadenopathy. *Radiology* 1984;153:181–188.
31. Hoane BR. Comparison of initial lymphoma staging using CT and MRI. *Am J Hematol* 1994;47:100–105.
32. Skillings JR. A prospective study of MRI imaging in lymphoma staging. *Cancer* 1991;67:1838–1843.
33. Tesoro-Tess JD, Balzarini L, Ceglia E, et al. Magnetic resonance imaging in the initial staging of Hodgkin's disease and non-Hodgkin lymphoma. *Eur J Radiol* 1991;12:81–90.
34. Bengel FM, Ziegler SI, Avril N, et al. Whole-body positron emission tomography in clinical oncology: comparison between attenuation-corrected and uncorrected images. *Eur J Nucl Med* 1997;24:1091–1098.
35. Tumeh SS, Rosenthal DS, Kaplan WD, et al. Lymphoma: evaluation with gallium-67 SPECT, *Radiology* 1987;164:111–114.

19

Melanoma

Hans Ch. Steinert and Rahel Kubik-Huch

The incidence of malignant melanoma of the skin, as well as death from melanoma, is increasing dramatically throughout the world. As with most cancers, the causes of malignant melanoma are multifactorial. Many studies have demonstrated that the development and progression of melanoma are based on increasing levels of cutaneous solar exposure, especially ultraviolet B radiation, in combination with the genotype, phenotype, and immunocompetence of the patient. Fortunately, nowadays most patients are diagnosed early, so that melanoma can be cured with surgical removal of the lesion. Histologic verification and accurate microstaging of tumor thickness are essential for treatment decisions and predicting the risk of metastases. The total vertical height of a melanoma (Breslow index) is the single most important prognostic factor in clinically localized melanoma. Once metastases develop, other prognostic factors must be considered. The number of metastatic nodes has a significant prognostic value. The high mortality of patients with melanoma is due to its early hematogenous spread. The mechanism of hematogenous spread and implantation of melanoma cells is poorly understood, and the location of metastases is unpredictable. The skin, subcutaneous tissue, and distant lymph nodes are the most common sites of distant metastases, but melanoma can metastasize to all organs. Because of the poor response to chemotherapy and immunotherapy, early detection and surgical excision are important in improving the prognosis. The number of metastatic sites is the most significant factor predicting survival in patients with distant metastases. Therefore, accurate staging is essential for the early detection of metastases.

Whole-body positron emission tomography (PET) using fluorodeoxyglucose tagged with fluorine 18 ($[^{18}F]FDG$) is clinically used for the staging of patients with high-risk malignant melanoma (i.e., Breslow thickness of greater than 1.5 mm or known metastases).

H. Ch. Steinert: Nuclear Medicine, University Hospital, CH-8091 Zurich, Switzerland.
R. Kubik-Huch: Diagnostic Radiology, University Hospital, CH-8091 Zurich, Switzerland.

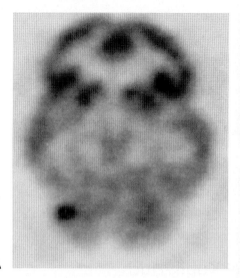
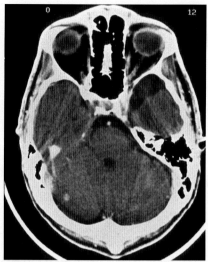

A   B

Figure 19-1. Surgically proven brain metastasis of a malignant melanoma in a 22-year-old man. **A:** Axial [^{18}F]FDG PET scan of the brain demonstrates a lesion with a markedly increased uptake in the right cerebellum. **B:** Corresponding contrast-enhanced axial CT scan of the brain.

WHOLE-BODY STAGING

For the staging of malignant melanoma, a combination of conventional imaging modalities is used, including chest x-ray, ultrasound (US) (of the abdomen and lymph nodes of the axilla, cervical region, and groin), and computed tomography (CT). However, these methods are intrinsically spot-imaging methods and better used to evaluate a given region rather than the entire body. Furthermore, identification of tumor tissue (e.g., in normal-sized lymph nodes) is difficult with these methods. If a lesion is detected, further procedures such as biopsies or follow-up examinations are necessary to confirm or exclude malignancy. [^{67}Ga] gallium citrate and immunoscintigraphy with monoclonal antibodies to screen for melanoma have been advocated, but false-negative scans are common.

Malignant melanoma shows one of the highest [^{18}F]FDG uptakes of all tumors (1). It has been demonstrated in several studies that whole-body [^{18}F]FDG PET is an effective imaging modality for screening for metastases from malignant melanoma (Figs. 19-1 to 19-5). In a study of 33 patients, our group reported a sensitivity of 92% and a specificity of 77%

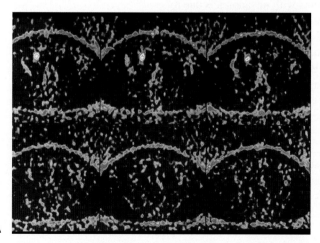
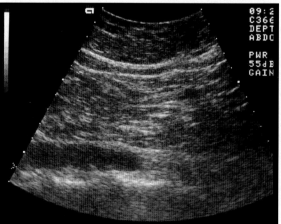

A   B

Figure 19-2. Surgically proven abdominal metastasis of malignant melanoma in a 51-year-old man. **A:** Axial [^{18}F]FDG PET scans of the upper abdomen shows a small lesion with increased uptake. **B:** Corresponding US of the upper abdomen shows no suspicious lesion. A reevaluation was performed 7 months later.

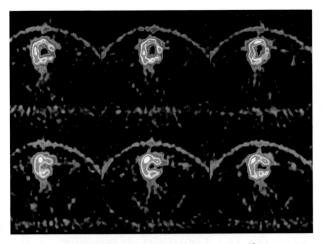

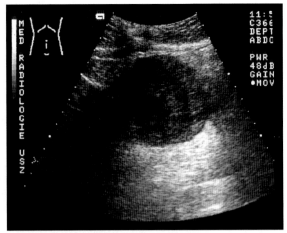

C

D

Figure 19-2. *(continued)* **C:** Axial [^{18}F]FDG PET scans demonstrate a large central necrotic lesion in the upper abdomen. **D:** Corresponding US shows a large hypoechogenic mass.

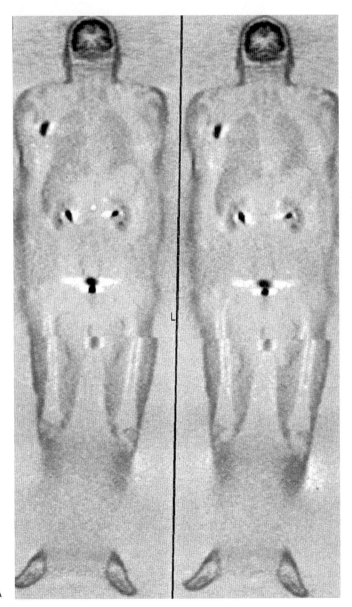

A

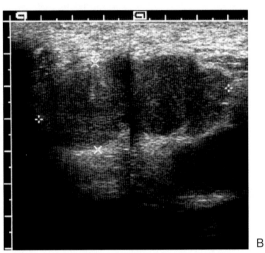

B

Figure 19-3. Surgically proven axillary metastases of malignant melanoma in a 72-year-old man. **A:** Coronal [^{18}F]FDG PET scans show a lesion with a markedly increased [^{18}F]FDG uptake in the right axilla. PET was performed after fine-needle biopsy of this lesion was inconclusive three times. **B:** Corresponding US of the right axilla demonstrates a large hypoechogenic mass.

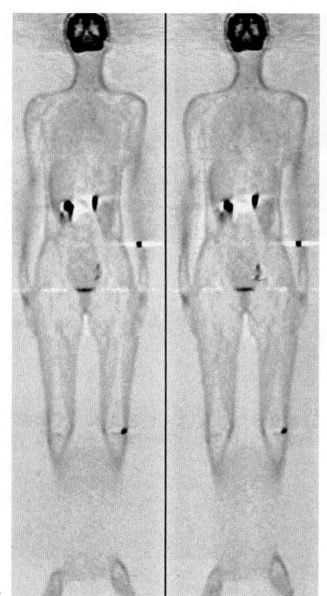

A

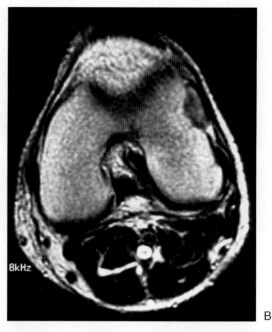

B

Figure 19-4. Surgically proven knee metastasis of malignant melanoma in a 39-year-old woman. **A:** Coronal [^{18}F]FDG PET scans show a lesion with markedly increased tracer uptake in the lateral aspect of the left knee. There is an injection artefact in the left lower arm. **B:** Corresponding MR image of the left knee demonstrates a metastasis in the left lateral femoral condyle.

for the reading of PET images without clinical information (2,3). Specificity improved to 100% when clinical information, such as location of biopsy sites or location of subcutaneous injections of interferon, were obtained. [^{18}F]FDG PET was also highly accurate in differentiating benign from malignant lesions. In six patients (18%), whole-body PET depicted previously unknown metastases. In four of these six patients, the metastases were surgically removed. The excellent results in staging high-risk melanoma patients with whole-body [^{18}F]FDG PET have been confirmed in larger patient series (4,5).

Recently, the cost effectiveness of whole-body [^{18}F]FDG PET in melanoma patients has been studied. Our group reviewed the treatment records of 100 patients with newly diagnosed malignant melanoma and a Breslow thickness greater than 1.5 mm or known metastatic melanoma (6). In patients with known metastatic disease, all metastases had been removed. Two staging procedures were defined:

Conventional staging consisted of physical examination, chest x-ray, and US of lymph nodes and the abdomen.
Any suspicious lesion after conventional staging resulted in additional CT scans and histopathologic correlation.

Staging with whole-body [^{18}F]FDG PET included inspection of the skin. Suspicious lesions were confirmed by biopsy or another imaging modality. The review found 172 staging protocols that could be analyzed for cost comparison. The total cost of conventional staging was SFr 257,224 (approximately $174,000), compared with SFr 261,650 (approximately $177,000) for PET, thus only 1.7% more. Among the 72 patients with metastatic disease, conventional staging costs were SFr 227,445 (approximately $154,000), while PET staging costs were SFr 201,414 (approximately $136,000). In this subset, the PET protocol cost 11.4% less than conventional staging. We and our colleagues concluded that a Breslow index tumor thickness of greater than 1.5 mm is a cost-effective cut-off for deciding whether to use PET, since these patients have a higher risk of metastases. Gambhir et al. (7) compared the cost effectiveness of imaging strategies using conventional staging alone, including body CT and brain magnetic resonance (MR) imaging, versus conventional staging with whole-body [^{18}F]FDG PET. Sixty patients with suspected recurrence from malignant melanoma were included in the study. The study also looked at survival using measures of life expectancy based on the literature, and savings due to changes in patient management resulting from the use of PET. The incremental cost-effectiveness ratio of the [^{18}F]FDG PET strategy compared with the conventional staging strategy was $3,000 to $8,000 per year of life saved, a figure far below the standard of $50,000 per year of life saved used by health economists in the United States to characterize a cost-effective intervention.

Imaging Protocol

Patient Preparation

Overnight fasting with no breakfast or fasting for at least 4 hours is required before [^{18}F]FDG application.

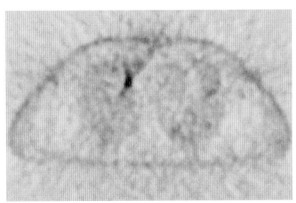

A

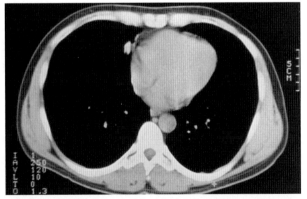

B

Figure 19-5. Surgically proven lung metastasis of malignant melanoma in a 38-year-old man. **A:** Thoracic axial [^{18}F]FDG PET scan demonstrates a lesion with a markedly increased tracer uptake on the right. **B:** Corresponding thoracic CT scan, soft tissue window: 2-cm-diameter paracardial mass. Differentiation between a vascular structure and metastasis is not possible. **C:** PET-CT image fusion of the thorax.

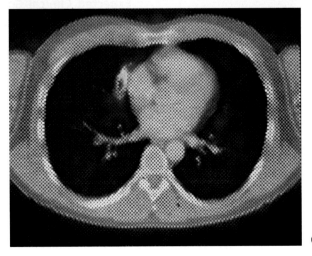

C

TABLE 19-1. *Appraisal/reimbursement status of PET in melanoma*

Disease	German consensus classification	USZ classification	Replacement potential	US reimbursement status: Medicare/BC-BS	Swiss reimbursement status
Melanoma staging (Breslow ≥1.5 mm)	1a	—	—	yes/yes	yes
Melanoma, therapy control	2b	—	—	yes/yes	yes

See page 8 for abbreviations and appraisal scheme explanations.

Emptying of the bladder is required before PET acquisition; lavage of the bladder, if required, is performed via a urinary catheter with 2 L of 0.9% saline solution during PET acquisition in the pelvis.

Data Acquisition

After a 45-minute postinjection uptake phase, the patient is placed in the camera with hands down.

Whole-body two-dimensional (2D) acquisition is carried out step by step from pelvis to head, and then patient is turned around for acquisition from proximal legs to feet.

Acquisition time is 4 minutes per bed position (axial field of view approximately 15 cm) for the emission scan.

Total whole-body acquisition time is 60 to 70 minutes; whole-body transmission correction not applied.

Additional 3D brain PET acquisition is carried out in patients at high risk for brain metastases (Breslow index >4 mm, neurologic symptoms, primary tumor located in the head); acquisition time is 20 minutes for the emission scan and 10 minutes for the transmission scan.

Image Fusion. Image fusion is usually performed for lesions less than 0.8 cm, if required for surgical resection.

Appraisal of Clinical Relevance of PET in High-risk Malignant Melanoma (Breslow ≥1.5 mm or known metastatic disease) (Table 19-1)

Primary Tumor. No indication for PET in the evaluation of primary malignant melanoma.

Secondary Manifestations. There is a very strong indication for [18F]FDG PET, as detection of lymph node metastases is improved.

Tertiary Manifestations. There is a very strong indication for [18F]FDG PET as the best single test for detecting distant metastases.

Expected Clinical Consequences from PET Findings. Surgical resection is the treatment of choice for regional lymph node metastases or a single distant metastasis. If multiple metastases are present, patients are referred to chemoimmunotherapy. In extended metastatic disease, only palliative symptomatic therapy is indicated. Patients with high-risk melanoma and without evidence of metastatic disease benefit the most from adjuvant treatment with recombinant interferon alfa.

Exceptions. [18F]FDG PET has a high sensitivity for detecting metastases. However, false-negative findings have been described for small metastases in the brain, liver, basal parts of the lung, and skin. Possibly, false-positive results are caused by infection and inflammation.

REFERENCES

1. Wahl RL, Hutchins GD, Buchsbaum DJ, et al. 18F-2-deoxy-2-fluoro-d-glucose uptake into human tumour xenografts. *Cancer* 1991;67:1544–1550.

2. Böni R, Huch-Böni RA, Steinert HC, et al. Staging of metastatic melanoma by whole-body positron emission tomography using 2-fluorine-18-fluoro-2-deoxy-d-glucose. *Br J Dermatol* 1995;132:556–562.

3. Steinert HC, Huch-Böni RA, Buck A, et al. Malignant melanoma: staging with whole-body positron emission tomography and 2-[F-18]-fluoro-2-deoxy-d-glucose. *Radiology* 1995;195:705–709.

4. Damian DL, Fulham MJ, Thompson E, Thompson JF. Positron emission tomography in the detection and management of metastatic melanoma. *Melanoma Res* 1996;6:325–329.

5. Rinne D, Baum RP, Hör G, Kaufmann R. Primary staging and follow-up of high-risk melanoma patients with whole-body ^{18}F-fluorodeoxyglucose positron emission tomography. *Cancer* 1998;82:1664–1671.

6. Steinert HC, Ullrich SP, Guillong E, et al. Staging of malignant melanoma: cost effectiveness of whole-body FDG PET versus conventional imaging. *J Nucl Med* 1998;39:94P.

7. Gambhir SS, Hoh CK, Essner R, et al. A decision analysis model for the role of whole-body FDG PET in the management of patients with recurrent melanoma. *J Nucl Med* 1998;39:94P.

PART V

Clinical PET Imaging of Inflammatory Diseases of the Body

20

Clinical PET Imaging of Inflammatory Diseases

Gustav K. von Schulthess, Katrin D. M. Stumpe, and Ivette Engel-Bicik

Imaging of inflammatory diseases of the body and their sequelae is very important clinically. Most frequently, the lung, musculoskeletal system, or the soft tissues are involved, but any organ can show signs of inflammation. Imaging of cerebral inflammation with positron emission tomography (PET) is dealt with in Chapter 8: Brain Tumors. When the involved structure is known, morphologic imaging is used to assess the pathologic alterations (e.g., inflammatory joint disease). However, diagnosis should be made so that healing can occur before the inflamed structure is altered; therefore imaging methods must be used that can show early effects of inflammation. The classic statement that inflammation manifests itself by *calor, dolor* and *rubor* (heat, pain, and redness) is due to local hyperemia (i.e., hyperperfusion and increased capillary leakiness in a region of inflammation). Therefore, imaging of regional blood volume and perfusion, which are nonspecifically increased in inflamed tissues, can be useful in the early localization of the site of an inflammation not accessible to diagnosis by clinical means. As a result, in the assessment of inflammation, dynamic scanning with contrast media is a key imaging procedure used in conjunction with computed tomography (CT) but mainly with magnetic resonance (MR) imaging and bone scintigraphy. It is noteworthy that the latter modalities cause no additional exposure to ionizing radiation when acquiring multiple images of the same structure during passage of the contrast-providing agent; they are therefore preferable for examinations involving dynamic scanning after contrast injection. Inflammatory-lesion imaging is frequently used in immunocompetent and immunocompromised patients with suspected inflammatory disease undergoing chemotherapy for the treatment of a malignancy. Respiratory tract infections are well assessed with chest x-rays and CT; skeletal and joint infections are imaged using x-ray, MR imaging, and bone scan; and soft tissue infections and infections of the visceral organs are most frequently imaged using ultrasonography, CT, or MR imaging. Gastrointestinal (GI) and genitourinary infections also are diagnosed with the morphologic imaging modalities, while infections of the GI tract are often identified by endoscopic means. Infections of the cardiovascular system, such as mycotic aneurysms, require cross-sectional morphologic imaging.

G. K. von Schulthess, K. D. M. Stumpe, and I. Engel-Bicik: Nuclear Medicine, University Hospital, CH-8091 Zurich, Switzerland.

All skeletal and soft tissue imaging with MR and with nuclear medicine techniques uses dynamic information to better characterize the nature of a lesion. Most often, the site of infection can already be identified clinically, but in some situations the focus or foci of infection cannot readily be found. This is definitely the case in a septic patient, in whom infection spreads hematogenously and can therefore lodge in any part of the body. While antibiotic therapy is successful in treating sepsis, not positively identifying the lesion with imaging may be dangerous, as abscesses requiring surgical rather than medical treatment may develop. As in tumor staging, the cross-sectional morphologic imaging methods are not ideal for finding lesions when there are no localizing signs and symptoms, and lesions showing contrast enhancement may turn out to be other than the infectious focus to be identified. Hence, false-positive and false-negative results occur. One example is the diagnosis of spondylodiscitis; it has become apparent that frequently not even MR imaging can distinguish it from erosive osteochondrosis. Morphologic imaging, particularly MR imaging, has become very widespread in identifying infectious foci in soft tissues and bone; nuclear medicine techniques are also widely used. The bone scan has excellent qualities for the search for bone and joint infections, antigranulocyte antibody scans have a definitive role in imaging of chronic osteomyelitis of the appendicular skeleton, and leukocyte imaging is still the "gold standard" for imaging infectious foci in bones and soft tissues in many institutions. However, the latter is a relatively involved and expensive procedure because a patient's leukocytes or, better still, granulocytes must be sampled, labeled *in vivo*, and reinjected.

Noninfectious inflammatory diseases including *collagen vascular diseases, rheumatoid inflammatory diseases,* and *granulomatous diseases,* such as sarcoid, may also require imaging in various instances. Depending on the manifestation, various imaging modalities are used, but predominantly x-rays, CT, MR imaging, and bone scans. Manifestations of collagen vascular diseases are evaluated using CT and MR imaging in most instances. Major imaging questions are the presence and activity of inflammatory tissues (i.e., the arteritides). Assessment of inflammatory changes in a given joint in rheumatoid inflammatory disease is most frequently accomplished using MR imaging. This is also the case for assessment of extension of pannus into a joint or the progression of joint destruction in a critical body region, such as the atlantooccipital joint. Late sequelae also are obviously seen on standard x-rays. If a survey of affected joints is needed or the diagnosis of a chronic polyarthritis cannot be made on serologic grounds, bone scan is a simple method for demonstrating all involved joints and therefore can yield a distribution pattern, which may be important for distinguishing osteoarthritis from polyarthritis.

In addition to the identification of foci, observing the regression of inflammatory changes under therapy is helpful, as it indicates whether the therapeutic regimen is adequate and whether it can be discontinued. Again, as in tumor imaging, the morphologic methods are less sensitive than one would desire them to be in answering this question.

STANDARD IMAGING MODALITIES IN NUCLEAR MEDICINE

Nuclear medicine offers a variety of methods for the diagnosis of infectious diseases. These include three-phase bone scintigraphy for bone infection, gallium Ga 67 scintigraphy, and scintigraphy using colloids, nonspecific immunglobulins, and labeled leukocytes (either with indium, technetium [Tc], or with Tc-labeled antibodies against leukocyte surface antigens). Indium 111–labeled leukocytes have been the "gold standard" for infection imaging (1), as this method has been shown to be highly sensitive and specific. ^{111}In-labeled leukocytes are excellent for demonstrating inflammatory processes in the soft tissues and in bone and joint disease. Except for the evaluation of associated tissue necrosis, encapsulated infection, or in spondylodiscitis.

The results of ^{99m}Tc-labeled antibody against granulocytic surface antigens are comparable to those obtained with labeled leukocytes, with the advantages of a lower patient radiation exposure and greater ease of labeling preparation (2). The physiologic differences in the mechanisms of infection labeling with these agents and direct leukocyte labeling are that the reinjected labeled leukocytes belong to the circulating granulocyte pool and ac-

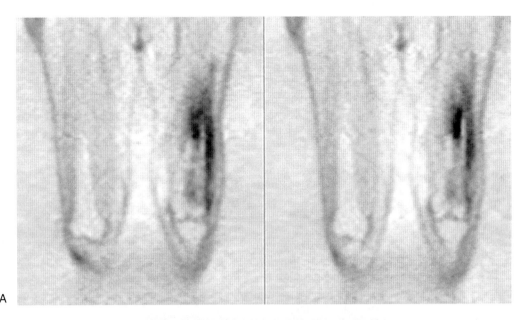

A

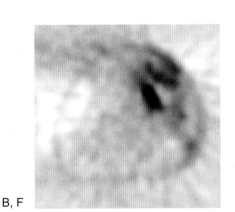

B, F

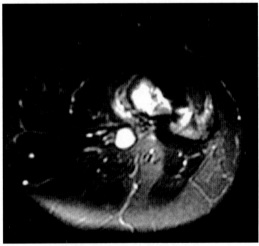

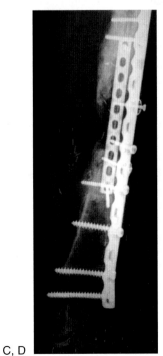

C, D

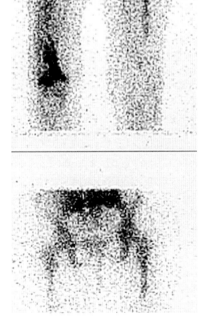

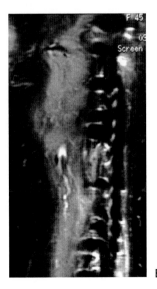

E

Figure 20-1. Osteomyelitis in a patient with a fibular transplant and osteosynthesis after open left femoral fracture. Coronal **(A)** and axial **(B)** [^{18}F]FDG sections through the thigh show intense linear tracer accumulation in the region of the fibular transplant and intermediate uptake in the surrounding soft tissues. **C:** Corresponding x-ray shows the osteosynthetic material and the fibular transplant in the left femur. **D:** ^{99m}Tc-labeled antigranulocyte antibody scintigram shows expansions of hematopoietic marrow in the proximal femora and intense activity in the distal left femur. T2-weighted coronal **(E)** and axial **(F)** MR scans through the left middle femur show metal artifacts in the left thigh and some signal enhancement in the region of the fibular transplant.

tively migrate into the infectious focus by diapedesis, while the antibody against granulocytes binds to any granulocyte encountered in the body and can also nonspecifically diffuse to the site of infection and bind to the granulocytes that are already there. Therefore, the latter method shows stronger accumulation in normal hematopoietic bone marrow than ^{111}In-labeled leukocytes. This makes the method less than ideal for the detection of infectious foci in the axial skeleton, which contains most of the human granulopoietic marrow. Clinical applications of ^{99m}Tc-labeled antibodies against granulocytes are comparable to those using ^{111}In-labeled leukocytes.

Pitfalls of ^{99m}Tc-labeled antibodies against granulocytes include the following:

Swallowing of activity from sinus or upper respiratory infections leads to bowel activity in the absence of any intestinal disease. To aid in interpretation, additional images of the head and chest, as well as repeated delayed images, should always be obtained (^{111}In-leukocytes only).

Physiologic bone marrow uptake in the vicinity of prosthetic implants is often disrupted and gives confusing information (Fig. 20-1).

In septic patients, leukocytes are activated and migrate physiologically into the marginated pool of the lungs, so that a lobar pneumonia cannot be diagnosed with certainty.

Poorer image quality of inflammations in the upper abdomen because of physiologic liver and spleen uptake.

Gallium 67 is not very specific, as it is used in tumor as well as inflammation imaging and cannot differentiate between the two (3). In addition, there are several other limitations. Gallium requires delayed imaging with delays of at least 24 to 48 hours, and it has a substantially lower spatial resolution and a high radiation burden than Tc-based nuclear medicine imaging.

Recent data, including data from our own group, suggest that PET using fluorodeoxyglucose tagged with fluorine 18 ([^{18}F]FDG) may be an excellent tool for identifying inflammatory foci and possibly also for evaluating response to antibiotic therapy (4–6). The pathophysiologic basis is that, when activated, granulocytes and macrophages experience a metabolic burst during which they use substantial amounts of glucose (7). The number of patients scanned for the detection of inflammatory foci is still relatively small, and much more experience needs to be gained before [^{18}F]FDG PET can be assigned a definitive place in the imaging algorithms for inflammation. The main reason that there is less experience with imaging of inflammation than tumors has to do with PET logistics. While a patient undergoing staging for a tumor can easily wait a few days for a scan, inflammatory disease imaging is often a relative emergency, requiring an imaging examination within 24 hours or less. This poses stringent requirements on the logistics of a PET center. In fact, only in PET facilities that can offer PET scanning throughout most working days will the method be considered a serious imaging option by referring clinicians. As this is the case at our institution, we have recently noted a substantial surge in unsolicited requests for infection imaging in a wide group of patients, such as candidates for heart transplantation and patients with unclear findings on MR imaging. Lack of definitive data in inflammation imaging is even more apparent for therapy monitoring, and to our knowledge, there are no substantial data on immunocompromised patients. In these patients, leukocytes are either absent or malfunctioning due to immunosuppression, and since [^{18}F]FDG accumulation is likely to occur in activated leukocytes, tracer uptake in these patients may be so low that lesions are not identifiable. On the other hand, it is possible that [^{18}F]FDG also accumulates in the infectious agent itself and therefore may still be a valuable imaging method. As [^{18}F]FDG is accumulated in inflammatory cells, noninfectious inflammatory disease also shows tracer accumulation, as documented by occasional reports (8,9). Hence, there is likely no specificity between infectious and noninfectious inflammation by [^{18}F]FDG PET. PET will thus probably serve as a search and localization methodology, guiding clinicians to the best biopsy site, and possibly as a method to monitor therapeutic effects. Therefore, this chapter discusses PET infection and inflammation imaging of the various organ systems jointly. The data presented are interesting and may suggest to readers to try some novel applications of PET; however, we must emphasize clearly that many statements and claims in this chapter are not yet fully substantiated in an adequate number of well characterized patient populations.

RESPIRATORY SYSTEM

Infections of the respiratory system are frequent and rarely need more imaging than a chest x-ray. If this becomes necessary, CT is the method of choice, but sometimes a definitive diagnosis cannot be made, and only follow-up imaging to assess therapy will yield the final diagnosis. Respiratory tract infections are relevant to PET imaging of bronchial carcinoma and other tumors, because not infrequently weak mediastinal PET accumulations are interpreted to be moderate inflammatory changes of the central bronchial tree or of lymph nodes in smokers with chronic bronchitis (Fig. 20-2). Furthermore, patients with a central bronchial carcinoma may show a poststenotic pneumonia that at times is difficult to distinguish from tumor (Fig. 20-3). Patients who have possible other infectious foci besides those identified in the lung may profit from the large field of view and the excellent signal-to-noise ratio of [^{18}F]FDG PET (10–13). With these capabilities, PET may show additional lesions that do not respond appropriately to an antibiotic regimen given to treat the pneumonia. Figure 20-4 shows a patient with bilateral pneumonia under antibiotic therapy who had little pulmonary [^{18}F]FDG accumulation but a very intense sternal focus that turned out

(text continues on page 236)

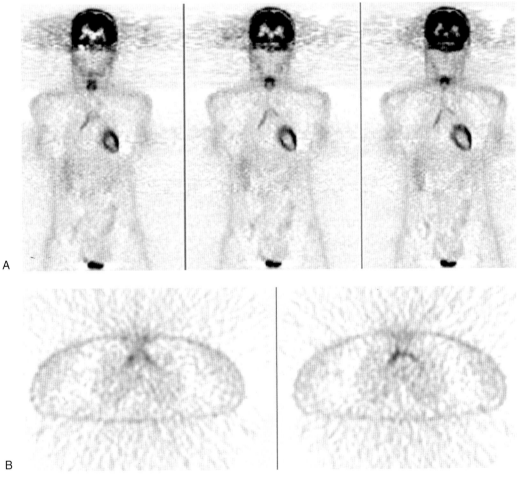

Figure 20-2. Chronic smoker's bronchitis. **A:** Coronal [^{18}F]FDG PET sections show increased intermediate tracer uptake in the lymph nodes along the main stem bronchi. **B:** Corresponding axial [^{18}F]FDG PET sections through the upper thorax.

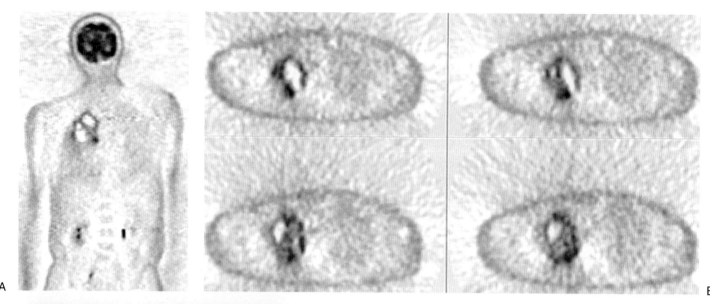

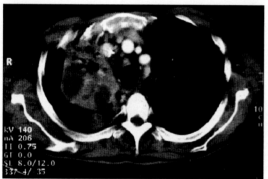

Figure 20-3. Pneumonia with central necrosis. Coronal **(A)** and corresponding axial **(B)** [18F]FDG PET sections demonstrate an increased circular tracer uptake with central photopenia in the right upper lung. **C:** Thoracic axial CT section above the aortic arch level shows an inhomogeneous mass in the right upper lung.

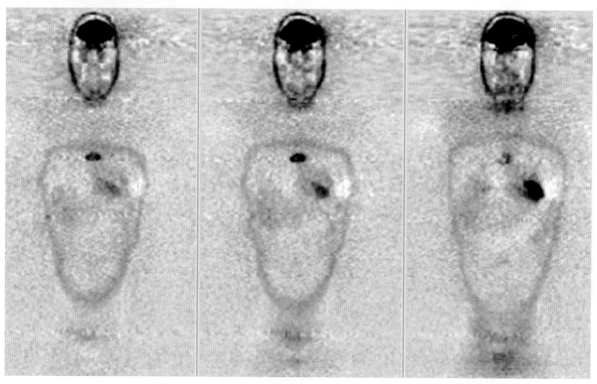

Figure 20-4. Sternal osteomyelitis. Coronal **(A)** and axial **(B)** [18F]FDG PET sections show intense focal tracer uptake in the sternal body.

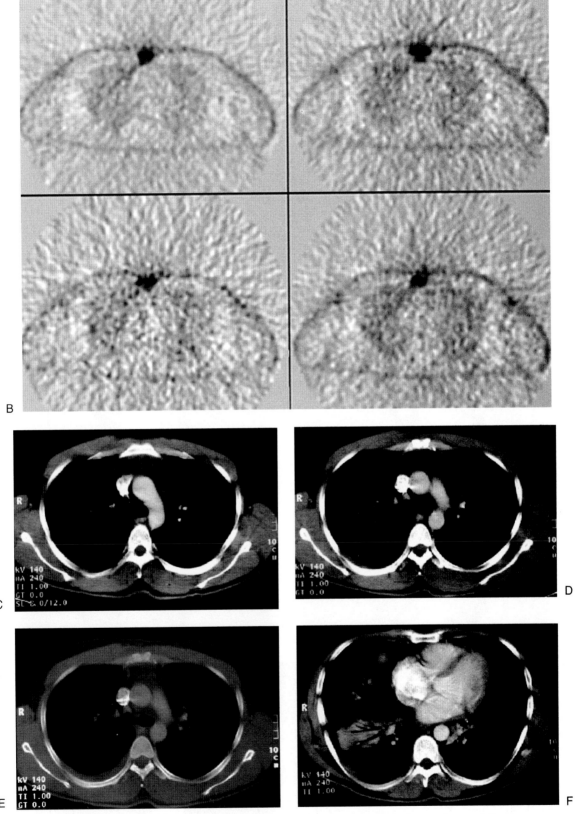

Figure 20-4. *(continued)* **C–F:** Axial CT sections through the upper thorax show soft tissue retrosternally, infiltrations in the basal parts of both lungs, and a right pleural effusion.

to be infected. Other inflammatory diseases, such as sarcoid or Wegener's granulomatosis, also show high [^{18}F]FDG uptake on PET scans (14,15). PET scanning in these diseases has currently no major role to play.

PET may also be useful in demonstrating sites of intense inflammatory change that would be preferred biopsy sites, as it appears to be better than other imaging modalities in distinguishing infectious foci from reactive processes occurring in their surroundings (Fig. 20-5). Another potential indication in these diseases may be monitoring of therapeutic response. From our experience with infection PET imaging, it is clear that distinguishing pul-

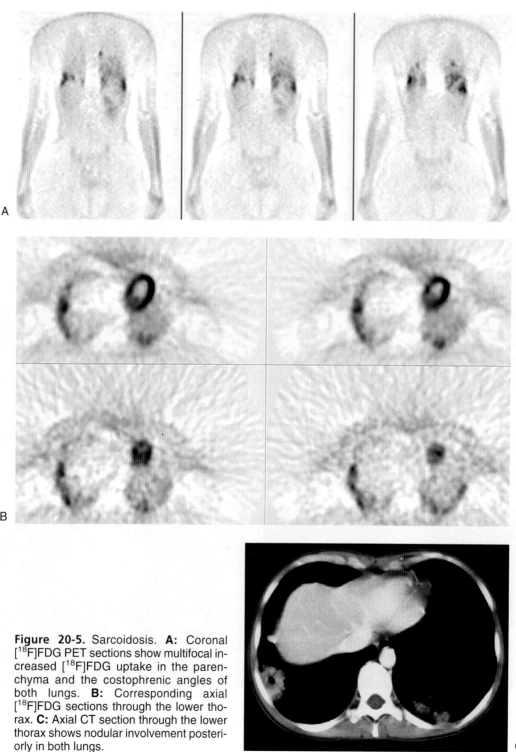

Figure 20-5. Sarcoidosis. **A:** Coronal [^{18}F]FDG PET sections show multifocal increased [^{18}F]FDG uptake in the parenchyma and the costophrenic angles of both lungs. **B:** Corresponding axial [^{18}F]FDG sections through the lower thorax. **C:** Axial CT section through the lower thorax shows nodular involvement posteriorly in both lungs.

monary inflammation from tumor is only possible using additional criteria, such as the distribution pattern of [^{18}F]FDG accumulation. This will certainly increase the specificity of infection PET imaging, but the differential between malignant tumor and infectious focus remains an issue affecting specificity. For example, when a solitary pulmonary nodule can be diagnosed with PET as having no [^{18}F]FDG accumulation, a malignancy can be ruled out. Conversely, when [^{18}F]FDG uptake is seen, this is likely to be tumorous, but an actively infected granuloma remains in the differential (16).

CARDIOVASCULAR SYSTEM

Physiologic accumulations of [^{18}F]FDG in the vascular system occur relatively frequently; most often they are noted in the lower extremities (see Chapter 7: The normal PET scan). PET may be helpful in some patients with vascular disease. In fact, there have been claims that PET may be able to identify atherosclerotic plaques when they are inflamed and that infectious agents may be partially involved in the generation of atherosclerotic plaque. While this is of high potential future interest, one major problem of using PET for plaque imaging is the currently insufficient spatial resolution.

The clinical issues in the imaging of cardiovascular inflammation are the identification and characterization of endocarditis, vasculitis, and vascular infections, such as mycotic aneurysm and infected hematoma. Evaluation of endocarditis cannot be made with PET, since the heart physiologically accumulates [^{18}F]FDG when a patient is not fasting, and furthermore quite often a fasting period of even 4 to 7 hours will not suppress cardiac glucose metabolism. Since one would expect endocarditis as an inflammatory disease to exhibit enhanced [^{18}F]FDG accumulation, this would be indistinguishable from normal accumulation in the myocardium. However, PET may play a role in better characterizing lesions in the vascular system suggestive of infection. Not infrequently, sterile aneurysmal lesions show contrast-medium enhancement on CT or MR imaging that thus can be misinterpreted as infection. Imaging of hematomas with the question of superinfection and of mycotic aneurysm is done using CT and, with increasing frequency, MR imaging. Since both techniques now have excellent angiographic capabilities, the morphologic alterations of the vasculature can be readily depicted. Infected blood shows alterations in its signal behavior on MR imaging, suggesting the diagnosis, and the addition of contrast enhancement further improves specificity. Still, [^{18}F]FDG PET of such structures may be more specific and more sensitive than the cross-sectional imaging modalities, as our experience suggests. PET scanning in this setting may be helpful because the lack of [^{18}F]FDG accumulation will probably rule out infection. Figure 20-6 shows a patient who had an abdominal aortic aneurysm repaired by a graft, which on CT and MR imaging showed contrast enhancement suggesting a graft infection. PET scanning showed not only no [^{18}F]FDG accumulation in the graft but also an abdominal accumulation subcutaneously, and some pus was noted to drain from the umbilicus. Thus, the diagnosis of a subcutaneous phlegmonous lesion was made. In another case, a subcutaneous enhancement of signal was noted on MR imaging in the left groin, with extension into the testicular sacs after an arterial puncture, as well as a thrombosis, of the superficial femoral artery (Fig. 20-7). [^{18}F]FDG PET imaging showed tracer accumulation in all these structures, thereby confirming the diagnosis of septic arterial thrombus with infected hematoma in the groin. In addition, this patient showed some pulmonary uptake, which was interpreted to represent septic emboli, although they were not confirmed.

The value of morphologic imaging of vascular lesions in collagen vascular diseases lies in confirming a suspected diagnosis (e.g., Takayasu's arteritis). With the advent of contrast-enhanced MR angiography, an increasing number of institutions no longer perform conventional angiography. Whether PET has any role to play in the diagnosis and management of collagen vascular diseases is open to question. By showing accumulation, it may add to distinguishing atherosclerotic from inflammatory stenosis, or it may eventually

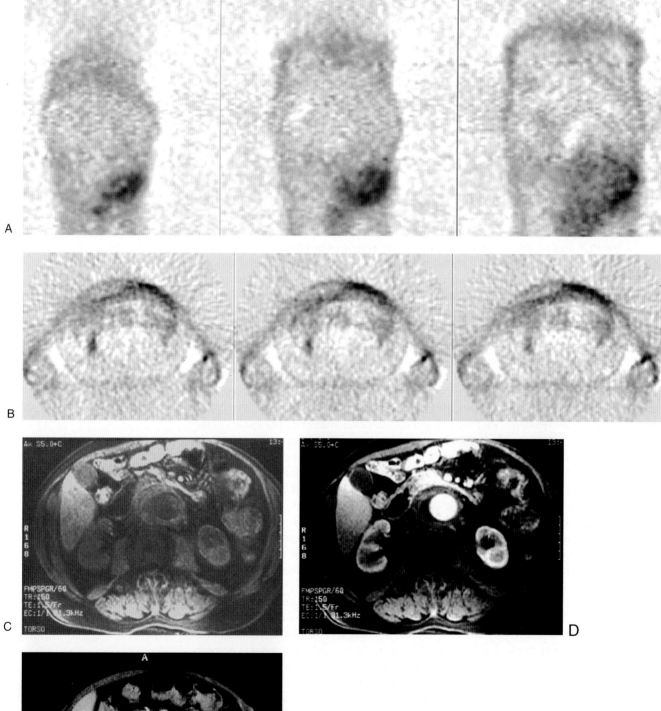

Figure 20-6. Graft replacement of the supra- and infrarenal aorta and a subcutaneous wound infection in the left abdominal wall. Coronal **(A)** and axial **(B)** [¹⁸F]FDG PET sections show diffuse subcutaneous activity in the left abdominal wall, but no accumulation is seen in the region of the aorta in the axial sections. **C,D:** Dynamic T1-weighted axial MR sections show contrast enhancement in the soft tissue surrounding the supra- and infrarenal aortic graft. **E:** Axial CT section through the lower abdomen shows soft tissue surrounding the aortic aneurysm.

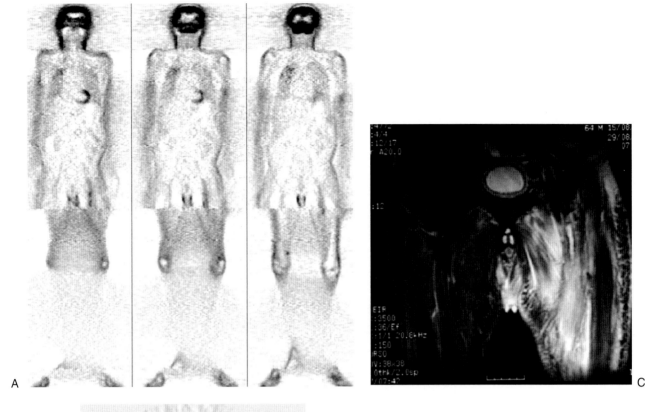

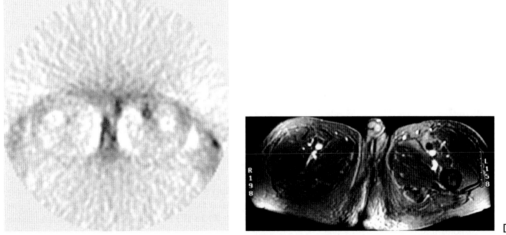

Figure 20-7. Thrombosis of the left superficial femoral artery. **A:** Coronal [^{18}F]FDG PET sections show linear increased tracer uptake in the course of the left superficial femoral artery, increased uptake in the scrotum, and diffuse intermediate increased uptake in the right upper lung. **B:** Corresponding axial [^{18}F]FDG PET section through the thighs shows focal tracer uptake in the region of the left superficial femoral artery. Coronal **(C)** and axial **(D)** T2-weighted MR scans demonstrate an intense signal in the proximal left superficial femoral artery and fluid accumulations in the adjacent muscles with extension into the scrotum.

have a role in therapy monitoring. Figure 20-8 shows a case of Takayasu's arteritis in which multiple moderate [^{18}F]FDG accumulations in the mediastinum correlated with stenoses noted on MR angiography.

GASTROINTESTINAL AND GENITOURINARY SYSTEMS

Inflammatory changes of the gut can be readily identified with PET imaging. In fact, nonspecific moderate- or even high-intensity [^{18}F]FDG accumulations of the colon can be

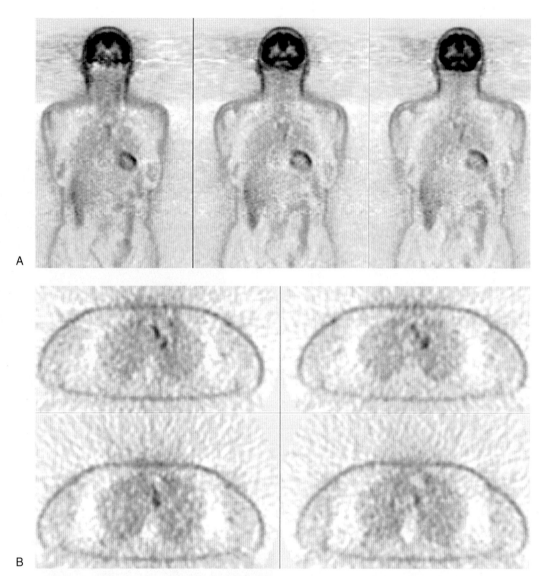

Figure 20-8. Takayasu's arteritis. **A:** Coronal [^{18}F]FDG sections show intermediate linear tracer uptake in the anterior mediastinum. **B:** Corresponding axial [^{18}F]FDG sections through the upper mediastinum. **C:** MR angiogram shows the typical stenoses of the large vessels leaving the aortic arch. Axial MR scans at a supraaortic level **(D)**, at the level of the aortic arch **(E)**, and at the level of the ascending aorta **(F)** demonstrate hypointense tissue thickening of the vessel walls.

seen relatively frequently in patients who have no history of intestinal disease. At this point, the significance of such accumulations is unclear, and therefore they are termed *nonspecific*, even though they may well represent important information. As the colon is a site where many bacterial species thrive, one can speculate that patients showing such accumulations during scanning for other purposes suffer from a transient bowel infection, an alteration in bowel bacterial growth due to antibiotic medication, early diverticulitis, beginning inflammatory bowel disease (IBD), or transient nonspecific inflammation. Thus, until further data are available, [^{18}F]FDG accumulation in the large bowel is of uncertain clinical significance, unless a specific pathology in the gut is expected. In a series of 27 patients with infectious diseases taking antibiotic therapy, we noted moderate to strong [^{18}F]FDG uptake in regions of the colon in six patients, while a review of 354 consecutive [^{18}F]FDG PET scans revealed tracer uptake in 110 patients.

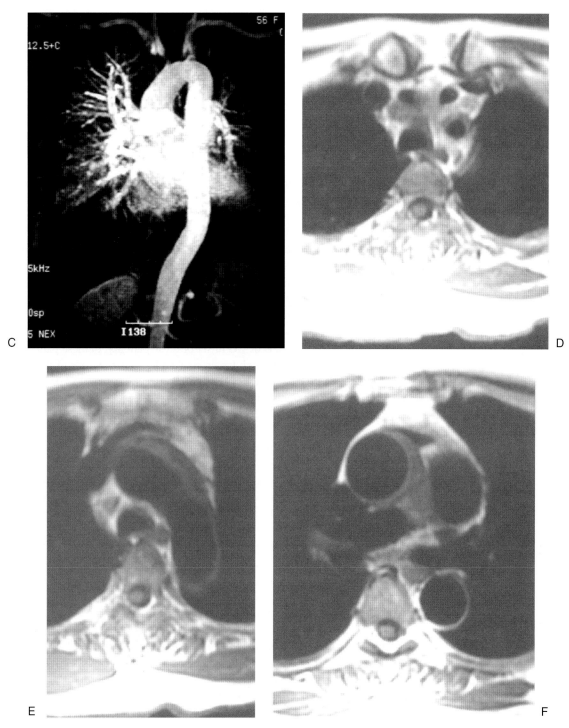

Figure 20-8. *(continued)*

There are more detailed data on [^{18}F]FDG PET in patients with inflammatory bowel disease (IBD). Management of patients with IBD requires information about the extent and activity of the inflammatory process. To estimate the activity, scores have been developed for Crohn's disease (CD) (17) and ulcerative colitis (UC) (18), since no single parameter for disease activity is available. In clinical practice, the Crohn's disease activity index (17) and the clinical activity index (18) for UC are the most often used scores. Although both scores have shown a fairly good correlation with endoscopic and histologic extent of disease, the tests are not very discriminatory of the various pathologic disease states. The "gold standard" for the evaluation of disease extent in both the colon and the ileum is endoscopy, which also permits obtaining biopsies (19). For detection of complications such as fistula or abscess in CD, CT or MR imaging is usually necessary. Although endoscopy is probably indispensable for primary diagnosis, a noninvasive method for long-term monitoring of the disease would be very useful (18).

After the initial diagnosis, management of patients with IBD aims at preventing relapse and recognizing complications. Disease extent and the clinical course determine the therapeutic activity. The timing and amount of reduction of maintenance treatment are chosen arbitrarily, based on empiric data rather than on individual parameters. Most often, therapy is reduced if a patient is doing well during a certain period of time. Unfortunately, reduction of therapy is often followed by an increase in clinical activity. Thus, low clinical activity during therapy does not predict the course of disease after the reduction of treatment. This might be due to the fact that clinical activity only in part represents histologic activity. However, histology requires endoscopy, and repetition of this invasive method is limited in chronically ill patients with IBD. Therefore, [18F]FDG PET may be a good alternative in the management of patients with known IBD.

In a pilot study performed at our institution, seven patients referred for routine colonoscopy were studied with [18F]FDG PET (20). Histology revealed active inflammatory disease consistent with CD or UC in six of these patients. In these patients, [18F]FDG PET demonstrated moderate to high tracer uptake in various regions of the intestine (Fig. 20-9). As expected, PET could not differentiate between CD and UC or between specific and nonspecific inflammation. The concordance of disease extent derived by histology and PET imaging showed a fairly good correlation. It seems that microscopic inflammation is at least equally well demonstrated by [18F]FDG PET as by endoscopy. Our preliminary data suggested that PET performs practically identically to endoscopy for disease localization. The best concordance between PET and histology was achieved in the ascending, transverse, and descending colon segments, because anatomic identification generally causes no problems. In the terminal ileum and the sigmoid, however, small, focal areas of [18F]FDG accumulation often could not be assigned to specific areas, resulting in underestimation of disease extent.

Although quantitative image analysis by means of regions of interest (ROI) offers no additional information regarding the discrimination between CD and UC, calculation of ratios between ROIs of intestinal activity and a reference region, for example, a vertebral body, could have some potential value. Especially in a setting of long-term monitoring of patients receiving treatment for IBD, quantification could be of value in measuring disease activity during therapy.

This pilot study demonstrated the utility of [18F]FDG PET for identifying active inflammation in IBD. The results were confirmed in a series of 25 patients. PET seems to be inferior to endoscopy with respect to assigning areas of inflammation to anatomic structures. However, this is less important if the initial diagnosis is made by endoscopy and is paralleled by a PET study. In this regard, PET could lead to a new, noninvasive imaging modality for long-term monitoring of patients with IBD. Therefore, PET results may permit adjusting treatment or monitoring new therapeutic approaches.

Limited data exist on inflammatory changes in other organs and structures of the upper abdomen. One study has appeared concerning the usefulness [18F]FDG PET for abdominal abscess detection (21). Most notably, there have been some studies claiming that pancreatic carcinoma and chronic pancreatitis can be distinguished on the grounds of a lower [18F]FDG uptake in the latter disease (22). More recently, some authors claim no longer to be able to rely on this method. Infectious involvement of the liver, the spleen, and the kidney has not been extensively examined with PET until now (23). One area of particular interest may be the diagnosis of pyelonephritis in children.

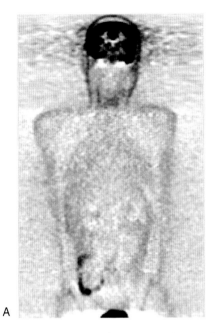

Figure 20-9. Crohn's disease. Coronal **(A)** and transaxial **(B)** [^{18}F]FDG PET scans show very extensive uptake in the terminal ileum and ascending colon. The axial image demonstrates tracer uptake in the gut wall but not intraluminally.

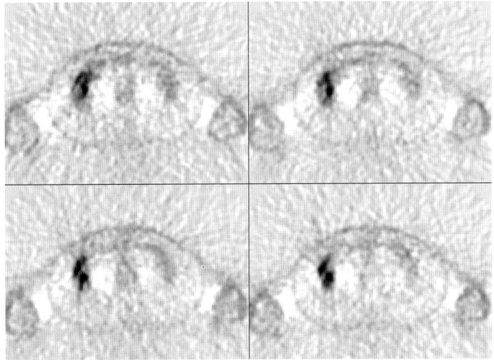

BONES, JOINTS, AND SOFT TISSUES

Imaging of bone and joint structure inflammation makes predominant use of MR imaging and bone scanning, with the latter being more frequently used when staging (i.e., identification of lesion dispersion) is required. Osteitis and osteomyelitis, including spondylodiscitis, are common diseases, occurring in all age groups. While children show mostly bone infections, which spread hematogenously, adults more often show localized infections, unless they have a generalized sepsis.

Bone infection is a common disease in children, readily diagnosed with bone scans. In the past decade, MR imaging has started to play an increasingly important role in the diagnosis and definition of the extent of osteomyelitis, although, like bone scan, it is not completely specific. Furthermore, many patients suffering from bone infections have undergone osteosynthesis after trauma and thus have metallic implants in the infected regions (see Fig. 20-1). This frequently makes MR imaging uninterpretable. In addition, the diagnosis of postoperative wound infections after cardiothoracic operations is often difficult, especially in patients with a subacute clinical presentation. To distinguish between superficial and deep infections, tomographic scan options are required. PET with its inherent tomographic capability is an excellent method of excluding osseous sternal infection in patients with suspected mediastinitis after thoracic operations (see Fig. 20-4).

Many institutions use labeled leukocytes as the "gold standard" method of identifying infectious foci, but, as stated at the outset of this chapter, this method is cumbersome and costly and definitive imaging frequently requires 24 hours. The use of antigranulocyte antibodies is increasing, as it is a simpler method of leukocyte imaging, but, the sensitivity of this method is inferior to that of labeled leukocytes. It is mostly useful in the peripheral appendicular skeleton, where there is no hematopoietic bone marrow, since radioactivity in leukocyte and antigranulocyte antibody scans shows the hematopoietic marrow prominently, thereby making the diagnosis of inflammation difficult in bones containing hematopoietic marrow. It is important to recall that in infectious states the hematopoietic bone marrow may extend into bones previously containing fatty marrow (i.e., femora and humeri). In this case, infection and bone marrow expansion may be difficult to differentiate from each other, particularly in patients whose bone anatomy has been altered due to trauma or chronic infection. Figure 20-1 shows this pitfall, with PET clearly delineating an infected fibular transplant in a region of bone destruction in the left femoral diaphysis. If early results are confirmed by controlled studies, PET may become an excellent imaging modality, particularly in patients with osteosynthetic material where the MR imaging artefacts are usually prominent, precisely in the ROI. As inflammatory cells only use [^{18}F]FDG when activated, [^{18}F]FDG PET may even turn out to be more specific than leukocyte scanning. The only other situation in which hematopoietic cells are also avidly metabolizing glucose is when the bone marrow is recovering after chemotherapy (see Chapter 7 and Fig. 7-13).

Imaging of joint inflammation also seems possible with PET. As inflammatory joint diseases (i.e., osteoarthritis and autoimmune joint diseases) all have a prominent inflammatory component, it is not surprising to find [^{18}F]FDG uptake even in patients with diseases unrelated to the inflammation being investigated. In a recent review of over 350 patients who underwent whole-body [^{18}F]FDG PET for tumor staging, a surprisingly large fraction of about 230 patients showed [^{18}F]FDG uptake into the acromioclavicular and the glenohumeral joints; this finding was clearly dependent on patient age (24). It is indeed the acromioclavicular joint that most frequently shows arthritic changes in a large number of autopsy cases (D. Resnick, private communication, 1998). To our knowledge, no study has appeared examining the use of PET in the evaluation of inflammatory joint disease, and it may indeed be a good but too costly examination, as the clinical imaging questions in joint disease are either geared to a specific joint, where high resolution MR imaging is needed, or to the search for affected joints, in which case bone scanning is quite adequate. Still, PET may eventually have a role in monitoring disease activity, which again should be most adequately reflected by local glucose utilization.

PET imaging of soft tissue inflammation has been used by a small number of researchers, and the early results are again extremely promising. Figure 20-10 shows the left lower extremity of a patient with a left lower leg fasciitis. PET appears at least equivalent to MR imaging and may be able to identify precise regions of inflammatory response. This is of interest particularly if the best biopsy site is to be found, but since PET is a whole-body screening technique, septic patients may well benefit from it because distant foci can also be identified. Very much as in tumor staging, PET may become the method of choice for searching for infectious sites in the soft tissues when a focus is not

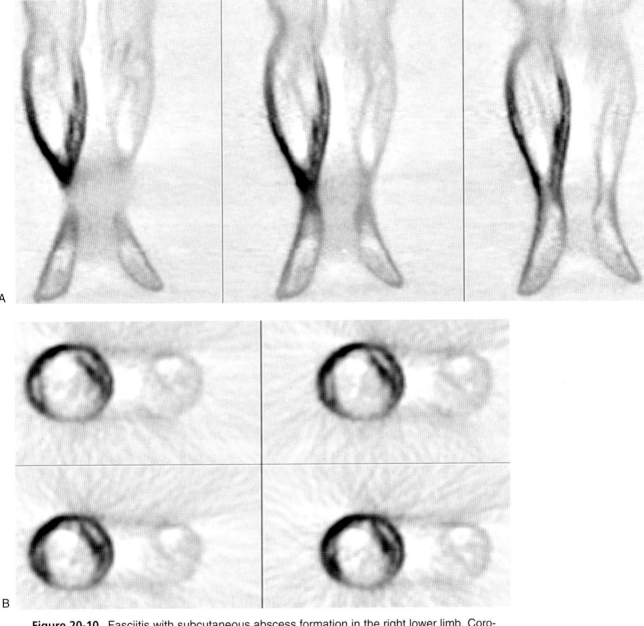

A

B

Figure 20-10. Fasciitis with subcutaneous abscess formation in the right lower limb. Coronal **(A)** and axial **(B)** [^{18}F]FDG sections demonstrate subcutaneous tracer accumulation of the right lower extremity, interpreted as fasciitis with subcutaneous abscesses and without involvement of the muscles. *(continues)*

evident clinically and on low-cost imaging studies. When the focus is found, morphologic imaging may then define whether an interventional or a conservative approach should be taken.

POSTTHERAPEUTIC CONTROL IN BONE INFECTION

It is well known that it is difficult on MR imaging to see a posttherapeutic response in time, as a bone marrow edema will last for a certain time. This is demonstrated in a patient with osteomyelitis in the left foot who was treated with antibiotics for 6 weeks (Fig. 20-11).

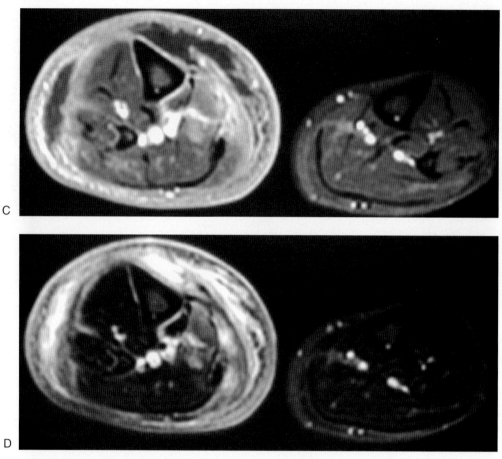

Figure 20-10. *(continued)* Unenhanced **(C)** and contrast-enhanced **(D)** T1-weighted axial MR sections show a fasciitis with subcutaneous abscess formation and contrast enhancement of the underlying muscles.

In the follow-up PET scan, there was no [^{18}F]FDG uptake in the left intermediate cuneiform. In contrast, MR imaging continued to demonstrate bone marrow edema after 6 weeks, without any reduction in signal intensity.

APPRAISAL OF THE CLINICAL RELEVANCE OF PET IN INFLAMMATION IMAGING—AND OUTLOOK

PET imaging of inflammatory foci has not received much attention, and unlike with PET imaging of the brain, the heart, and tumors, no consensus conference on inflammation imaging has taken place to appraise PET's relevance; therefore, a "not classified" status is found in Table 20-1. While our experience with the initial imaging of inflammation suggests that PET performs excellently—thus the high grades—the number of follow-up studies has been so limited that we cannot confidently classify the method. No reimbursement is available for PET inflammation imaging in any country.

PET identification of sites of inflammation and monitoring of inflammatory disease activity are very new and extremely promising fields of clinical PET application. At the moment, the number of published papers on this subject is still very small. Despite this, our experience with over 100 patients with some kind of inflammation makes us very optimistic. We are certain that PET will eventually play an important role in finding unknown inflammatory foci and defining disease activity in situations where a good parameter for deciding on discontinuing therapy is needed. Furthermore, the use of PET in patients with

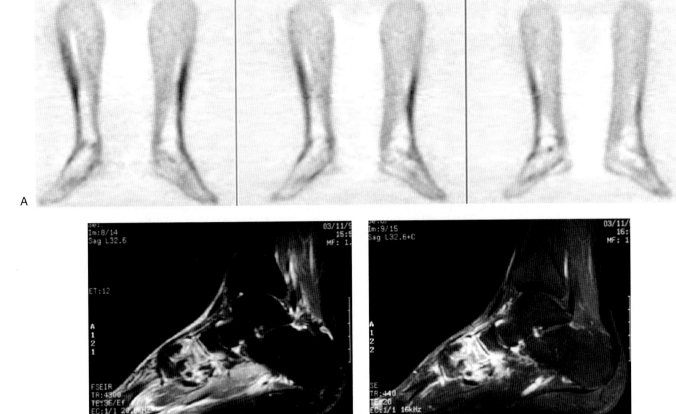

Figure 20-11. Posttherapeutic scan in a patient with osteomyelitis in the left intermediate cuneiform and a suspected septic arthritis in both talotibial joints. **A:** Coronal [¹⁸F]FDG PET sections show intermediate-intensity circular tracer uptake in the right talotibial joint and no uptake in the left intermediate cuneiform. T2-weighted **(B)** and contrast-enhanced T1-weighted **(C)** sagittal MR scans show signal intensity in the left intermediate cuneiform and in the dorsum of the left foot.

infection and osteosynthetic material may become widespread. Obviously, the cost of PET is high, but the therapeutic consequences of mismanagement can be enormously costly, and precise information on the inflammatory status of a lesion is needed. As pointed out initially, inflammation PET imaging poses the highest logistic problems for a PET center, as imaging of inflammation is frequently an emergency procedure requiring virtually around-the-clock availability. While this is unrealistic with PET, some centers are now able to run clinical PET examinations 5 days a week from early in the morning until late afternoon.

TABLE 20-1. *Appraisal/reimbursement status of PET in inflammation*

Disease	German consensus classification	USZ classification	Replacement potential	US reimbursement status: Medicare/BC-BS	Swiss reimbursement status
Soft tissue infection	—	4	3	no/no	no
Bone infection	—	4	3	no/no	no
Infection of osteosynthesis mat.	—	4	3	no/no	no
Fever of unknown origin	—	4	3	no/no	no

See page 8 for abbreviations and appraisal scheme explanations.

REFERENCES

1. Seabold JE, Forstrom LA, Schauwecker DS, et al. Procedure guideline for indium-111-leucocyte for suspected infection/inflammation. *J Nucl Med* 1997;6:997–1001.
2. Becker W, Palestro CJ, Winship J, et al. Rapid imaging of infections with monoclonal antibody fragment (LeukoScan). *Clin Orthop* 1996;329:263–272.
3. Seabold JE, Palestro CJ, Brown ML, et al. Procedure guideline for gallium scintigraphy in inflammation. *J Nucl Med* 1997;6:994–997.
4. Ichiya A, Kuwabara Y, Sasaki M, et al. FDG-PET in infectious lesions: the detection and assessment of lesion activity. *Ann Nucl Med* 1996;10:185–191.
5. Sugawara Y, Braun DK, Kison PV, et al. Rapid detection of human infections with fluorine-18 fluorodeoxyglucose and positron emission tomography: preliminary results. *Eur J Nucl Med* 1998;25:1238–1243.
6. Stumpe KDM, et al. PET imaging of infectious foci with fluorine-18 fluorodeoxyglucose (abstract). EANM and Radiological Society of North American 1998.
7. Gutowski TD, Fisher SJ, Moon S, et al. Experimental studies of 18-F-2-fluoro-2-deoxy-d-glucose (FDG) in infection and in reactive lymph nodes. *J Nucl Med* 1992:925[abst].
8. Wahl RL, Fisher SJ. A comparison of FDG, l-methionine and thymidine accumulation into experimental infections and reactive lymph nodes. *J Nucl Med* 1993:104[abst].
9. Yamada S, Kuboto K, Kubota R, et al. High accumulation of fluorine-18 fluorodeoxyglucose in turpentine-induced inflammatory tissue. *J Nucl Med* 1995;7:1301–1306.
10. Jones HA, Clark RJ, Rhodes CG, Schofield JB, Krausz T, Haslett C. *In vivo* measurement of neutrophil activity in experimental lung inflammation. *Am J Respir Crit Care Med* 1994;149:1635–1639.
11. Bakeheet SM, Powe J. Fluorine-18-fluorodeoxyglucose uptake in rheumatoid arthritits-associated lung disease in a patient with thyroid cancer. *J Nucl Med* 1998;39:234–236.
12. Jones HD, Clark RJ, Rhodes CG, et al. Positron emission tomography of 18FDG uptake in localized pulmonary inflammation. *Acta Radiol Suppl* 1991;376:148.
13. Taylor IK, Hill AA, Hayes M, et al. Imaging allergen-invoked airway inflammation in atopic asthma with 18F-fluorodeoxyglucose and positron emission tomography. *Lancet* 1996;347:937–940.
14. Lewis PJ, Salama A. Uptake of fluorine-18 fluorodeoxyglucose in sarcoidosis. *J Nucl Med* 1994;10:1647–1649.
15. Brudin LH, Valind SO, Rhodes CG, et al. Fluorine-18 deoxyglucose uptake in sarcoidosis measured with positron emission tomography. *Eur J Nucl Med* 1994;21 297–305.
16. Desan NA, Gupta NC, Redepenning LS, Phalen JJ, Frick MP. Diagnostic efficacy of PET-FDG imaging in solitary pulmonary nodules: potential role in evaluation and management. *Chest* 1993;104:997–1002.
17. Best WR, Becktel JM, Singleton JW. Development of a Crohn's disease activity index. National Cooperative Crohn's Disease Study. *Gastroenterology* 1979;70:439–444.
18. Rachmilewitz D. Coated mesalazine (5-aminosalicylic acid) versus sulphasalazine in the treatment of active ulcerative colitis: a randomised trial. *BMJ* 1989;298:82–86.
19. Modigliani R, Bitoun A. Endoscopic assessment of inflammatory bowel disease. In: *Inflammatory bowel disease*. London: Chapman and Hall, 1991.
20. Bicik I, Bauerfeind P, Breitbach T, et al. Inflammatory bowel disease activity measured by positron-emission tomography [Letter]. *Lancet* 1997;350:829–831.
21. Tahara T, Ichiya Y, Kuwabara Y, et al. High (18F)-fluorodeoxyglucose uptake in abdominal abscesses: a PET study. *J Comput Assist Tomogr* 1989.
22. Bares R, Klever P, Hauptmann S, et al. F-18 fluorodeoxyglucose PET *in vivo* evaluation of pancreatic glucose metabolism for detection of pancreatic cancer. *Radiology* 1994;192:79–86.
23. Shreve PD. Focal fluorine 18-fluorodeoxyglucose accumulation in inflammatory pancreatic disease. *Eur J Nucl Med* 1998;25:259–264.
24. Stumpe KDM, Dazzi H, Schaffner A, et al. PET imaging of inflammatory lesions. *Eur J Nucl Med* 1998;25:908[abst].

Appendix

Appraisal/reimbursement status of PET for various diseases: a synopsis (July 1999)* (See page 8 for abbreviations and appraisal scheme explanations.)

Disease	German consensus classification	USZ classification	Replacement potential	US reimbursement status: Medicare/BC-BS	Swiss reimbursement status
Brain Imaging					
High grade glioma					
Grading	1b	3	2	no/no	yes
Tumor recurrence	1a	4	4	no/no	yes
Tumor residual	1b	4	4	no/no	yes
Determination of best biopsy site	1a	4	4	no/no	yes
Grade change	–	4	4	no/no	no
Low grade glioma					
Grading	1b	4	4	no/no	yes
Tumor recurrence	–	1	3	no/no	yes
Prognostic criteria	–	3	3	no/no	no
Grade change	–	4	3	no/no	no
Other tumors					
Grading	3	3	2	no/no	yes
Tumor recurrence	–	3	2	no/no	yes
Prognostic criteria	–	–	–	no/no	no
Grade change	–	–	–	no/no	no
Brain inflammation	–	2	2	no/no	no
Focal epilepsy					
Temporal lobe FDG	1a	3	3	no/yes	yes
Extratemporal lobes FDG	1b	3	3	no/yes	yes
Focal epilepsy Flumazenil	1b	–	–	no/no	
Cerebrovascular disease					
Acute stroke	2a	–	–	no/no	no
Chronic CVD (before surgery)	2b	3	3	no/no	yes
Dementias	1a	3	3	yes/yes	yes (<70y)

continued

APPENDIX *(Continued).*

Disease	German consensus classification	USZ classification	Replacement potential	US reimbursement status: Medicare/BC-BS	Swiss reimbursement status
Heart Imaging					
Coronary artery disease (CAD); unclear other investigations	1a	3	3	yes/yes	no
Before heart transplantation	–	4	3	yes/yes	yes
Hibernating myocardium	1a	4	3	yes/yes	yes
Coronary three vessel disease	–	4	3	yes/yes	yes
Tumor Imaging					
Nonsmall cell lung cancer NSCLC					
NSCLC, mediast. lymph node staging	1a	4	3	yes/yes	yes
NSCLC, recurrence	1a	4	4	yes/yes	yes
NSCLC, distant metastases	2b	4	4	yes/yes	yes
Therapy control NSCLC	2a	4	4	yes/yes	yes
Solitary pulmonary nodule (high risk)	1a	3	3	yes/yes	yes
Melanoma staging (Bresl > 1.5 mm)	1a			yes/yes	yes
Melanoma, therapy control	2b			yes/yes	yes
Multiple myeloma	–	1	0	no/no	no
Malignant lymphoma, initial staging	1b	3	2	yes/no	yes
Malignant lymphoma, residual tumor	1b	4	4	yes/no	yes
Malignant lymphoma, restag./recur.	2a	4	4	yes/no	yes
Malignant lymphoma, therapy resp.	2b	3	3	yes/no	yes
Diff. thyroid cancer, neg 1–131, el. TG	1a	4	3	no/no	no
Head/neck cancer: unknown primary	1a	2	2	no/no	no
Head/neck cancer: staging (II or more)	1b	3	3	no/no	no
Head/neck cancer: local recurrence	2a	4	3	no/no	no
Esophageal cancer	–	3	3	no/no	no
Gastric cancer	–	–	–	no/no	no
Colorectal cancer: staging, CEA>30	2b	–	–	yes/no	yes
Colorectal cancer: recurrence	1a	4	4	yes/no	yes
Colorectal cancer: therapy contr.	2a	–	–	yes/no	yes
Liver cancer	–	1	1	no/no	no
Pancreatic cancer: primary	1a	2	2	no/no	no
Pancreatic cancer: local recurrence	1b	–	–	no/no	no
Pancreatic cancer: NM staging	2b	–	–	no/no	no
Renal cell carcinoma: recurrence staging	2b	3	3	no/no	no
Breast cancer: local recurrence	2a	3	4	no/no	yes
Breast cancer: lymph node staging	2a	3	2	no/no	yes
Breast cancer: distant metastases	2a	3	3	no/no	yes
Breast cancer: therapy control	2a	3	3	no/no	yes
Ovarian cancer: recurrence	2a	2	2	no/no	no
Ovarian cancer: primary, dist. mets., therapy control	2b	2	2	no/no	no
Other gyn. cancers: endometrial, cervix, vagina, vulva	2b	–	–	no/no	no
Germ cell ca.: non-seminomatous Therapy control (excl. diff. Teratoma)	1b	3	3	no/no	yes
Germ cell ca.: non-seminomatous Lymph node- and restaging	2a	3	3	no/no	yes

APPENDIX *(Continued).*

Disease	German consensus classification	USZ classification	Replacement potential	US reimbursement status: Medicare/BC-BS	Swiss reimbursement status
Germ cell ca. non-seminomatous: Teratoma	2b	2	2	no/no	yes
Germ cell ca. seminomatous	2b	2	2	no/no	no
Prostate cancer	–	1	1	no/no	no
Prostate cancer: recurrence	2b	–	–	no/no	no
Bladder cancer: lymph node staging	2a	–	–	no/no	no
Bladder cancer: local recurrence, dist. Metastases, therapy control	2b	–	–	no/no	no
Neuroendocrine tumors	2b	–	–	no/no	no
Neuroendocrine tumors: dedifferentiation	–	4	4	no/no	no
Inflammation Imaging					
Soft tissue infection	–	4	3	no/no	no
Bone infection	–	4	3	no/no	no
Infection of osteosynthesis mat.	–	4	3	no/no	no
Before heart transplantation		4	3	yes/yes	yes
Fever of unknown origin	–	4	3	no/no	no

REFERENCES

1. Schwaiger M, et al. Indikationen für die klinische Anwendung der PET in der Kardiologie. *Z kariol* 1996; 85:453–468.
2. Bartenstein P, et al. Konsensus-Neuro-PET. *Nuklearmedizin* 1997; 36:46–47.
3. Reske SN, et al. Konsensus-Onko-PET. *Nuklearmedizin* 1997; 36:45–46.

Subject Index

Page numbers followed by f refer to figures; page numbers followed by t refer to tables.